Clinical Studies in Psychiatry

By HARRY STACK SULLIVAN, M.D.

Conceptions of Modern Psychiatry
The Interpersonal Theory of Psychiatry
The Psychiatric Interview
Clinical Studies in Psychiatry

Prepared under the auspices of

THE WILLIAM ALANSON WHITE PSYCHIATRIC FOUNDATION
COMMITTEE ON PUBLICATION OF SULLIVAN'S WRITINGS

Mabel Blake Cohen, M.D.   Dexter M. Bullard, M.D.
David McK. Rioch, M.D.   Otto Allen Will, M.D.
Helen Swick Perry, *Editorial Consultant*

HARRY STACK SULLIVAN, M.D.

Clinical Studies
IN
Psychiatry

Edited by
HELEN SWICK PERRY, MARY LADD GAWEL,
and MARTHA GIBBON
With a Foreword by DEXTER M. BULLARD, M.D.

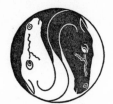

W · W · NORTON & COMPANY · INC · *New York*

PRINTED IN THE UNITED STATES OF AMERICA
FOR THE PUBLISHERS BY THE VAIL-BALLOU PRESS
2 3 4 5 6 7 8 9

Contents

Editor's Preface

MUCH of the work of preparing this book for publication has centered around making a representative selection from the clinical lectures given at Chestnut Lodge. There were over a million words in these 246 lecture-discussions, given over the period from October 1942 to April 1946. Only about 130,000 words have been included in this book, mostly material contained in lectures given between April and November 1943.

It seems appropriate to trace briefly the process by which we arrived at this selection. When we began work, there was little to guide us through this mass of material. There was no notebook of Sullivan's to serve as a guide to organization, as there was for the lecture series used for the other two posthumous books, *The Interpersonal Theory of Psychiatry* and *The Pyschiatric Interview*. And only about half of the lectures had been transcribed from the recordings. It proved impractical for several reasons to have all the lectures in the clinical series transcribed so we might make our selection from the transcriptions. There were, of course, the realities of time and money; but in addition, it was actually easier to judge the value of a lecture by listening to the recordings themselves. Sullivan's spoken word did not always carry over well to verbatim transcripts. Therefore, we first undertook the task of listening to practically all the recordings, and then writing summaries and evaluations of each lecture. These summaries gave us a kind of bird's-eye view of all the material, and made it easier to delineate the problems implicit in making selections.

Three main problems presented themselves: (1) We did not wish to select material which had already been covered essentially in published books and articles, since there were so many unpublished lectures with new content available. (2) Since the lectures covered a three-and-a-half year period during which Sullivan's ideas expanded and changed steadily, we did not wish to treat the whole lecture series as a unit, and organize the best material on a given subject into one chapter irrespective of the time at which the lecture was given. In fact, such an approach soon appeared to be quite impractical. In this series of lectures particularly, Sullivan depended on his small audience for the refinement of his theory, and this in itself resulted in modification of terminology as he went along. And finally, we faced the problem of somehow maintaining a systematic, coherent, and full theoretical statement on mental disorder, while at the same time trying to include the best of the clinical lectures. That is, Sullivan approached mental disorder in terms of its interrelation in a coherent theoretical system, and this point-by-point development of a system of thought seemed a necessary ingredient for the book.

As a nucleus for this book, the lectures from 50 through 99 seemed most successfully to meet these criteria. Perhaps a word should be said about the lectures which have been omitted. The first 49 lectures cover, in general, the developmental approach to mental disorder and the psychiatric interview; these have been omitted since they repeat somewhat the material in the other two posthumous books, although their formulations are earlier. The lectures from 100 through 246 include many brilliant discussions of particular problems in therapy, often growing out of actual clinical problems presented by the group; for the most part these lectures have not been used in the book, although a few illustrative discussions of clinical problems have been selected for inclusion. The wide range of topics covered—for instance, the doctrine of the will, the self-system of the therapist, the handling of dream material in the therapeutic setting, and hospital management of mental illness—prohibit organization into a unified book.

Within the main block of lectures making up this book—50 through 99—the major omissions have been part of the discussion of hysteria and the lectures on psychosomatic disorders. These omissions have been made in order to devote more space to those areas in which Sullivan himself felt that he had most to contribute. Other omissions have been made to eliminate repetition or digression, and certain substitution from contemporary material has been necessitated by record failures.

With the publication of the present book, the three major theoretical approaches used by Sullivan are in print: the developmental eras as a frame of reference, from the 1946–47 lectures (*The Interpersonal Theory of Psychiatry*); the theoretical statement of the significance and the handling of the psychiatric interview, from the period of 1944 and 1945 (*The Psychiatric Interview*); and, in this book, the theoretical statement of the genesis of mental disorder, from lectures given in 1943. If isolated lectures are published subsequently, they may thus be viewed in terms of this time sequence and in the context of the over-all theoretical formulations.

In any such undertaking as this book, the final result is the work of many people. We should like to make particular mention of the contributions made by each member of the Committee. As already noted in the preface to *The Psychiatric Interview*, we are particularly indebted to Otto Allen Will, M.D., for his preliminary assessment of the value of the clinical lectures in general and his detailed evaluation of those transcriptions which were available. We should also like to mention the valuable suggestions made by David McK. Rioch, M.D., who delineated areas of the working manuscript of this book which needed further enrichment from other lectures. And finally, we would like to give tribute to the Chairman of the Committee, Mabel Blake Cohen, M.D., who has played a major role in expediting this entire project and who made many valid and constructive criticisms of this book at each successive stage. In addition to the help of the members of the formal Committee, we should like to make special mention of the assistance of Stewart E. Perry, who is largely responsible for the selection, transcription, and reworking of case illustrations, particularly in the section on obsessionalism.

Of necessity there has been some division of labor among the editors of this book. Including the preliminary task of assessment, the work has been in progress for over three years. Mary Gawel has been largely responsible for an intensive check of the transcriptions used in this book against the recordings themselves; this process included a preliminary editing and cutting of the transcriptions—a painfully slow job in which the involved procedure of translating the spoken, informal word into communicative readable sentences was begun. My main task has been to select the connective material necessary to make these lectures into a book. To Martha Gibbon fell much of the task of the final editing and internal cutting required to strengthen the book and make it a unified whole.

In the preparation of the manuscript for publication, we are particularly indebted to Philip A. Holman and Sadie J. Doyle, staff members of the journal, *Psychiatry*. For careful and conscientious assistance in typing, checking, rechecking, and correcting, much of which was done under pressure, we are indebted to Verna Breese, Marguerite Martinelli Brockway, Sterline Cushman, Clara Mae Lewis, and Ann Salzman. And finally, we would like to make mention of the valuable assistance of Colleen Chassan during the stage of galley proof.

HELEN SWICK PERRY

March 1, 1956

Foreword

It has been over ten years since I heard Harry Stack Sullivan give the lectures at Chestnut Lodge from which this book is made. As I read them over in book form for the first time I find myself again responding enthusiastically to the continued pertinence of his ideas. At times I can visualize the scene and recapture the moods of both Sullivan and the group, which included Mabel Cohen, Edna Dyar, Frieda Fromm-Reichmann, Douglas Noble, Robert Morse, David Rioch, Alfred Stanton, Edith Weigert, Ben Weininger, and Mabel Wilkin. The setting was the recreation room of my house, on the grounds of Chestnut Lodge. The staff would assemble after lunch, before an open fire in cold weather; the great Dane would lie down on the hearthrug, and Sullivan would begin. In warm weather, the sounds of the lawn mower sometimes came through the open windows, and Sullivan's irritation would mount visibly when he had to wait to continue his point. At times the dog would be used to illustrate a point, and on these occasions Sullivan might take time out to pat his head, as if asking his opinion too. Needless to say, there were times when the discussion became as spirited and acrimonious as, may I say, learned. Sullivan's mood varied markedly and so did that of the rest of us. Sometimes we would marvel at a brilliant *tour de force* of Sullivan's, but at other times we would object vigorously to a seeming inconsistency in his presentation. It is a matter of record that no one ever went to sleep—one did not when Sullivan held the floor.

A brief history of the genesis of these lectures will perhaps be useful in evaluating their contents. After the publication of his *Conceptions of Modern Psychiatry* in 1940, Sullivan had always intended to expand his concepts of personality development and to show how failures and misfortunes in the developmental eras are subsequently manifested in psychiatric disorders. But with the outbreak of war in 1941, he dropped his other work to devote all of his time to acting as psychiatric consultant to the Selective Service System. When this work terminated, he began to explore the possibilities for expanding and developing the *Conceptions*, and I invited him to lecture for an indefinite period to the medical staff of Chestnut Lodge and to use the staff for an exchange of ideas as he developed his concepts. He accepted and arranged to come to Rockville twice a week.

The program as conceived was a happy one for both lecturer and audience. Sullivan began with his ideas of personality development and his concepts of empathy and autistic thinking, and gradually progressed into his now well-known theory concerning the stages of personality growth. The lectures quickly turned into discussions; and since no time limit had been set in which a topic must be finished or the series must terminate, the material was developed both fully and leisurely. A talk of an hour would be followed by a half-hour of discussion, with all members of the group participating. Questions were raised about the topic of the day or about previous material, and only when a subject had been temporarily exhausted would the next one be taken up.

From this early leisured interchange at Chestnut Lodge emerged the more formal statement of personality theory which was presented later in the form of lectures given at the Washington School of Psychiatry and posthumously published in 1953 as *The Interpersonal Theory of Psychiatry*. The present book omits for the most part the earlier statement of theory of personality development and concentrates on the clinical observations from which the theory grew. Since the wealth of clinical material presented in the Chestnut Lodge lectures was too great for inclusion in one book, the Committee on Publication of Sullivan's Writings of the

William Alanson White Psychiatric Foundation has authorized the selection for publication of those clinical problems which he delineated most ably and which are deemed of particular importance to those interested in both the theory and practice of psychiatry.

Sullivan's development of a theoretical position and the attendant therapeutic maneuvers to influence a patient's achievement of increasing insight are masterpieces of close reasoning. Of particular interest is his development of the concept which he variously refers to as "dynamisms," "interpersonal dynamisms," and "dynamisms of difficulty." These are processes of interaction occurring between people which foster or hinder the establishment or maintenance of satisfactory interpersonal relations. Most of the dynamisms discussed in this book are concerned with the maintenance of security, in contrast to the pursuit of satisfactions. Among those selected for inclusion are the process of selective inattention, the obsessional dynamism, the development of the paranoid way of thinking—culminating in the paranoid attribution to others of unacceptable personal traits—and the phenomena pertaining to dissociation. Grief as a normal process of compensating for loss—and its failure to function in the service of avoiding the self-accusations of melancholia—is covered in considerable detail. Throughout the book, the schizophrenic modes of thinking are explored carefully, since they constituted Sullivan's major interest in the field of mental disorder. Although these subjects have been dealt with by most writers on psychiatric theory and treatment, Sullivan's exceptional capacity to understand the inferences of schizophrenic communication throws a much clearer light on many of these processes and hence is of major significance in formulating therapeutic maneuvers. This is especially well illustrated in his delineation of the paranoid problem and its relation to homosexuality.

As clinicians, we continue to find that his ideas are of the greatest practical usefulness in the therapy of the more serious disorders, as well as a stimulating frame of reference for the continual testing of new hypotheses. This applies particularly to his formulations of the obsessional, paranoid, and schizophrenic processes. Although the book lays down no dogmatic rules for treatment, careful study will increase the psychiatrist's capacity for formulating an over-all therapeutic strategy in approaching the problems of the treatment of the psychoses.

DEXTER M. BULLARD, M.D.

Medical Director, Chestnut Lodge

President, The William Alanson White Psychiatric Foundation

PART ONE

Dynamisms of Living and Their Misuse in Mental Disorder

The Interpersonal Theory of Mental Disorder

IN APPROACHING the subject of mental disorder, I must emphasize that, in my view, persons showing mental disorder do not manifest anything specifically different in kind from what is manifested by practically all human beings. The only exceptions to this statement are those people who are very badly crippled by hereditary or birth injury factors. There is probably no particular difficulty in grasping this notion except when the disorder picture includes the reappearance of processes that properly pertain to late infancy and early childhood. From my viewpoint, we shall have to accept as a necessary premise that what one encounters in various stages of schizophrenia—the odd, awe-inspiring, terror-provoking feelings of vastness and littleness and the strange strewing-about of relevance—are part of the ordinary experience of these very early stages of personality development in all of us. Most of us, however, experience these processes in later life only as strange fragments carried over from sleep or in our fleeting glimpses of what I call anxiety.

The way in which these primitive types of mental operations become separated from our awareness is in the development of the self-system. The tracing of that development through the various eras of personality growth is absolutely essential to an understanding of my approach to mental disorder and I have already dwelt on it at some length.[1] The self-system is struck off in the personality because of the necessity for picking one's way through irrational and un-understandable prescriptions of behavior laid down by the parents; in other words, the child has to be educated to a very complex social order, long before the reason and the good sense of the whole thing can be digested, long before it becomes understandable—if it ever does. And the self-system comes to be the organization that controls awareness; all the operations that are not primarily of the self go on outside awareness. That can be observed very clearly, however difficult it may be to reason it out with pellucid simplicity.

Early in the process of education and socialization, the self-system begins to emerge in personality; and from then on the diffuse referential processes of an early period usually begin to recede from awareness. From the time that the self-system begins to emerge, three aspects of the personality process can be rather readily distinguished: first, the waking and thoroughly active self; second, the part of the personality which is not readily accessible to awareness—the rest of the personality, which in another context can be considered as the whole personality with the self as the eccentric part; and finally, the period spent in sleep, in which the self is relatively dormant and many things are done which cannot be done when the self is functioning actively.

Now, in avoiding or minimizing the anxiety that is inherent in the unceasing struggle to protect the self-system from the diffuse referential processes that cannot be admitted into awareness, various specific processes, the dynamisms, come into play. In the following series of lectures I shall consider

[1] *Editors' note:* In the first 40 lectures (unpublished) of this series of clinical lectures, Sullivan traces the development of the self-system through the various eras—infancy, childhood, the juvenile era, preadolescence, early and late adolescence. For Sullivan's latest statement on this approach, see *The Interpersonal Theory of Psychiatry*; New York: Norton, 1953.

these dynamisms from this tripartite viewpoint as unitary abstractions that are useful both in thinking about what a patient is showing and in observing what is going on within ourselves. I use the word dynamism, you will observe, where other psychiatrists often use the term mechanism. Mechanism has never suited me because it always suggests a Diesel engine. And the one thing we are sure of in interpersonal relations is that there are processes which are dynamic; they are not static, mechanical entities. These processes have something in them of the element of energy and they are very apt to go on until something in the way of a goal, a terminal state, is reached, whereupon they cease for the time being and show no trace until they are next called forth.

When I speak of dynamisms of difficulty [2] I mean those processes which, although they are a part of every personality, are at the same time the particular parts of the personal equipment that are often misused. In other words, these dynamisms go into action in situations or in fashions that do not achieve a goal, or that, at best, achieve only an unsatisfactory goal. As a result they tend to go on and on. Their frequent recurrence or their tendency to occupy long stretches of time characterizes the mentally sick as distinguished from the comparatively well.

[2] *Editors' note:* Sullivan later abandoned the term "dynamisms of difficulty," although he did not abandon the concept: "In further commenting on the critical opposition of anxiety and the self-system to favorable growth in late adolescence, I would like to call attention to the parataxic processes concerned in avoiding and minimizing anxiety. These processes extend from selective inattention—which to a certain extent covers the world like a tent —through all the other classical dynamisms of difficulty, to the gravest dissociation of one or more of the vitally essential human dynamisms. And incidentally, while I once liked the rubric, dynamism of difficulty, it has lost its charm over my years of attempting to teach psychiatry, because the conviction grew among some of the people who encountered this usage that these dynamisms represented peculiarities shown by the morbid. On the contrary, I believe that there are no peculiarities shown by the morbid; there are only differences in degree—that is, in intensity and timing—of that which is shown by everyone. Thus whenever I speak of dynamisms I am discussing universal human equipment, sometimes represented almost entirely in dreadful distortions of living, but still universal." *The Interpersonal Theory of Psychiatry;* pp. 304–305.

It is the extraordinary dependence of a personality on a particular dynamism that is, I suppose, the fundamental conception to have in mind in thinking of mental disorder. The schizophrenic patient, for instance, is often a person who has in the past persistently shown the dynamism which we call dissociation as a means of resolving the conflict between powerful needs and the restrictions which the self imposes upon the satisfaction of these needs. That is, people who have dissociated anything as powerful as lust, for example, are in great danger of schizophrenic collapse.

We shall consider these dynamisms in an order roughly following that in which they appear in the evolution of personality. First, we shall discuss sublimation, which appears quite early in life, and then we shall take up the obsessional dynamism, which comes into being with the learning of language. Both of these dynamisms have a relation to the protection of the self-system from the appearance in consciousness of types of referential process, thought, or revery closely related to the schizophrenic-like processes of late infancy and early childhood; and we shall pause from time to time to consider their relationship to these earlier referential processes. In the juvenile era, the vast body of processes for controlling awareness which I refer to as selective inattention first becomes an important dynamism. From there we shall consider a number of other dynamisms, all part of the human paraphernalia for protecting the self-system from the minor but effective manifestations of anxiety and the more threatening possibility of the collapse of the self-system. And finally, as the last step in this survey of the dynamisms of difficulty, we shall consider the dissociative processes themselves and their relation to major personality disorder. We shall then be in a position to move on to the therapeutic implications and possibilities in terms of the major patterns of difficulties—the so-called clinical entities.

In considering the various dynamisms or processes of living we shall have to keep in mind that they are what has to go on from the very character of human nature in interpersonal situations. The situation exists because the tendency, the potentiality, or the possibility of the processes not only exists but has force; and this force shows in the tendency integrating the situation. Thus under certain circumstances, people are pulled together, situations are created so that something can work itself out. These situations may be integrated (1) by single, that is unitary, tendencies; (2) by several tendencies which are congruent and which can work in a unitary situation without peculiar things happening; or finally (3) by conflicting integrating tendencies. It is only now and then that one is lucky enough to find a situation that is simple, that is the product of *an* integrating tendency, instead of two or more congruent integrating tendencies or conflicting ones. In the event that there are congruent integrating tendencies, the processes are apt to be rather successful in the sense of all concerned coming out rather better than they went into the situation. When there are conflicting integrating tendencies, on the other hand, many things happen which in essence make up pretty nearly the sum total of human misery. So it is that complex situations and complex processes can be both pleasant and unpleasant, successful and quite otherwise.

Now I should like to consider the problem of where we look for information about these integrating tendencies. What are the basic ideas in attempting to define them?

Integrating tendencies may be defined, first, in terms of their goals, so that one might say that an integrating tendency is that sort of nature in two or more people which causes them to engage in reaching such and such an end state, which incidentally sets up the situation in which such processes can occur. For instance, the goal of the tendency to seek human intimacy, which I shall deal with as if it were a simple tendency at the moment, might be said to be reflected in all those situations in which two or more people tend to understand each other better, to come to a clearer grasp of their particular little differences of views, impulses, and so on. Thus the term, goal, however dubious philosophically, is quite an adequate term for describing this process since the culture is organized to think in terms of what you are doing this *for*, and *for* implies a goal. Time is another consideration here. Time reaches from here into the future and, in a somewhat imaginary way, into the past; and a vast number of plans and operations going on now are clearly foreseen to lead to something in the future which we may quite properly describe, I think, as the goal of the activity without becoming too much preoccupied with more recondite problems of chance.

An even more striking approach to defining integrating tendencies, motives, or drives is in terms of what so-called 'individual' people *feel* about these goals. All of you know that at times you feel hungry, at times some of you may even feel a little bit lustful, quite often some of you feel angry, and at other times some of you feel very kindly, in fact, positively loving. This felt component of the integrating tendencies that create situations with other people and move toward goals is so intimately related to what we term hunger, lust, anger, love, affection, and so on, that it is quite proper, if you do not get confused as to your unique individuality, to relate these terms that everybody knows to the integrating tendencies to which they pertain. For instance, in a situation in which love is the active force, the participants feel what they call love. One can indeed label integrating tendencies by the feeling that accompanies them—their 'emotional' representation within awareness. The only trouble with that particular attempt to define them is that many of the integrating tendencies are not represented in awareness by any feeling; and very often integrating tendencies that are sometimes represented in awareness by feeling are very effective without any such representation;

in other words, they are working unconsciously or externally to awareness. Thus integrating tendencies can be active and situations can exist without the participants *feeling* emotion.

And finally, and somewhat more obscurely, integrating tendencies can be defined in terms of the factors that they make relevant or—and this may sound a little paradoxical—in terms of the factors that make *them* relevant. In other words, since integrating tendencies pertain to the very tissue of life—to what goes on between people—you can understand that we can define them in terms of what the people concerned take seriously when the integrating tendency is in effect, or, to express it another way, what the closely related factors in people are which lead them to be integrated into a particular situation.

In this attempt to define integrating tendencies, you will observe that the field of effort is never perfect because it is so extremely complex; but it is also never utterly obscure. And it is by this variety of approaches to such a complex area of study that we can, I believe, get clearer and clearer on what we are talking about, what we are thinking about, and actually what we are living.

Whichever way you approach a classification of integrating tendencies, you are on much safer ground if you consider two great general goals of the situation. These two grand divisions of goals have come into being from the most fundamental aspect of humanity itself—namely, that humanity and the human beings that make up humanity are extraordinary evolutions of very capable animals. Human beings are not animals, but they start as animals. And these animals are converted into human beings instead of merely members of the species *homo sapiens* by assimilating and becoming part of a vast amount of *culture*—culture being all that is man-made in this world, everything from scientific views and informal cultural and social organizations of people to the most holy traditions and institutions such as the state and the nation. All of these things are 'remains' of human life that has been lived; but all of them are also an active living part of a lot of people. It is in the process of getting from the status of being born a vastly gifted animal to the status of being a person living with other people, and losing any such neat biological individuality as the infant *homo sapiens* had, that a great quantity of the traditions, principles of life, and what not that have been worked out by others in the historic period and that have been wished on us by our parents, teachers, companions, and so on, get into us and become in many ways the most striking thing about us. And it is in that process by which the human animal is converted into a human being—a subject of psychiatric interest instead of merely a subject of biological interest—that there comes about a great differentiation of the goals of behavior and therefore of the integrating tendencies that characterize interpersonal relations. This differentiation I shall discuss in terms of *satisfaction* and *security*.

We never have a chance of discovering what a human animal who did not become a human being would be like, because human animals cannot live without help, and the help proceeds to bring them culture. And so, as you might surmise, this brings us to the other group of integrating tendencies—those which pertain to something markedly influenced by culture. This division of integrating tendencies is *not* clearly indicated in the biological heritage of the human animal; instead they are called out by the processes and are particularly relevant to the situations which are concerned with being a person in contradistinction to being an animal. They are, then, more clearly derivative of culture, of the assimilation of the man-made which has gone into one's education and so on; and when we have studied these, we find that they can be quite adequately placed under one heading—*security*. In contradistinction to the pursuit of satisfaction, these integrating tendencies of prevailingly cultural or educational origin pertain to the pursuit of security, or the maintenance of security, or the avoidance of insecurity. Each of you, when you think about it, will see that you have had experience in the past—and the effects of that experience are still manifest in the present—in which you were esteemed by somebody as good, important, worthy, or you were considered in an unfavorable, derogatory, or depreciatory way. The most general term I have ever found for the states which are attendant upon being valued, respected, looked up to, and so on, is a feeling of personal security; and the term, insecurity, works out even more impressively when one looks for a general term to encompass all the states and all the processes that are called out by situations in which that is not the case.

This differentiation between pursuits of satisfaction and the maintenance of security—that is, the avoidance of anxiety—is, I think, one of the most important classifying principles in all that we will have to say about living.

CHAPTER
2

Sublimation, Obsessionalism,
and the Early Referential
Processes

In attempting to formulate any of the important dynamisms
of personality, we must always have some highly refined statement of the abstraction that we are dealing with. As I have
already noted, one such device for viewing the intangible realm
of process is found in the tripartite view of personality—the
self-system, the total personality, and sleep. The first of these
three major places to look—the self-system—is the one about
which the person can tell you something, for it concerns what
occurs within awareness. What he can tell you must always
be viewed as the manifestation of experience of complex dynamic processes within the self-system. In other words, while
the processes within the self-system don't rattle off statements, the statements that come forth imply certain patterns
of process. In some cases these patterns are of great complexity and are intensely interesting to study, as, for example, the
additional processes in the self-system by which dissociation
is maintained.

Perhaps still another abstraction that may be useful to keep
in mind is that there are many gradations in the level of refinement of referential operations. At one end of the scale are the

referential operations of very early life in which there is no precise delineation of what is really relevant and important in achieving a satisfaction which is itself unknown or very dimly realized; such a state of mind might be described as a vague and global feeling of unutterable turmoil. Through many gradations, the level of thought operations is increasingly refined by an ever more exact realization of what is actually relevant to the result that one is after. And, correspondingly, the amount of life that can be encompassed in referential operation becomes smaller and smaller until finally, at the quintessence of evolution of the thinking faculty, we find ourselves in the region of mathematical logic, in which the necessary relationships of ideational operations themselves are the subject of thought.

The schizophrenic process is of a piece with the referential operations of very early life, at the beginning of this scale. There is not the most rudimentary discrimination between what is relevant and what is irrelevant in a vast total situation that is impinging upon one's end organs. Correspondingly there is an extreme lack of clarity as to the action which reaches the goal, if it is reached at all, and nothing like cause-and-effect thinking as to why the goal is or is not reached.

Thus here are two poles, although the pole at the beginning of the scale is, in a sense, imaginary—that is, we never reach it, within awareness; we only see it in the schizophrenic, when communication doesn't click, so far as we are concerned. Between these two poles there are unnumbered refinements. Only the upper few of these refinements are admitted to our awareness, and this arises clearly, it seems to me, from the history of the self. At an early age of development, the child uses obscure, autistic, unrefined thinking operations in communicating with his parents, and eventually the parents come to feel, "People won't understand Willie; these statements of his don't make sense." So gradually Willie gets to know that he must always make sense, or sound like people who think they make sense. And so awareness is simply relieved of these uncommunicative processes; there is no sense in paying attention to these more primitive types of mental operations, and finally they are just confused puzzle books. But they continue to go on outside of awareness, and the time when we know they go on, from our personal experience, is when we are asleep, for some fragments of them are carried over into waking life as remembered symbolic operations in sleep.

The Dynamism of Sublimation

We shall start out with sublimation, a dynamism which has enormous place in the earlier phases of education or socialization, and which therefore serves good purposes for many people in many situations throughout life, including the purpose of enabling them to maintain mild maladjustments instead of experiencing more severe mental disorders. I define sublimation as the unwitting substitution of a partial satisfaction with social approval for the pursuit of a direct satisfaction which would be contrary to one's ideals or to the judgment of the social censors and other important people who surround one.[1]

Now, in saying that sublimation must be unwitting, I am not just being overprecise and unduly restrictive. I have arrived at this statement by the method of inference, in which you take what you have observed, as well as what you have never observed, and feed it into the hopper of the mental analytic machinery of deductive and inductive reasoning. To follow my reasoning about why it must be unwitting, you must think of the self as the 'apparatus'—the bundle of processes, selected memories, knowledge of relationships, and so on—that is struck off the very rich and capable human personality by the necessity for feeling secure in contact with

---

[1] *Editors' note:* At a later period, Sullivan defined sublimation as "the unwitting substitution, for a behavior pattern which encounters anxiety or collides with the self-system, of a socially more acceptable activity pattern which satisfies part of the motivational system that caused trouble." *The Interpersonal Theory of Psychiatry;* p. 193.

others, long before one can possibly analyze and make reasonable sense of the cultural prescriptions of behavior—what is
right and wrong, what should be said and done, and so on. If
you think of the self as something other than that, then I do
not know how I can make plain, by deduction and induction,
why sublimation must be unwitting. The self is primarily a
very elaborate bundle of memories, processes, perceived relationships, and past experience, understandings of the course
that events follow in hanging together—all in the interests of
making one feel competent to deal with other people without
becoming aware of the myriad threats to one's self-esteem that
are implicit in almost any interpersonal situation. All these
things that have such pomp and circumstance in one's own
known mental operations represent a special modification of
human potentialities, developed historically from the need to
become acculturated too fast, for we don't live long enough
to take it reasonably in our stride.

The steps by which I reason that sublimation must be unwitting are the following. The self controls awareness, and
this is perhaps well demonstrated in the very disappearance
from awareness of all the earlier and more broadly referential
types of thinking. That these earlier referential operations
exist—in fact, that life utterly depends on them in most contexts—is not too hard to realize. You know very well that how
you get where you do in your thinking in many cases—what
your interests are, what occurs to you, and so on—is not a
tedious ticking off of logical thinking. Part of the mythology
or perhaps truth of psychoanalytic training is that one gets
nearest to these earlier referential processes by the free association method of psychoanalysis. But even there the psychiatrist
seldom encounters things that are not pretty crude abstracts of
logical thinking or ordinary report; if he does get beneath
these, he doesn't know what is going on, and the patient doesn't
know either. We just are cut off from our early methods of
thought as ingredients of awareness, and the reason is not very

far to seek, because a great part of the education in mid- and late-childhood is to bring language habits into conformity with the requirements of communicative speech. Such conformity is very important, for the person who says extremely obscure things which he cannot explain is strongly suspected of suffering mental disorder—an indication of what bad prestige these more primitive types of referential operation have as compared with logical thinking in words, and particularly as compared with consensually valid statements that are built up with careful reference to a censor so that they will mean to the other person what they were intended to mean.

So far, I have tried to show that the self controls awareness. But what about this business of sublimating? Let us say that a person has a need for satisfaction that has gotten him into trouble; and he wishes he could do something about it, but knows that he can't. Let us say that somebody else comes along and tells him, "I'm afraid, my good man, that you would have to have a special universe in order to proceed directly to get this satisfaction. It just isn't done; it's going to make a lot of trouble. But why not do so-and-so, which will really come quite close to giving you satisfaction, and *is* done, and is socially approved?" Then the person is perfectly justified in saying, "I'm profoundly grateful to you. That, of course, is extremely good advice. I shall follow it." And we'll say that he does. Now it might seem that in the course of events the person would become so habituated in doing this socially approved thing for partial satisfaction of his needs that it would be almost the same as direct complete satisfaction. If he lived long enough, that might be the case. But for a very long time he would have to remind himself that, while this is not quite what he wants and is really a good deal more work, it is the only way that he can get part of his satisfaction and feel secure too. In other words, he will have an awareness of frustration, of dissatisfaction, because what he is doing is not the direct and simple thing that he really wants, but is what he has to do to feel secure. And this is not the sort of thing that makes a person feel very proud of himself, very sure of himself, and very well pleased with life. It means that he has to be careful to choke off every impulse for direct satisfaction, and drag in this partial satisfaction pattern that has social approval, and make the most of what he gets out of it. Now this is what would happen if sublimation could be within awareness.

The unwitting character of sublimation is magnificently demonstrated in the course of early education, when people learn that however great the tensions in the rectum may be, they have to go through certain preliminaries of finding the right kind of thing to sit on, getting the right garments down, and so on, before they relax. There is no business in that, you know, of thinking, "Well, now, this is the thing that is done; if I relax too soon, it will be most unfortunate"—there is no thinking of what the laundry will charge, and so on. One begins immediately to find the right sort of thing to sit on when the tensions become pretty strong. That is the way sublimation works. You don't get immediate relief in the tensions, but by going through a lot of motions, you get what really is ever so much more satisfactory in the long run. But the joker about it is that the satisfaction isn't complete, and the incompleteness is this: I don't believe that there will ever be, in any of us, an entire absence of envy for the unimportance that such a thing as emptying the rectum has, for example, for my dog— and even she is pretty highly cultured; she wouldn't do it on the rug, for instance. All the social restraints, habits of clothing, peculiar ideas about particular odors, and what not —all this great pile of artifacts of human life is eternally reiterated to us by these very necessities of finding the proper toilet equipment for relieving our bowels, or hiding in the woods if we happen to be in transit by car.

Thus all sublimatory things are more complicated than the direct satisfaction of the needs to which they apply. But they entail no disturbance of consciousness, no stopping to think why they must be done or what the expense connected with direct satisfaction would be. There is simply no consciousness of the need for the direct satisfaction—it is all very suave and efficient. And that is just the opposite of the case where you tell a person in rational terms, so that he has it within awareness, to "sublimate" something. In successful sublimations, where you find a person showing an extraordinarily efficient handling of a conflict between the need for a satisfaction and the need for security, it is always done without perturbations of awareness; you never find this efficiency in any of these reasoned solutions. The path is laid down in the region of mental process from which we are denied anything like ready access in adult life, and since all operations in that region are relatively without disturbance—unless mental disorder is entailed—it works just as smoothly as if we had nothing to do with it, as if there were no complex process involved.

So when a person is having a bad time with something that is intensely unsatisfactory to him about himself, if he happens on what we, as psychiatrists, will afterwards call a sublimation, it brings him great relief; without his noticing it this strain and stress that he has been suffering disappears, and life thus becomes richer and fuller. It may be that he doesn't get quite as much rest from his sleep, but that is the only real rift in the lute—and nobody is any too clear, when he wakes up, about what happened while he slept. Perhaps I have now said enough to emphasize why the process has to be unwitting if it is to be sublimation; otherwise it is a sort of chronic headache.

Now I am attempting to tackle this thing from a three-point observational pattern. Insofar as we can define this dynamism —call it something that will become familiar and useful to us —our first observational point is, What must be necessary in the self-system of a person in order that the appearance of this thing that we are talking about as a dynamism is conspicuous? From this viewpoint, we find—and this is what is really behind the definition and happens to be this very "must" that we are talking about—that quite unwittingly the person has passed out of a severe struggle between an unsatisfactory desire and a wish for social security, you might say, into some new activity in life which is very rewarding in terms of satisfaction and security. So we say that in sublimation there must be this element of unawareness of what has been done; there must not be a clear connection between the new way of life and the conflict-provoking impulse that gives it its chief energy.

Our second observational point is, What does this set up in living—that is, in the total personality? (I am for the moment talking as if personality existed in a vacuum.) Obviously, when sublimation takes place, there must be in the total personality what is left over, you might say, in terms of incomplete satisfaction, even if such a trifling thing as habits about defecating is concerned. What is to become of the remaining need for satisfaction? Where do we look for it? Do we, when sublimating, pile up tensions for the rest of our life? Obviously we don't. We get rid of the tensions, and the dynamism works, when it is not overloaded. Therefore, we must realize, first, that since the whole thing must be excluded from awareness, there must be a continuous process in the self which avoids anything that would readily break down the unconscious character of the performance. Second, there must be certain tensions representing the frustration and the partial character of the satisfaction, and so on. And third, something must happen to these tensions, because they don't accumulate. Thus we have to look for the time when the complexities in the self-system are naturally rather in abeyance, when we are theoretically really detached quite completely from any threats to our security, and that is in sleep.

So we come to our third observational point—sleep. The odd things that go on in sleep, and sometimes leave traces into the next day, are ways of keeping us living—in other words, keeping us comfortable. So we look to the dream-world to see the satisfactions of any large part of the tensions which are being sublimated. Sometimes the needs that are unsatisfied in waking life cannot be handled by symbolic operations in sleep. For instance, an adolescent may have an eternal gnawing fear that he is "homosexual," whatever that means to him. If the conviction ever becomes complete, then he goes into panic and a great part of his life is spent in avoiding a thing which he cannot sublimate. This is so critical a situation that the self manifests itself even in sleep and the person is not able to have a frank homosexual dream—that is, one which comes within his notion of homosexuality.

Thus we cannot say that sleep is the time characterized by the total absence of the self-system as a functional entity; but it is the only time in life when the activities of the self-system are vestigial most of the time. Therefore, needs that cannot be satisfied in waking life can, if there is no very large tension connected with them, be satisfied by symbolic operations in such a way that they don't make trouble. If it were not for that, we would all blow up early in life and the human race would become extinct, for the social order is such that unnumbered needs for direct satisfaction have to be more or less thwarted, postponed, or something of the sort. We succeed, however, in discharging the urgencies of things by operations in sleep. And the way that we can maintain even the semblance of comparative mental health in the waking state is often by these extraordinarily complex, more or less continuous operations that I call the dynamisms of difficulty. But I want to remind you that they are part of the equipment of the best adjusted, in many cases, although they also are often seen as the explanation of very serious trouble.

Early Referential Processes and Schizophrenia

A dynamism which is, perhaps, even older in the life history of each of us than sublimation is the appearance in consciousness of types of referential process, thought, or revery [2] which most of us leave behind us when we pass into the state of education in verbal communication, but which in schizophrenia, contrary to ordinary experience of most of us, appear in consciousness in waking life.[3] We have every reason to suppose that the very young have referential processes. They do learn. They make adjustments to sometimes extraordinarily complex situations created by their parents, uncles, grandparents, brothers, sisters, and so on. And yet we are perfectly certain that they do not have the clear, concise, precise, and very limited type of referential operation that we have when we, for example,

[2] Revery and thought are practically synonymous with me, except that I prefer to use revery when I refer to the earlier types of things—the less clearly consensually valid sort of symbolic operation. Thought is traditionally more or less associated with referential processes that are at least somewhat adapted to communication with someone else, instead of merely to serve the direct purposes of a person.

[3] *Editors' note:* In another series of about the same period as this lecture, Sullivan has discussed the origin of the schizophrenic process as follows: "What do we have to infer about the 'private mental state' of infancy, to use the old jargon? We must necessarily infer what we can about the infantile mental state, if only because we see almost intimidatingly obscure phenomena in certain people much later in life. And if we have a somewhat scientific attitude toward reality, it is much easier for us to presume that a very obscure phenomenon that we observe in a person of 17, for instance, has a history than it is to assume that this obscure phenomenon is some strange intervention of a personal devil, either a member of the theological hierarchy or a form of disease called mental illness. We have with us always a group of people who are said to suffer schizophrenic disorders. There is good reason for assuming that there are mental states before speech; and either we have to get absolutely mystical in our thinking about the schizophrenic processes, indulging in obscure autistic reveries on the subject, or we have to accept some of the schizophrenic phenomena as simply evidence of these early types of thought. If we view them from the latter standpoint, the schizophrenic processes are not unprecedented, unutterably obscure, and un-understandable. Thus before we plunge into the wilderness of the autistic revery of the schizophrenic, it is a good idea to wonder if these things are unprecedented in the history of the person; and the moment that we look closely at them with this respectful attitude, we discover that in many of the most obscure processes of the schizophrenic illnesses we are probably seeing regressive reactivation of processes which make up the mental life of the infant—which are, however, covert and implied rather than observable."

make a scientific statement. What goes on in their revery or thought processes is much more diffuse and less circumscribed as to the precise meaning of what is symbolized; and that is, in some ways, highly advantageous at a time when the young have practically no information about the culturally given or socially given world that they have to learn about. If they couldn't do much of anything until they had gotten quite clear on the relation of a particular event to their past experience, it would take several centuries to learn enough to put on such a performance as I am somewhat uncertainly doing just now. So, clearly, these rather diffuse and anything but precise implicit referential processes are extremely handy in getting one's first grasp on living. And if only from the principle of simplicity, we can presume that there is no time in subsequent life when some of these relatively primitive or early types of processes might not also be very handy. This can be seen in sleep. Let us say that a personality is loaded up with a great variety of interlocking frustrations, and the somatic organization is full of tensions; if the person had to do any scientific formulation of the situation in sleep, he would have to sleep for a century or two. But instead, he has recourse in sleep to these much earlier types of process and may dispose of his troubles more or less successfully in a good night's sleep.

Now, we do not have to appeal to any slightly puzzling latency period to account for the disappearance of these types of referential process from full awareness—from consciousness, as it is ordinarily called. Insofar as these things get themselves invested with words, the words are the highly autistic language of the uneducated child; the words have meaning, but the meaning is intensely personal and sometimes extremely difficult for someone else, even another child, to in any sense approximate. These autistic words of childhood are not very useful in an attempt at precise, consensually valid communication. However, insofar as these vague, relatively unpurposed symbolic operations use words, these highly autistic, personal words are just the thing, because the processes themselves are very personal. They are not intended for teaching one how to do solid geometry; they are intended for grasping the almost ungraspable complexity of social life and fitting one into it somewhat.

In the process of the child's acquiring our possibly most valuable social tool—our native tongue, and the ability to use it with considerable satisfaction among our fellows—the parents and teachers and other representatives of the social order have to suppress this autistic speech and beat into the child a very considerable respect for what might be described as the dictionary meanings of verbal terms. And since children have the stupendous capacity of the human being for learning and for making connections and seeing relations, imaginary or otherwise, they do not cultivate their autistic words into new words; the things just disappear, like a great many correct and erroneous notions that we have had in the past. They do not leave us; they presumably continue to be available for appropriate types of referential process or thought process, but, at least, they disappear from awareness. It would be very awkward if, as I was attempting to say something, some of the words I used revived in themselves the meaning they had for me when I was five. I am afraid that this would be even more complicated for my hearers.

So, of course, in the process of learning the language, and learning to behave as people are supposed to behave, all these essentially very useful—personally useful—but socially useless types of rather diffuse, generalized reference are gradually utterly forbidden awareness, where they would just confuse and harass us. And, as I say, you do not have to drag in any conceptions except that of acculturation and learning in the special field of language and the expression of one's so-called mental states to account for the fact that the self-system comes gradually to exclude from awareness all of these earlier types of mental process. Thus if and when we have to have recourse to them in the midst of the waking life, we go into a state of abstraction, which is ordinarily called a brown study, in which we literally are not particularly in touch with the environment and are entirely out of touch with what is occupying us. And when these rather general processes have done their work, then we rise into full awareness again and find that we have an idea, a hunch, or something or other which is quite clearly the product of these more or less early types of process.

Now the schizophrenic is, so far as I can discover, essentially characterized by the fact that his self-system has lost control of awareness, so that it cannot exclude these earlier processes and restrict awareness to late, highly refined types of thought. By the time one becomes schizophrenic, the self is in such a critical position that these much earlier types of mental process receive more or less the same clear representation in awareness that they did in late infancy or early childhood; but that does not remove from them all the values—crazy, impractical, and so on—which have been attached to them in the early years, and which are the reason for denying them consciousness whenever possible. This gives us the very curious picture of a patient who, part of the time, is as lucid and as skillful in formulation as we are; who, in fact, every now and then unhorses us by the pellucid perfection of his inference about things which we are struggling with—you see, he has been less handicapped with other people's explanations as he went along. But this same patient at other times thinks in these more or less global terms of very early life, to his great chagrin and our utter confusion. The rapid and unpredictable shifts in levels of consciousness in schizophrenia depend, from a theoretic standpoint, on this very business of what disadvantage the self-system is working under. If the disadvantage suddenly becomes great, then the schizophrenic processes flow in and engulf all clear formulations. In other words, at times when the self is not readily able to carry on its function and is operating comparatively inefficiently, awareness includes these earlier processes, which are ingredients in all of us, but which, once we have left early childhood, we never ordinarily encounter except in sleep.

The problems, the life situations confronting the schizophrenic, are of great complexity and are highly individual in the sense of strikingly autistic, because they haven't been well socialized in his history. Moreover, the situation confronting him is of the greatest urgency, often amounting—once awareness has extended to these earlier processes—to a feeling of cosmic threat, of literal world disaster, terrifying beyond the capacity of words to readily depict. So one can see why the self—which is invented, evolved, tooled, and refined for the purpose of making us feel secure among our fellows, getting what we want from cooperation with them, and avoiding their more open hostilities—has neither any vast place in fending off this enormous threat that the schizophrenic feels nor any particular probability of utility in that connection. Its inadequacy to maintain security in the face of this tremendous threat from within, and apparently from without, shows itself in this failure of one of its most striking adult functions—namely, the restriction of awareness of one's mental processes to those which are more or less clearly valid in communication. Thus the schizophrenic state is, I say, essentially one in which this restriction of awareness of the types of mental process going on has broken down, and the person is much more in touch with all that is going on in his personality as symbolic operations than the rest of us are, except in our dreams. Incidentally, the fact that the self-system has failed to maintain this very important control of awareness of implicit process does not mean that the self-system disappears. Its functional efficiency is somewhat a function of the momentary situation; so when there is no great pressure, the schizophrenic is in much the same mental state as we, and the implicit processes that he notices are those more or less capable of communication. But then if there is an increase in threat, an increase in tension—a severe anxiety caused by the schizophrenic's seeing, or seeming to see, either that he is about to involve himself in something which horrifies him, or is having something horrible thrust on him—at that time the self-function is minimal in controlling awareness; and the types of mental process which he experiences within himself, and often outside himself, are of the very much earlier type, which most of us have experienced in unpleasant and very obscure dreams.

So schizophrenia as a dynamism is in a strange way a statement of the failure of the tripartite division. But you must also remember that all the dynamisms at certain times represent failures, and the very act of failing to maintain a crazy adjustment often reveals how it was done as long as it worked. And schizophrenia is an adjustment in the sense that, despite the unnumbered incursions of more primitive processes into awareness, all schizophrenics part of the time carry on adjustive efforts which are very reasonable, considering how little ease adjustment has for them. This is perhaps another reason for saying that we are all more simply human than otherwise.

PROJECTION

As I have said, these processes, at least the very early ones, are highly autistic and extremely personal. They deal with other people only in the sense that I might be said to deal with the birds that seem to be so unaccustomed to cars that they stay on the road too long to get away safely, so I slow the car down a little. I suppose children's primitive thought processes deal with others much as I deal with the birds. In such circumstances, as in all of life, the refinements and complexities of the operation are probably more or less adequate to the more or less dimly foreseen goal of the operation. In a great many of these early situations, it is not necessary nor yet possible for the child to be quite clear on the demarcation between I, myself; mama; her nipple; the dog; the inanimate Teddy-bear; and so on and so forth. The boundaries between such things impress our adult awareness a good deal, because we hang clothes and one thing and another on them, and thereby sometimes improve the impression that we make on others. But the child knows nothing of all this and just hasn't developed the capacity that we adults have of making an awful lot of verbal noise about just where our fingertips end and the unoccupied air begins. As a result of this, a good many of these primitive processes (and I do not mean by "primitive" that they are particularly savage, or anything like that) lack anything like precise separation of "thee" and "me"—of what is within and what is perhaps a few feet without. That characteristic combines with some of the many idiosyncrasies of our distance reception—in other words, the means by which we actually do keep track of events rather clearly outside us—to make it quite difficult for the schizophrenic to be very clear on which is he and which is somebody else.

Thus, just from the nature of the thing, projection, as we solemnly talk about it in psychiatry, does not need to be so terribly mysterious in the beginnings of the process. Among the distance receptors, it just happens that the sense of hearing, which is a very instant link of contact with circumambient reality, has at least a tenuous relation to what is so essential in learning—namely, speech. And so when the types of operations based on the auditory reception of events are of this primitive level, there is a lack of certainty as to whether a given thought went on in one's own head, or is a remark that somebody else made, or is a thought that has in some strange fashion been put into one's head. This uncertainty is not so terribly difficult to sympathize with, for occasionally some of you may have experienced auditory hallucinations in the moments of falling asleep or waking up. And if so, you have really been very, very close to the recurrent state of an actively disturbed schizophrenic, except that you, slightly better off than he, immediately felt fairly sure that this had happened 'in' you. But it was very moving and impressive. It had all sorts of rather unearthly emotional tones, perhaps threat or awe, or various other emotions that we do not ordinarily associate with anything anybody says to us. If you have had such an experience, you almost certainly can recall the almost lightning-like speed with which the self gained control, and you were awake and very intent indeed on whether or not anything strange was happening—showing with what vigor the presence of these earlier types of processes is excluded from our ordinary waking consciousness.

The Obsessional Dynamism

The obsessional dynamism, which is extremely fashionable in the morbidities of the American people, can appear and is certainly founded pretty early in life. As the child becomes increasingly adept at the use of language, he learns to say things which have still an exclusively personal reference, but which are taken by papa, mama, and the various other censors as adequate adjustive efforts. A very simple example is the child-training by which little Willie, having taken a clap at baby sister, is upbraided for this unseemly and ungentlemanly conduct and is directed to say to little sister, who doesn't talk yet, that he is sorry. The statement that he is sorry seems to have very considerable power, in that the social censors became more tolerant and he perhaps escapes a licking. And later on he may discover in school that a soft answer to the teacher, couched in terms of certain of the values which are at the moment popular, turneth away much wrath and perhaps gets him a good deal of unjustified consideration.

And if, in the education of this person, there is at least one parent who is a past master at appealing to noble ethical principles with which to confuse issues about performances which are more self-centered than hostile, then the child has a great deal of experience—not only personally, but by proxy—with the strange power of certain formulae to suspend, nullify, or greatly change what he begins to sense as the simple and natural course of events. It is not at all strange, then, that a good many people show—as one of the moderately useful, but also somewhat maladjustive types of patterns that persistently appear in their lives—a preoccupation with thought of a more or less consensually valid type, but thought which, when you study it carefully, is not communicative to you of anything like what it means to the person who is doing the thinking. I am inclined to say that the essence of the obsessional dynamism is that the self-system is occupied at times of stress, tribulation, tension, and so on, with not very complicated and singularly stable— in the sense of unshifting, unprogressive—preoccupations that sound like words of adult speech, although they are not communicative as such.

The obsessional neurotic, as it were, plucks out of the tissue of autistic speech of early childhood certain words, phrases, or sentences, and uses them as the points of preoccupation, at least, if not as the actual content of preoccupation. In other words, in the pursuit of security, the obsessional person regresses in certain cognitive operations—knowing operations— to the stage of quite autistic speech. This is by no means a massive and uniform regression, because all that is needed is that one will be able to achieve, by the magic of this preoccupation, an immunization to social threats. But it is a real regression in the sense that these more primitive formulae stay; they continue to exist in a person who can be very intelligent indeed in appraising many problems which happen not to touch on this realm of security. And they are relatively fixed, in that they do not undergo much change over a period of time.

Much of the obsessional thinking and many of the obsessional rituals sound all right, or can be talked about all right. But you can understand anything from them only when you realize that these things, as a prop to adjustment, were fixed in childhood when the referential meaning of words was much more autistic, much more difficult to grasp, and that what these people think really is anything *but* as obvious as it may sound or look. Once you realize that it isn't as simple as it seems, the obsessional's communication provides almost a theater in which you can see the supplementary processes in the self by which a dynamism is maintained. And this dynamism in essence consists of extraordinarily free satisfaction of needs, made possible because security is maintained by a somewhat magical autistic performance. As a result, except for rather well-focused attacks on the security of an obsessional neurotic, the dynamism is quite adequate to meet the ordinary run of life events, and therefore the person does not suffer any great accumulation of anxiety from any great accumulation of tensions and unsatisfied needs, nor any great onslaughts of anxiety from acute insecurity. The load on the sleep mechanism of the rather obsessional person therefore is, contrary to first-blush expectancy, quite low; the obsessional sleeps very peacefully in his bed at night. As long as by these rather primitive operations one maintains a jittery security among one's fellows, then, of course, there is not a constant conflict between one's less elevated needs and one's feeling of insecurity. Thus you will find obsessional personalities doing hostile, aggressive, and even frank sexual things with the most charming simplicity—something that you encounter in no other branch of the dynamisms of difficulty. But, as you would necessarily expect, the self-system is so busy with operations which add up to security for the obsessional —which we call obsessional processes—that it is very hard to get the obvious formulated in working with them, which is that there is a good deal of satisfaction in their lives and that satisfaction sometimes comes easier for them than it seems to for the healthy people among whom they have their being.

We have here taken only a brief sideswipe at the obsessional dynamism. We shall consider it more at length as we go along.

Manifestations of These Dynamisms in Ordinary Life

Now all of these processes have a 'normal' manifestation in ordinary life, a regular and useful place in every personality. I would like to stress, especially about sublimation, that you often see it when it does not require psychiatric treatment.

A great part of the acculturation of the young is a sublimatory process, in essence. It works beautifully, and in some cases leaves rather significant areas of life that are dealt with only in sleep. The people who accomplish these sublimations are very useful citizens, and do not know that they are any more handicapped than anybody else; they certainly would, I think, be justified in shooting any psychiatrist who wanted to disturb their living.

The obsessional dynamism may also be useful. To connect this process more thoroughly with ordinary life, let me comment on the things that all of us do which are obsessive in the very mildest sense, and why some of them are even useful. All of you have, on occasion, found that a song or a license number or something of that kind has gotten to be on your mind to the point of nuisance. And if you have paid any particular attention to this experience, you have probably gotten more and more puzzled as to what on earth this tag, or song, or visual information about the highway had to do with anything on earth. There was simply no spread of meaning; you didn't get answers. What had happened was that the words of the song or the numerals of the license plate, which were actually communicative, had for some reason or other caught onto some autistic context which was beneath the level of awareness maintained by yourself in the process. You just could not get to this autistic context because you were awake.

For some people, if not for all, when it is untimely to abolish full awareness—as we do when we go into the states of abstraction and brown study—the next best thing, in order to have time out for the subterranean processes, is to occupy awareness with one of these obsessional tags. That, I think, is an extremely helpful clue to the whole business of the substitutive reactions. Perhaps you have sometimes gone out for a drive when you had a serious professional problem on your mind, and can recall, if you search yourself, getting preoccupied with your speedometer reading, or something of that kind. You have found it rattling around over and over again in the most classical obsessional fashion, for no earthly end— you didn't want to remember it; it was utterly useless information. But presently you found yourself moving back to thinking on the problem that had been on your mind when you set out, and it was clearer. Thus it seems that giving the self something to fool with, as it were, is about the only way we can rest when we are thoroughly awake and are in circumstances such that we simply cannot become abstracted— for getting really abstracted while driving a car is a pretty desperate risk, especially in heavy traffic. And so the next best thing may be this recourse to consciously meaningless preoccupation with some tag or something, which perhaps has all its meaning in that it is convenient; it is something to roll around in your mind while the genuinely cognitive processes are proceeding on a more primitive level of symbol operation, beneath or outside of awareness.

Thus if we look at the obsessional dynamism, not in its full-blown misuse but in its simple everyday manifestation, it is completely describable as the replacement of adjustive process by referential process which is adequately explained as a substitute, as a way of avoiding or temporizing with events. And its normal manifestation, its regular place in every personality, seems to be just that—it keeps one busy while more useful referential processes run somewhere else; and when these potentially more useful processes have gotten well under way, the substitute process disappears.

To consider the dynamism of schizophrenia from the viewpoint of its useful manifestation in ordinary life, let me recall our definition and what this must imply about the self-system —schizophrenia represents a failure to control awareness of ordinarily unwitting levels of thought. Certainly, those ordinarily unwitting levels of thought are utterly necessary for human life, and certainly the ability to admit them into awareness in very fragmentary and very carefully selected areas could be occasionally useful. If we were not taught to be afraid of these things, to feel that they were so queer and so unearthly, I surmise that we would be much better acquainted with the sort of thing that schizophrenics are painfully well acquainted with. But unfortunately our system compels us to lose touch with reality in the sense of time, and the people around one, and so on—to go into a brown study—before we have recourse to these more primitive, wider referential types of mental process. If these more inclusive referential processes were accessible to awareness, then you could entertain them and still keep track of such things as time and your friends— even lay these processes down for the moment and make a polite remark often enough, without first going into a sort of trance state. And so, while I cannot recommend schizo-phrenic processes, still all of us use the same thing, but we just are not equal to the shock of being quite clear on what they are.

The Relation of Sublimation and Obsessionalism to Schizophrenia

The utility of setting up all these modal points is lost if one thinks of them as stages in transition to something else. It is really much more valid to think the other way—that the in-creasing complexity and adaptive expense of these dynamisms is a measure of the character of the problem that faces the person. In other words, it is a question of the degree of neces-sity. At one end of the scale, the necessity may be one that we handle in our stride: we are annoyed by something, but then a beautiful solution comes along; perhaps we toss off a con-ciliatory remark, which is a sure way of sublimating the other fellow, so to speak. But at the other end of the scale, because of a long, long, long, historic course of events, one meets the final intolerable calamity in which the efficiency of the self is destroyed to the point where it cannot control awareness, and one is flooded with all sorts of panicky, primitive mental processes which have the disastrous results on one's behavior, one's attitude toward other people, and so on, that lead to admission to mental hospitals.

Now the general frame of my approach has tended to obliterate one important point about sublimation: If one attempts to sublimate the major portion of satisfactions for the genital dynamism, it is fairly certain that the sublimatory machinery will break down rather quickly. The process cannot handle things of that magnitude. And the way it will break down is fairly certain to be excitement. The sublimatory activities will be pushed more and more wildly, and anxiety will become a more and more conspicuous accompaniment of the hyper-activity, so that a psychiatrist will diagnose an excitement. And excitements very often have schizophrenic accompaniments and eventuate in schizophrenic disorder. Thus when we talk about sublimation, we are abstracting a very typical process from a continuum in which, at a certain point, sublimation may take very frankly schizophrenic form. In this, as in a great many other complex fields, we facilitate our thinking by conceptualizing as if abstractions plucked at certain points were real entities—even though the human manifestations of these abstractions show vast variations and overlappings and so on. Actually such abstractions are just extremely convenient devices for reducing the overwhelming individuation and complication of nearly everything in life.

With regard to the obsessional dynamism, major dependence on it nowadays precedes the appearance of frank schizophrenic phenomena often enough so that one can assume a relationship. But let me invite your attention to the fact that about 20 years ago no less a person than Adolf Meyer said that the presence of a neurosis practically precluded the appearance of a more severe disorder, and illustrated this by saying that the obsessional neurosis was never observed to proceed to schizophrenia. I am not saying that Meyer was wrong. Meyer was a terribly careful observer, although you can't always be too sure of just what he meant by his terms. But I think that the type of cultural problem that people have to deal with has changed, and that what might have seemed to be a very important insulation against schizophrenia 20 years ago is quite obviously not an insulation now. This means, of course, that it was not really an insulation then; it was just that the types of problems that occurred in the culture 20 years ago were well handled by an obsessional neurosis. While that may be true in some cases now, it is not in others. For a period of over 10 years, I was able to keep myself almost continuously worried to death with a group of patients who showed a prevailingly obsessional way of handling life, but who, under pressure, would have episodes of frank schizophrenic handling of life; but then as the pressure was dissipated either by my work or by a fortunate course of events, they would drop back to an outstandingly obsessional picture. Thus these dynamisms are so clearly related today—although they did not appear to be 20 years ago —that I manifest a tendency to consider them always together. But that may be confusing at this particular stage in our attempt to get things clear and organized, and so I am trying to look at them as fixed points stuck here and there in the possibilities of human life. Our expectations are such that it is easier to make sense of the thing, in our thinking and in our therapeutic attack, if we put a person where he outstandingly fits, at one of these modal points, or midway between them.

I am discussing things that interest the psychiatrist in their morbid manifestations, and perhaps failing properly to insist to you that this preoccupation with them as morbid entities, or as hypotheses which explain what we see in very sick people, should not obscure the fact that sublimation, for instance, is a complete success in a great deal of the early education. Since sublimation in the vast majority of instances is just as smooth and useful as can be, it becomes a dynamism of difficulty only by definition, because it happens to be of a piece with pathological sublimation. Thus, instead of calling sublimation a way-station, I would call it a way of life. And I would not call it a way of staving off something more serious, for anything that works is a way of staving off failure, and we are really sort of straining the language to say that success is a way of staving off failure.

Nor do I want anyone to become too preoccupied with the notion that schizophrenia is the finish in the progression of dynamisms. We will be ever so much clearer in our minds if we study the progressive overcomplication of attempts at living from the standpoint of the pressures that lead to the overcomplication, rather than if we think of it as a natural progression of dynamisms. In discussing these dynamisms, I can scarcely avoid ticking them off one after another, which may make them sound more or less like stepping stones, implying a logical progression of dynamisms. But when they work, they are fine. When a dynamism doesn't work, something else follows; the preceding one has failed because of greater pressure, you might say. The thing that follows it does give a speciously logical picture of the first having served to delay the second. But the answer is really in the magnitude of the stress in the personality. I have a fear of people getting to thinking that if they try to clear up a person's obsessional neurosis, he will develop schizophrenia, or thinking that there is any risk of a person's becoming schizophrenic who has spent 20 years being a pretty classical obsessional nuisance to all and sundry. If a person has spent 20 years with a good working dynamism, the chances are rather immensely against his becoming schizophrenic, because the longer he lives, the less the pressures that are going to provoke a serious illness.

There is an ideal way of life, in which a situation calls for action, the action is immediately and simply forthcoming, and the situation dissolves and a new situation follows. A great deal of living is made up of such simple, direct activity. When everything has become frightfully difficult for an obsessional patient, I spring this on him: "I suppose you drink coffee safely in the morning? For God's sake, don't start thinking about that. Otherwise you'll drown yourself." We psychiatrists are apt to overlook the fact that there are simple, direct, and utterly inexpensive dynamisms. When they are not simple, they are apt to be, under certain circumstances, our ethical business. And the greater their complexity, largely in terms of the machinery called out in the self, the greater the chance of their being the official business of the psychiatrist. Now let me add one thing: I suppose some of you psychiatrists, if not all of you, have had patients who were still schizophrenic leave the hospital as social recoveries and do very nicely for years. They had learned that it wasn't perversity or hostility in the environment that made the environment regard them as crazy. So they patched up an imitation of normality—they stopped attempting to communicate the primitive material which is the essence of schizophrenia— whereupon the environment was no longer worried about them and everything went beautifully. They still had access to levels of thought processes which we would call schizophrenic, but they were no longer psychotic in the sense that their actions and attempts at communication had disastrous effects on the particular environment. This is only an example of the fact that we may see these same dynamisms in situations where they are not a psychiatrist's business. We should keep that in mind rather than rattle off, as is ordinarily done in the text-books: "This is a mental disorder, characterized by so-and-so."

CHAPTER
3

Selective Inattention

WHEN YOU consider the opportunities for learning implicit in the various developmental eras of personality, you may well wonder how in the world we can pass through such a great variety of educative experiences—experiences which, as one looks at the pattern of things, would almost certainly tell an intelligent creature something—without any effects from such educative experience whatever. How is it that after we finally get to the point where we think we may now be able to get by—in other words, we are more or less going concerns—we do not learn more from there on? To be more specific, how is it, in the realm of the psychiatrist, that our patients will have an experience that can well be described as bumping their heads against a stone wall, and will do it several times a day, with considerable pain and one thing and another, but never learn a single thing by it?

The explanation, I believe, is to be found in a universal bit of human equipment—selective inattention—which to a great extent enables us to stay as we are, despite remarkable experiences that befall us, simply by keeping the attention on something else—in other words, by *controlling awareness* of the events that impinge upon us.

Concentration as the Focusing of Awareness

In an attempt to verbalize this process which I call selective inattention, I shall first consider a type of experience that is commonly referred to as concentration. Some of you, I suppose, suffered psychiatry in the days when concentration was a fashionable preoccupation of educational psychology and everything was explained in terms of alleged difficulties with it. Having had an eccentric childhood which gave me a chance to escape the necessity for knowing everything too soon, I have never been quite satisfied with that explanation, and in the course of forty years or so I finally got around to thinking about something that seems to make more sense— that is, that concentration is one part of the whole process of selective inattention.

Beyond any controversy, there are situations in which the content of consciousness—what one is aware of—is extremely narrow and focused. How intense concentration can be may be beyond your personal experience unless you have at some time had an interest such as long-range marksmanship, for example. Thousand-yard rifle-firing necessitates telescopic sights to have anything like a satisfactory view of the target, and brings into play judgment that sometimes borders on the uncanny; this judgment has to take into account, for example, the mirage—disturbances of refraction caused by the sun falling on a considerable part of the area in between you and the target on a cloudy day—the air currents to which the warm earth gives rise, the wind velocity, how wide the wind's front is, and how uniformly it is passing over the transectory of the bullet, which you may get a hint of by noticing such things as the movement of trees or grass along the course. Furthermore, the sights on a gun are such that they aim somewhere else than where you are looking, and the whole trick is to get them so ranged that you see the target when you are aiming at something else that happens to have just the proper relationship to the transectory, so that the bullet will hit the target. Thus very complex judgment is involved in determining when to fire and what to fire at. And people who are very deeply interested in that sort of thing, and who are, at least part of the time, very good at it, cannot be reached when they are getting ready to fire.

I have literally been so much of a scientist as to stick a pin into a very, very dear friend of mine on one such occasion. And sure enough, as I had expected, it was only after having fired that he reached around to the injured area and gave me the devil. Literally, on the rifle range, things are suspended from any disturbance of one's consciousness until it is time to notice them.

The reason for this is not far to seek. The performance is one that calls for so many exquisitely refined referential processes, which must be properly related to one another on the basis of previous experience and general understanding, that there is no chance of a person's making sense of it if he remains in contact with concomitant events which, however impressive, are to that purpose utterly irrelevant. The rifleman just lets those things ride until he is through with this very complex process. Then, having fired, he picks up the unnoticed nuisances that have impinged on him during the period of concentration.

We would call this a superlative use of the capacity, if you please, to separate attention from awareness—in other words, to restrict that which is in the focus of awareness very rigidly, and let the dust and leaves that blow in on the side wait until one has time to brush them off. When we have something to do that requires the use of a large part of the available analytic synthetic apparatus that biology has provided us with, we can get this all more or less focused on an extremely small context—the highly relevant events—for a short time. To maintain intense concentration of that kind for more than a short time would, I imagine, be profoundly exhausting and would rapidly lead to complete inability, because it would load up the sleep mechanism beyond any chance of its restoring itself.

Restriction or Suspension of Awareness in Emergency Situations

In meeting extreme emergency situations, we all show some ability to restrict or suspend awareness. Perhaps we can get a good many clues on how this operates if we study this process in the schizoid person. The schizoids are notorious for meeting emergencies, critical situations, with great calm. And, of course, calm in the face of extremely disconcerting events is a restriction of awareness, or concentration, if you please, on activities that are required for the meeting of the emergency. These people are very much like my friend who deferred suffering the pin-prick until he had fired his bullet. The schizoid person who has met an emergency is compelled, when on the other side of it, to notice some of the things that have been suspended—fear and nausea and all sorts of things. Although these people will tell you that they met something extraordinarily disconcerting to them as a matter of fact, once they have been through the crisis, they feel sick, and so on. In some of them who have continually to meet severe rebuffs and remain unaware of it, we see digestive spasms and other disturbances. So we know that while much that has personal significance can be deflected from awareness so that it does not disturb the state of mind at all, it does impinge on the personality. It just isn't missing; it has happened, it is experience. But it is experience generally external to awareness; and to keep it external to awareness, quite a few of the things that are connected with emotional experience in awareness have to be routed differently. For example, in most people when they are angry there actually is a marked increase of skeletal tone, on which physiologists can build brilliant hypotheses about preparedness to fight; but when the markedly schizoid person, or the person for some other reason intensely concentrated on some performance, encounters a situation which would normally make him thoroughly angry, instead of having an increase in skeletal tone, he has a great increase in visceral tone.

And this kind of restriction in awareness has a tendency to unwind. In other words, just as my friend reached around to the injured area after having done what he was really engaged in doing, so there is a tendency in all these things that are sidetracked out of the vision biologically, you might say, in the interest of special aspects of living, to return from their resting place when the time is ripe.

Fortunate and Unfortunate Uses of Selective Inattention

Now I want to address myself to the distinction between selective inattention that works to our good and selective inattention that works to the maintenance of a complex type of life. Whenever we have to do anything very difficult, such as long-range rifle work, or even things that are less complicated than that, we have to be inattentive to a great deal of the somewhat significant course of events in which we are immersed. If we could not shut out materially irrelevant events so that we could maintain a fairly compact organization of awareness and of preparation for action, we would just not get much of anywhere with a great many of the complex things we have to do. And of all the complex things we have to do, I suppose there is no category that approaches the maintenance of a feeling of personal security. So you might say that whenever one's feelings of security in relation to another person are at stake, awareness is rather sharply focused on the particular warnings in all the things that are happening to us, the particular possibilities that are before us, and so on, that need action to restore some measure of feeling of security and self-respect.

The thing that determines whether this is done well or ill, from the standpoint of long-range results for the person, is how smoothly the control of awareness excludes the irrelevant and includes the relevant. If it does not exclude things that are not really relevant and important at the time, then the outcome in action is apt to be poorly directed—what the person is trying to do will be somewhat confused. Even if his action does get the result, it is likely also to get some unpleasant irrelevant concomitants. On the other hand, it is quite important that what is relevant shall be almost immediately seized upon, and everything else be subjected to this selective inattention—or that it be "repressed" or "suppressed," or whatever you want to call it; at any rate, the result is that the irrelevant is not in awareness, although we know it is somewhere because in certain cases it makes its presence felt most of the time. For effective action there not only has to be a restriction of awareness to the relevant aspect of the situation; there also must be a certain restriction of recall, so that one recalls the past experience which is relevant to understanding the situation. Thus there is a remarkable amount of restrictive control necessary for meeting any complex situation.

But selective inattention interests us, as psychiatrists, not when the irrelevant is excluded from attention, but when the significant is not attended to. What about the peculiarity by which people who have serious life problems overlook, and assist the psychiatrist in overlooking, highly illuminating aspects of events that happen almost every day? Why is it that all of us learn so very little from a reasonably illuminating event which would entail some distinct shift in our personality? How does it come about that a patient, let us say, will give the psychiatrist an account of some current event in his life which is plausible enough to impress the psychiatrist as adequate, so that he goes on to the next topic, but which omits something very illuminating about the very problem they are supposed to be dealing with? This illuminating aspect of the event not only is not mentioned by the patient, but the performance is such that the psychiatrist doesn't even suspect that something is left out. That is what I really want to talk about here because it is vaguely related to the somewhat miraculous trouble of the schizophrenic in the opposite sense, you might say. The schizophrenic has lost some part of the control of what will enter awareness from the totality of implicit processes in the person. Everybody—practically everybody that we see—manifests an extraordinary amount of control as to what is noticed of the relevant role which he lives, and shows in some cases almost as much distress as the schizophrenic does when his 'morbid' control of the contents of awareness is disturbed. The thread that connects all of this is the fact that all of us are very much perturbed if anything goes wrong with the control by the self-system of any of the ingredients of awareness.

Two Clinical Illustrations of Selective Inattention

I once had a patient who provided me with a more elegant illustration of selective inattention than I ever hope to encounter again. He was an awfully well-reared young man, a chemist with some promise, the son of an ultra-distinguished musician and a socially correct mother. I think I heard him recount two or three hundred times, each time as a sort of prelude to the hour, an amazing event that had immediately preceded the hour. He came to my office by train from his place of activity, which was a considerable distance from mine. And time and again this young man, riding the train on the way to my office, had been astounded to discover himself entertaining markedly sadistic fantasies about other passengers. Each time, for the first two or three minutes, this amazing experience would be recounted. I had heard it perhaps two hundred times when one day, for some reason or other, all the factors added up in my mind and I interrupted before he finished. After he had recounted his fantasy of kissing some man and then biting a piece out of his ear I said, "And you were amazed!" He said, "Yes, what do you mean?" And I said, "Why, I just gave the rest of it." He said, "Yes, but why did you? I *was* amazed. But why did you say so? What do you know about it?" "Why, only that you have told me the same story two or three hundred times, except for trifling differences of detail." There was no immediate realization on his part that this was a tragically recurring amazement to a tragically conventional experience of his on the train. He did not remember the instance from the day before, and from the day before that, and so on ad infinitum. Now this disturbance of awareness to which I give the term selective inattention differs here only in degree from what is almost always happening, not only in many of our patients, but in all of us. Like all the other dynamisms of which I speak, selective inattention is universal human equipment, sometimes represented almost entirely in dreadful distortions of living, but still universal.

You see instances like that of my train-riding patient in which this restriction can apply in a curiously obscure way, so far as results are concerned. One might say, remembering that this person is under treatment for very obscure and extremely disabling personality problems, that the current event in which he entertains strikingly hostile, frequently masked, but often pretty blatantly sadistic revery processes about innocent bystanders who happen to be in the same conveyance is pretty highly relevant. It sounds very much as if the psychiatrist is being provided with pertinent data. And the event gets itself mentioned. But notice the rather exquisitely clever trick, if you please, that is played. There is no recall of the fact that this same thing happened and was recounted the day before. The patient hasn't an amnesia, for when finally I decide to strike the gong and go over the many times that I have heard it before, then the curtains are drawn back and he is astonished but remembers very clearly, "My God, yes!

Why I've told you that so many times! How in the world could I have overlooked it!" This is quite different from hysterical amnesia, where you practically have to arrange for the universe to fall on a person before recall can be effected. In selective inattention, the event is just so neatly cut off that everything is novel, it just has no purpose, you might say. Thus it is undergoing very much the process that I say is necessary in a great part of life—namely, it is being made almost irrelevant. Here is a bizarre event, but one is just astonished; it has nothing to do with oneself. Just imagine that such a thing could have happened!—that is the way it is greeted, instead of its being recognized as one of the outstanding peculiarities of one's life. So much for an instance which is almost a caricature of the process of selective inattention.

Let us consider another case in which selective inattention operates as an interference with recall of an event so that while the event impinges and may be picked up presently, it is prevented from flowing into relationship with the situation or with past experience. In this case, which is less striking, the patient—a very attractive young man—moves through life with the following peculiarity: He has singularly few relationships of any material intimacy with men; although men do not dislike him, everything in his relationship with them is superficial, and he has no particular friends. And his life is full of grand passions for women. He has fallen deeply in love with one woman after another for years and years past but, shockingly enough, nothing has ever come of it, not even those indoor sports which nowadays are so apt to accompany grand passions between the sexes. That is the story that is laid before the psychiatrist, and it is very mystifying to the patient; he doesn't understand it. He has been amazed at how many times he has been profoundly in love with somebody who seemed to like him; they would grow quite intimate in

the sense that they would spend a good many evenings together, and they liked the theater and one thing and another,
but it never got anywhere. He knew better than to propose;
there wasn't any chance. The girl would sort of gradually lose
interest in him. What lusts he had were pecuniary arrange-
ments with ladies who had prices, and had nothing to do with
these great love affairs.

Here was a person who gradually got more and more impressed with the fact that something was distinctly wrong
with his life. He was intelligent enough and sufficiently in
touch with his experience so that he could say later, "This
pattern about women occurs again and again." It absolutely
baffled him. Women seemed to like him, and he felt that they
meant a tremendous amount to him, and yet it never came
off. I should say that is just about as clear as most of the problems which are presented to the psychiatrist. It almost cries
aloud that there is something else he could tell you. And suppose you ask the critical question, "Well, what is it that you
do that warns the love object, in one of this long series of love
objects, that you aren't available, and so on? How is it that
they are discouraged? What do you do that is discouraging
to them?" Whereupon he would be amazed and would answer, "Why, nothing. I'm just all out in love. I'm terribly in
love again and again!" Well, to make a long story short,
there must be something in his relationship with these women
—something in the pattern of his behavior toward them—
that makes each love object unwilling to continue to be a
love object, much less to go on to some supposedly consum-
mating arrangement. But prod him as we may, we learn nothing, and after this happens a dozen times, let us say, we realize that there must be something very peculiar indeed about
the information that he picks up from his relation with his
love object. Clearly he must overlook something very important and very highly relevant in the relation. It is this
mysterious capacity for eternally overlooking things—things

that would abolish the mystery—that has impressed me with the profound theoretical significance of selective inattention.

Selective Inattention and the Self-System: Clinical Considerations

To make anything sensible in my system of ideas of psychiatry, one must first have, as I have said before, a pretty fair picture of the dynamics which occur within awareness or with very easy access to awareness. What can the person know about a given event? What can he experience? What can he observe if he centers attention properly on the thing? In other words, what are the characteristic peculiarities of the self-system concerned in this phenomenon of selective inattention?

Let us first consider the second patient, who is so attractive to women and so sterile of results. Instead of thinking too much about how beautifully free association will solve everything in the course of time, if there is that much time, I would settle with such a patient on what I think to be an overwhelmingly probable hypothesis. The hypothesis is that he acts toward each of this succession of love objects in a fashion which makes it impossible for the other person to take the love situation, the love episode, or whatever you want to call it, seriously. That is an extremely probable hypothesis, I believe. Now since, as he is getting older, he is getting more and more oppressed by the fact that he is no nearer marriage and raising children and all that sort of thing than he ever was, why should that hypothesis not occur to him? If the same pattern works out badly quite a number of times, and if careful scrutiny shows no negative instance, it would seem pretty natural for a person to think, "Ha, it's something *I* do," and to scrutinize one's performances in the next case that comes along. But that isn't the way it usually works, and it does not work that way in our young man who is getting more and more oppressed with his problem.

So we settle down with this patient and want as much as we can get of what he can recall of the current events in his relationship with the love object. In other words, we set a problem, which is, you might say, an exercise in reporting. The next problem we will set is an exercise in observing, but it will have a slight change that is of considerable interest to a psychiatrist: after we have had enough of his observations reported, then we will ask him to put himself somewhat in the position of the love object, of the other person, and observe and report the almost overwhelmingly probable effect on the other person of the things that he observes. And when we get to that, we may, for example, find that this man works so diligently at investing each of his feminine love objects with rare and desirable qualities which she obviously does not have and devotes so much attention to expressing his profound admiration for these qualities which she does not have that she cannot overlook the fact that she is not the person that he is in love with. She just happens to be someone on whom he has hung an ideal.

After getting moderately clear on the fact that this is about the situation with the current love object, we have him look back at some other instances. And we discover that, strangely enough, he has found in one love object after another, not a particular pattern of virtue which they did not have but, instead, a series of patterns of virtues which they did not have. Then we notice some things that are not too difficult to see when one is looking for them. We realize that this man is not working out a parataxic identification on one love object after another and happening to get lemons whom it doesn't fit. Rather, he has a way of discouraging each love object about any illusions that she may have that she will do, and he fits the practice to the personality. For example, if the woman is very docile and self-effacing, he will find in her the fine aggressive certainty of herself which is so very dear to him. And if she is quite domineering, then he will find in her an extraordinary consideration for other people's feelings; and her willingness to learn and to follow the lead of others is very dear indeed to him.

The joker in the thing is that it is classically an operation in the security realm; clearly it isn't a method of getting lustful satisfaction. The self-system, I repeat, is invented for facilitating the acquisition of a feeling of security, for success in dealing with others. Here is an exquisite piece of analysis and fraud, if you wish—that is, the self-system must have been right in the center of things all the time to provide anything like this skillful realization of what would hold each woman immunized from taking herself as the genuine love-object, so that she would gradually, feeling that he was an awfully nice idealistic person, put him in the class of brother and pass on.

Clearly, you see, this is not an activity of some dissociated system. It is activity of the self, and just as he has never observed that he is doing this—although he is doing it with the thing that ordinarily controls awareness—he also doesn't know that he is quite subtle at observing people to the point of being fairly sure what type of pattern they just cannot believe fits them. In other words, he draws a character so sharply pointed that it lets them out; they cannot fool themselves into believing that they are what he is in love with.

Thus selective inattention is very impressive when one observes that it could not possibly act so suavely, and so eternally at the right times, unless there was a constant vigilance lest one notice what for some obscure reason one is not going to notice. Selective inattention is the classic means by which we do not profit from experience which falls within the area of our particular handicap. We don't have the experience from which we might profit—that is, although it occurs, we never notice what it must mean; in fact, we never notice that a good deal of it has occurred. That is what is really troublesome in psychotherapy, I suppose—the really bland way in which people overlook the most glaring implications of certain acts of their own, or of certain reactions of theirs to other people's acts—that is, what they are apt to report as other people's acts. Much more tragically, they may overlook the fact that these things have occurred at all; these things just aren't remembered, even though the person has had them unpleasantly impressed on him.

So this is what I mean by selective inattention as a dynamism which deserves a place in psychiatric explanation. The process here passes out of the realm of the utterly necessary adjustive business in the course of concentration which precludes useless distraction, and reaches over into the realm where, although something always goes wrong, we just do not see the implications, the very highly probable, necessary concomitants and personal meanings of these events. The events themselves get into a class which is most natural and most striking in the peculiarities of recall which affect people when they get somewhere near my age—namely, that they can rattle off rather vivid recollections of events that occurred when they were, let us say, 20 or 23 years of age, and have a heck of a time trying to figure out what the course of events was yesterday—whether they did or did not stamp a letter before mailing it, and so on. I suppose that may be regarded simply as new testimony to the fact that they are getting on toward the terminus. But a much less startling and more probable explanation is that the longer we live, the more habitual many things become which were at one time quite novel and interesting things that counted. There would not be very much sense, you know, in overburdening our exquisite biological equipment with a lot of emotional concomitants that would give the recollection of events more vividness, when these events no longer are any more important to us than whether it rained lightly or very heavily when we were driving along the road in a closed car.

The point that I want to draw your attention to is what selective inattention does to a good many of these highly illuminating details of everyday life of people who have serious mental problems. Again it looks as if the highly significant things just weren't worth remembering, you see; they are just totally unimportant, just details of life that one is perfectly clear on, and they leave no record. The power of the process for difficulty and morbidity is suggested by my patient who was shocked at the horrible character of his fantasies, beautifully, day by day, month by month, year by year, and still these events retreated from his awareness as if they were utterly familiar trivia of life. If you know that every time you are on the train you have quite sadistic fantasies about your companions, then you know something about yourself. But if you are eternally amazed when such a thing happens, that is almost as if you were saying, "Well, this isn't me! This is something strange, isn't it? A great novelty!"

This is one of the very important warps of the textiles out of which mental illnesses are built. As psychiatrists, we encounter it when a patient discusses current events in his life or even sometimes when he recalls highly significant events in the past, yet quite generally fails to serve the great purpose of the process because he selectively inattends to certain aspects of these events. And the selective inattention is so suave that we are not warned that we have not heard the important thing in the story—that it has just been dropped out. This is the thing that so often baffles us: that we know we have a context that is within the patient's grasp and that the patient is headed in the right direction toward improving mental health; and we ask for anything that comes to mind in the way of history that would give meaning to the event that is being discussed, and we get it, and yet the thing does not jell. From my experience with the human mind, the reason it does not jell is that the important thing has been overlooked, very suavely, so that we just do not notice the gap where it belongs. Thus we have to be very clear on the extreme ease with which crucially important details are overlooked before we can properly attack the evil effects of selective inattention.

I may never have happened to say how ridiculous I feel about one of my most valuable roles in the world—namely, being allegedly somewhat useful as a chronic consultant on the treatment of a patient. I feel mildly ridiculous about it because I have really extremely little to offer to the patient or to the physician; but that extremely little is a whole series of simple facts that our elaborate educational system has not stressed sufficiently, which may again be an instance of selective inattention. And one of these simple facts is the value of the pychiatrist's saying in certain circumstances to the patient, "But that is not an adequate account." The patient has stopped before reaching the conclusion, or he has left out something very important in getting to the conclusion of his account.

It is because of the suavity with which communications showing specific inattention are produced and because of the delicate way in which we adjust our shifting parataxical relations with another person in conversation that the quite inexperienced interne writes a reasonably plausible life history on a patient, much of which is very badly confused in time element, so that the obvious significance of a number of the events just is not there at all. The patient has told the interne some of these things, and the interne has not enough frame of reference to place them certainly in time—to place them in the developmental growth of personality—and many of the significant things hinted at have been hinted at so smoothly that the interne just does not know that anything has happened, and proceeds to the next topic with the feeling that everything is going beautifully.

So also with many of our difficulties with patients. They tell us something that has happened and we just don't get it. Let us consider an utterly fictitious case of a patient who comes in and says to the psychiatrist, "My God, I have a horrible headache. I've had it ever since I had a quarrel with my wife about whether we should continue to eat ground beef or accumulate our ration points for a steak." Even though the psychiatrist may be rather weary of these damned family squabbles about any and every thing, the patient has perhaps this time given him a peculiarly lucid and meaningful account. That is, this time a somatic symptom is clearly connected to an unpleasantness with a significant person. In dealing with patients, psychiatrists generally have to be suspicious of a remark that seems so perfectly clear; that is, the psychiatrist would have to judge such a remark in terms of the course of the therapy. Sometimes such a remark may call for the psychiatrist's hurrying over the comment, giving the impression that he understands what the patient is saying and so does the patient. But in those instances in which I feel that the patient has communicated something here, however inadvertently, I might say, "Oh so? Well, now, let me see, what was said in this quarrel with your wife?" And if the patient seems bored with the idea of wasting time in telling me about the quarrel, I might then say, "Well, let's make it simpler. After precisely what remark did the headache manifest itself?" And sometimes that remark means something and is a clue in the therapy. I may let pass unnumbered such remarks, of course. The addition and subtraction and multiplication and division which decide when I will do something in therapy is terribly, terribly difficult to run in as a marginal note at this point in the development of the theory.

The Relation of Selective Inattention to Diffuse Referential Thinking and Schizophrenic-Like Processes

We may conclude, at least provisionally, that the manifestations of selective inattention are instances in which, surprisingly enough at first glance, we have dealt with something in the more diffuse referential manner, by which I refer to levels of reverie that are not admissible to awareness. Thus we may anticipate finding situations in the self-system that amount to a marked reduction of touch with the environment, so that there is no putting of the important details into the subsequent account of it because, so far as the self-system is concerned, there scarcely were such important details. One was relatively absorbed, you might say, in a mental state in which no notice was being taken of the course of events. All of us recall what we experience when we are trying to avoid having somebody impinge on us, yet know that we cannot just thrust the person out of the world without damage to his feelings. Our feeling that we have almost blotted out or almost stopped the process of interpreting what we heard, lest it distract us from something else we are doing, is the shift in awareness, the bending, you might say, of the level of self-consciousness to the point where this business dropped into the lower levels, as we do quite massively when we go into one of these periods of absorption customarily called brown studies. This is the thing that people struggle to put into words when they speak of stopping their ears against distraction, of filing some distractions for subsequent study, of blindly looking at things without seeing them. All those things are struggles to formulate in words the experiences which are, you might say, just the reverse of the classical schizophrenic experience, in which the prohibition of awareness of primitive processes fails, so that you are right among them, they are in awareness, here. In this reverse situation, attention is drawn in, away from all these somewhat distracting things, and one is not clearly conscious, one is not fully awake in connection with them.

Now it is at this point that I think we can see a little of the relationship between the extreme concentration on an exceedingly difficult performance and this drawing-in of awareness to a small mental content, leaving these important, but to be unattended to, events sort of in a marginal, shadowy, not-quite-complete condition. The situations under which this selective inattention—which, I insist, is a really remarkably frequently experienced dynamism—comes into being are of two orders. First, it appears when you are engaged in something extremely difficult, which, if you turn your back, will fall into nothing again and have to be done all over; and so you simply must not have irrelevancies impinging on you. Second, it appears in a situation which pertains to the stability of the self-system itself. Now with the marksman, it is the former. With most of our patients, it is the latter. They do not attend to highly significant details in events and they gloss over the hole in the account where each detail fitted because that is the simplest device for avoiding anxiety. If the same thing happens to you a hundred times a month, but you never quite notice it—it is not permitted to mean what it would have to mean if you noticed it carefully—then you do not have to get anxious about it. You see, the whole personality—all that has happened to us that we have digested, all that we have been, and so on—never has to get anxious about anything. Anxiety is the symptom, you might say, of all threats to security, particularly threats from unwelcome dissociated impulses which are part of the entire personality; and the hint of anxiety is the signal ordinarily for the self-system to control the spread of awareness.

So it is almost saying the obvious to tell you that we are here touching, in discussing this control of attention, on a dynamism which we may of course expect to be very prevalent in life, because it is through it that we most easily, with the least disturbance of our peace of mind, remain about what we always have been. In other words, it is the way we avoid having to change as a result of the experience that we have had with others. And I stress it as the simplest and easiest way, because, you see, it does not require the experience of anxiety and the considerable discomposure which anxiety always implies. I trust, however, that you will not work on to the conclusion that you are hearing a whole explanation of the people to whom we sometimes refer as anxiety-proof. This very suave manipulation of attention, it is true, can be conspicuous in people who seem never to experience anxiety, but there is more to the story than this one dynamism accounts for.

Nevertheless, I think I may say with reasonable safety that one of the great ways of struggling through life with calm is to shift the level of consciousness in an upward direction, you might say, make it contain less, be more concentrated on *a* train of process, *a* particular object, so that the other events go into the dark, not unnoticed, but without being attended to as to their implications and personal meaning. You know these events happened, when your attention is called to them, but the chances are you are not going to do very much elaboration within awareness on your own initiative, because that would produce anxiety or perplexity or something else very unpleasant.

Thus the patient—with all good intentions (as everybody always has) and in clear manifestation of what I insist is the powerful drive toward mental health—tells you something that might have been very profitable to deal with if you had been there and had seen all that happened, but leaves out the thing that would lead to some good use of the time. When he does this, he is simply avoiding distress, avoiding anxiety, just as he avoided it at the time that the thing impinged on him. So far as his awareness is concerned, he has given you an adequate account of what happened; the things unattended to were irrelevancies that would merely complicate the story. He doesn't think of what they are; he just knows that there were some irrelevancies that should not be brought in. And because all of us are almost always plausible, it sounds all right. But if you pay rather strict attention to what is concerned, there are indices of when it is pretty sure that the important thing is being left out.

Function of Recall in the Self-System [1]

In talking about what goes on in the self-system in selective inattention, we have seen that there is a sort of record in the self of an impinging event, even though the person has selectively inattended it; so if instantly you say, "What happened then?" the person will be able to tell you. In other words, you will have destroyed the process and put the person's attention under pressure to notice the data. But so far as the self-system is concerned, this identification of events without any development of their personal implications is all that happens, and the events pass by rapid transit into memory. They are available for recall, but not very easily available because a great deal of our recall is done by the facile flow of what we call association, which really means the aspects of a momentary pattern convenient for the recall of past events. When things go by rapid transit through awareness into memory without the development of implications, those undeveloped implications are not there for the purpose of recall. So while the experience that impinged on you, which you noticed and hurled into history, can be recalled, it is not anywhere near as handy as it might be, because it is not well tied into the general tissue of your life. That doesn't mean that it is 'repressed' or 'suppressed.' It just means that there is a much larger element of chance as to whether it can be facilely recollected or not. But under certain circumstances, it is susceptible to recall, despite the very great interference with getting the connections that will recall it. It is still available, if anyone is clever enough to pull the trick, but it certainly is not facile to recall.

---

[1] *Editors' note:* For a more detailed discussion of the function of recall in the self-system, see *The Psychiatric Interview;* 116*n*–118*n*; New York: Norton, 1954.

The Rest [Remainder] of the Personality, and Sleep

So far, I have been talking mainly about what goes on in the self-system in selective inattention. Now what must be the case with the total personality—in other words, what else, much harder to get at, must be going on? And what is left over to be dealt with in the strange interludes of our life when we are asleep, when the self-system is comparatively at rest because our security is automatically guaranteed?

It is quite clear that, particularly in the case of a person who has a fairly serious mental disorder, selective inattention which leaves important details out of so many experiences must apply to aspects of events, or events themselves, which are essentially anxiety-provoking—that is, which are productive of insecurity, of a feeling of uncertainty and relative helplessness to deal with significant people. Thus the condition which must exist as a result of this dynamism of selective inattention, so far as the whole personality is concerned, is that there is a building-up of processes in the pursuit of satisfactions—most of these things pertain to satisfactions—which amounts to dissociated or almost dissociated systems. This, in turn, means that one tends more and more to have these experiences to which one does not attend, and to that extent the level of insecurity slowly mounts. The patient, as it were, is getting more sick as a result of this very suave process, or he shows dissociated activity. And that in its turn means one of two things for the sleep area of the patient's life. In the first place, the sleep may become increasingly disturbed until there is grave risk of the eruption of a schizophrenic state; or in the second place, if the patient is becoming more and more the victim of dissociated activity, there may be no noticeable strain that has to be reduced by operations during sleep, and sleep may be relatively untroubled. It is theoretically perfectly possible for a person to live part of the time fairly clear on what the devil he is doing and to live the rest of the time charmingly oblivious to what he is doing. The greatest risk to such an adjustment is that somebody else is always prodding you at the wrong time, and saying, "Now why on earth do you do this?" And that question is a direct attack on a person's security, unless he knows what he is doing and why or at least has a beautifully plausible and highly respectable explanation handy. What I am saying here is that we do not need to assume that a person who shows a great deal of selective inattention is necessarily getting sicker. But we must assume that if he is not getting sicker, and if his sleep is not being disturbed, then he must be showing more and more clearly and abundantly dissociated activities which are fairly crudely meaningful. What is not complicated by the pursuit of security is usually distinctly more meaningful, more unvarnished, than what is; this same principle is true of the obsessionals who can pursue their satisfactions with the blindest disregard of what other people think of them, because they have another way of dealing with security problems.

When selective inattention is functioning rather adequately, it represents, you might say, the antithesis of the schizophrenic business. In schizophrenia, relatively primitive, broadly referential mental processes—instead of exquisitely specific referential mental processes—complicate awareness, and greatly complicate consensually validated forms of thought. But in selective inattention, lots of things which are initially in awareness drop out, because the level of attention is simply lifted above them. They are too unimportant, they are sort of brushed away, you might say.

A NOTE ON INTEGRATING TENDENCIES

Perhaps here I shall be able to add a little flesh to one of the skeletons in the conceptual framework I have tried to set up—namely, the development of integrating tendencies. Surely you know that every time you adjust the spark plugs on your car, you are, other things being equal, somewhat more expertly certain of what you are doing and what the considerations are. And so it is with every recurrent performance; we get something from the experience we have had. And the fact that an event impinges on us implies that we have receptors for such events and that the events have some at least rudimentary meaning in our living. And so, having made a rapid transit through the self, an event that has been selectively inattended is as much experience as are events that we have attended to minutely. But, clearly, its experiential value —the extent to which it is something important we have lived or undergone—is not in the self. In other words, you cannot tell somebody about it very easily; you do not know about it; you have literally been inattentive to it; you do not have data. But still, you are aware of it, and it can be recalled under the right circumstances. And, as we might well expect, the impinging of this event more or less facilitates the impinging of a similar event; it shows the same effect as any experience, whether attended to closely or not.

When a serious problem of living can be handled by so inexpensive, so easy a process as simply keeping the attention on something else, it is fairly natural that a very prominent feature would be its use to maintain a feeling of self-respect and worthiness, and so on, by just hurrying through evidences to the contrary. But the 'unworthy' tendencies which are treated in this somewhat cavalier fashion are experience; and this experience somewhat facilitates the recurrence of integrations which will satisfy the same tendencies. Thus, by being inattentive, one becomes all the more expert at doing the things to which one has to be specifically inattentive; and it thus comes about, as we often notice, that it is almost a miracle to anybody but the patient that he can overlook the obvious meaning of something about which he has a sort of sketchy awareness. The meaning becomes more and more relatively unmistakable to innocent bystanders because it does not have to be attended to by the patient.

Like sublimation, selective inattention can be very useful; to get anything done, one has to be pretty generally inattentive to a great many things. If, however, one attempts to treat certain of the fundamental needs of personality by selective inattention, then some very curious things happen very suddenly; we may discuss some of them when we consider hysteria.

As far as sleep is concerned, selective inattention is of quite a different order from sublimation. In sublimation, accumulated tensions resulting from unsatisfied needs are handled in sleep. But one does not selectively inattend in order to frustrate needs, but only to maintain security. How much insecurity accumulates depends on the relative significance of the tendencies treated in this fashion. Maintaining security is what the self is for; so as long as the self will not deal with these things, it is a safe bet that the reason the self will not deal with them is to maintain self-respect and security with others. But if this process is applied to too grave a risk confronting the personality, then sleep is very seriously disturbed, because the nonself part of the personality is so loaded up by the continuous necessity for suave avoidance through selective inattention. Then the tendency system becomes really threatening, and the time when such systems can threaten is when the self is inadequate to maintain security and the person comes really to be pretty close to the eruption of a schizophrenic state. The field in which selective inattention is probably most risky is the field of the very heavily loaded schizoid personalities who come to blow up. This is very much like sublimation, which is most heavily loaded in people who have an extremely irrational element in their inhibitions about genitality, and so on; that does not sublimate well, and they are apt to go off in excitements. The unfortunate outcome of the most pathological uses of selective inattention arises from its cultivating things inacceptable to the self without building any particular machinery in the self to hold it down. Thus it can be extremely risky if it happens to hit something that is a fundamental and unalterable threat to self-respect and a feeling of security.

Suppression, Repression, and Dissociation: Some Conceptual Relationships

Against the background of selective inattention, I want to discuss briefly the concepts of suppression, repression, and dissociation. I have largely discarded the concepts of suppression and repression from my thinking, although I continue to use the concept of dissociation.[2] Yet the question that I have to ask myself at such a juncture is this: Is my description of selective inattention merely a way of thinking, in very complicated language, about suppression and repression? I think not. It seems to me that the hierarchy of things that can happen about awareness of events begins with selective inattention and goes on to dissociation of events, with various degrees of awareness between, controlled largely by substitutive processes.

In considering these concepts, I shall use the terms suppression, repression, and dissociation somewhere near the sense, so far as possible, in which they are most frequently used.[3] The term repression is used in referring to contexts of life experiences which have been, as it were, excluded from the self by something which the psychoanalyst calls 'resistance' and which are very hard to get back into the self. And the concept of suppression was formulated, at least in part, to make clear the magnitude of the process of repression.

Both repression and suppression, as I understand them, refer

[2] *Editors' note:* See Sullivan's 1946 Foreword to *Conceptions of Modern Psychiatry* (p. ix) [New York: Norton, 1953] for a later evaluation of the concept of dissociation; there he notes that in his earlier formulation, as in this group of lectures, he may have given "undue importance" to dissociation as an explanatory principle.

[3] *Editors' note:* See Leland E. Hinsie and Jacob Shatsky, *Psychiatric Dictionary* [New York: Oxford University Press, 1953], for definitions.

to processes which are at least alleged to apply to motives; and when I talk about selective inattention I am not talking about motives at all. I am talking about things which you notice but never attend to—and they can be sentences or all sorts of things. The most general statement I can make of the 'motives' involved in selective inattention is the following: We selectively inattend either (1) to concentrate the ultimate limit of the great human adaptive capacities on a particularly difficult task, where one just cannot waste any resources on irrelevancies, or (2) to avoid anxiety by one of the less risky, if somewhat risky, methods that the human personality finds it possesses. Surely neither of those 'motives' can be suppressed or repressed; the terms do not apply to such things at all. And so I do not believe that there is much real danger of confusion between the thing that you may choose to think of as the process of suppression and what I have been discussing under the term selective inattention.

Selective inattention is suave and effortless; we just never do any thinking about something that we know happened. But the term suppression, in its classical usage, referred to instances in which one was more or less constantly under the necessity, certainly in significant situations, of avoiding anxiety by some sort of mental process that could not be trusted; there was a feeling of effort, a feeling of necessity, connected with it. And as to repression, once something was repressed, it was gone. That is all there was to it. You could walk around on the surface over it, and give the strongest kind of suggestions about it, but all that happened was a disturbance of physiologic process, and so on. Nothing appeared in consciousness. I have not encountered anything as simple and as comprehensive as the repression of orthodox psychoanalytic theory. Yet certainly I have observed instances of selective inattention which closely approximate the classical definition of repression. A great many things which have been subjected to selective inattention may ordinarily exist in such a fashion that they cannot be recalled. Even pretty closely parallel events may not provoke their recall. In these instances, the events show up with a strange vagueness which sometimes literally makes it impossible for the person to be sure whether he had such an experience or whether he only dreamed of such an experience. The recollection is singularly uncertain. In my patient who had the eternal sadistic fantasies on the train, for example, the experience did not provoke the recall that the same thing had happened the day before and on many days before that. I would say that recall of the sadistic fantasies of preceding days was strongly opposed. And that condition comes awfully close to the classical definition of repression. But what I hope I have made clear is that such a case is only an extreme instance and is no different in kind, but only in degree, from the most everyday instances of selective inattention. So it is that when one tries to formulate, in terms of my theory of selective inattention, the probable meaning of a thing like repression, one either encounters an extreme example of selective inattention or one runs flatly into what I call *dissociation*.

I very much prefer to speak of dissociation of major integrative tendencies rather than what is sometimes called the repression of such tendencies, for I do not think that repression actually describes what happens. What happens is that the personality manifests these tendencies, but the self-awareness never by any misadventure is concentrated on the events when these tendencies are being manifested. And there again, we have to expect that there is some machinery connected with this; how is it done? Tracing the way it is done, as I see it, tells a great deal about what it is like to have a dissociated system. All of us have some dissociated integrative tendencies; all of us have certain impulses which have not been provided with any reasonable channel for development by the culture. In other words, Western culture does not use part of our impulse equipment, if you please, part of our adjustive potentialities. It is because there are such things that Freud was led into what I feel is the flat mistake of assuming that the unconscious is largely the habitation of the primitive, the infantile, the undeveloped, and so on. There are indeed some impulses which are choked off in large measure very early in our education to be socialized human beings. But they are not choked off utterly—it is probably impossible to do so. Like the trees growing at the edge of the Grand Canyon, something happens, however terribly distorted.

So when it comes to a thing as essential to being human as a major integrative tendency, it is not going to be utterly ablated, or utterly cut off from the development of any stage of growth. But if a major integrative tendency gets very little place in socialized life, so that it has no material satisfaction in the operations of the self-conscious person, then all that happens is that it is never, in any way, represented in the self-system. It is not in the self-system; and it does not take any great machinery to keep it out, for it never was any part of the self-system. It is a separate organization of processes, and it runs on, in and out of season, when the self-system is not making its presence felt. As I have said, we all manifest some dissociated impulses; but we have never known of them, and we have never attended to the things that show them. No one has ever formulated them for us with such consummate skill that we could become clearly aware of them and they could become part of the self.

But what about the situations in which things that *have* enjoyed attention—that have been manifested within the self-system—cease utterly to be known to the person and vanish into this region in which we do things that we never notice, things that we would never accept as ours? What I am talking about is massive dissociation of impulse systems later in life; when I say later in life, I am still referring to something that ends before adulthood, because people with massive dissociated systems scarcely can proceed to what we define as adulthood, speaking in terms of personality development. We shall later consider how this skillful cancellation of experience takes place; but at the moment it is more important to discuss the growth of knowledge from experience. In other words, let us first consider what happens when an event *is* given a full measure of attention.

Let us say that we encounter a somewhat novel event and that we are highly alert, free from all the complex things we call fatigue, boredom, and so on. The awareness of this event consists of a recognized pattern of sensory input—recognized in that it falls readily into connection with some past experience which has been run through the perceptual mill. Let us say, for example, that I have been hit with a ripe tomato, which means that a great many things are impinging on the distance receptors, and so on, with lots of reference to past experiences in terms of color sense, consistencies, splash, and all sorts of things. Almost the next thing that happens is the response of implicit processes to the event: "How come this tomato? Has it fallen on me by accident or did somebody throw it at me? And if the latter is the case, am I the natural target? Was I intended to be hit? Or am I just an innocent bystander, and someone whose aim is bad has hit me instead of the person he was throwing at?" All these questions are almost automatically asked. This is so because, almost from the cradle to the grave, it is extremely important for us to know whether people are expressing contempt, praise, dislike, like, or what not, for us. This is the source of our security and of our insecurity; and the self-system was invented for that business—for providing us with some skill in the almost impossible task of living securely among other people who are equally victims of a somewhat unfinished culture. Thus when anything happens that might have personal reference to us—that is, might represent an attitude of another person or persons who come along—the natural thing is first to identify the event in the sense of, you might say, physical geographical terms, its secondary attributes, and one thing and another, and then to go on and elaborate the implications of this event with respect to our security. What does it call for in terms of security? But before you can say what it calls for, you have to have some sort of notion of what it implies, what it means. Keeping to this example of the ripe tomato, it calls for changing your clothes as quickly as possible, because many people might be tickled to death to see that you had been splattered with a tomato, and anyway it would be indecorous to go about in such a condition. But this is not the primary activity of the self; the self is primarily concerned with what you do about the impulse that broke loose in the person who hurled the tomato at you. How is that to be dealt with? How is one to avoid such gross, offensive attacks on one's dignity and propriety?

This is what I mean by the automatic growth of implications. This growth of implications is not carried to the same end by everybody, or even to the same end by the same person under different circumstances. It is a function of one's eductive operations, which Spearman [4] made a very considerable effort to formulate. The classes of what he called eductive operations can be, in turn, converted into tests of the capacity to see relationships—which I rather think is the single most significant intelligence test that has ever been worked out.

I have tried to give you an impression of what a staggering number of things happen very swiftly in regard to an event which is given the full measure of attention, clearly within awareness—that is, within the self-system. A pattern appears in awareness marked with recognition in terms of other experiences in the past that are closely related to this, which give it, as it were, its identification, from there on until one

[4] Charles Spearman, *The Nature of 'Intelligence' and the Principles of Cognition*; London: Macmillan, 1923.

is through with it. But in selective inattention you will observe that the pattern appears, is recognized—that is, falls into meaningful reference to the past—and the process ends. That is the essence of selective inattention from the standpoint of the self—that is what can be observed.

Now something which I have not stressed very much, but which is axiomatic, is that we do not experience things which have no precedents. It takes a terribly long time to discover what happened to us if we have no past experience to which this thing can be attached. And there is a constant growth of experience, in the sense of reactive tendencies which show the benefit of past contact with similar situations. This is very generally true with anything that you can get a report on, and so we are certainly entitled to suppose it is the universal case, whether it happens in the self or outside it, until something comes along that proves the contrary—and, I might add, I have never heard of anything that even suggested that the contrary could be proved.

So when we see a person moving through life with a striking type of selective inattention, like the boy who every day had sadistic fantasies on the train but never remembered having had them before, we are justified in assuming something like this: that if we had a full record of this boy's sadistic fantasies, day by day, we would see in this record certain continued stories, certain elaborations, and so on, which would literally represent a development of the skill, detail, and refinement of his sadistic fantasies. There would be a growth in refinement and increased specificity of the impulse to injure innocent bystanders, insofar as that is the meaning of his having these fantasies. Thus I am saying that everything that I have observed, as well as the principle of the minimum complexity of hypothesis, is in favor of the assumption that everything that happens to us that gets any sort of notice from us—conscious or unconscious, witting or unwitting—fits into the theory of the development and refinement of integrating tendencies, or interpersonal processes, which characterize us. So we have to assume that such things as dissociation—which go on quite suavely, but entirely exterior to the personal awareness of the creature that is showing them—also become elaborate and refined. Thus what may start out as a rather clumsy dissociated activity may finally become a performance which is strikingly and exquisitely refined—in the sense of showing a vast amount of experience—even though the person is blissfully unaware of it.

A fantastic and possibly much too complex illustration of that appears in automatic writing—a dissociated activity which most people think of when they are getting used to the term. A very large block of the somatic equipment of the person—including, in this case, a large area of the cortex, and a great many connections, and a huge body of muscle tone—can move out of personal awareness and perform as if it were part of another person. That is a classic and spectacular demonstration of dissociated behavior.

But the dissociated behavior that I think is of principal interest to the psychiatrist is much less dramatic and does not entail anything so strikingly suggestive of hysteria as a major segment of the body's breaking loose and performing by itself, as if it were part of another person. The dissociated behavior that I am talking about begins, if you please, historically, in various movements, postures, and so on, of early life. David Levy, who has been very, very useful to me in providing observational support for theoretical necessities, found in studying peculiarities of posture and movement that some of the strikingly individual attitudes and movements at certain times were reproductions—often quite imperfect, with a good many details dropped out—of nursing attitudes of the individual.[5] The time when these things were most apt to be observa-

[5] *Editors' note:* At the request of the editors for appropriate reference to published writings on this subject, Dr. Levy has sent us the following information: "A few notations on the work Sullivan refers to can be found

ble and uncomplicated by whatever else was going on in the
person was when the person was tired, sleepy, and getting
somewhere near sleep. At that time, the posture was often a
rather accurate reproduction of the conventional nursing
posture at the mother's breast. Thus here are rather elaborate
patterns of nerve, muscle, the kinesthetic business of bone
geography, and so on, that have apparently survived with
very little change from very, very early in post-uterine life.
They have changed some; I suppose if you made a careful
study of photographs of people falling asleep, taken at six-
month intervals, you could see the gradual elimination of
things which are awkward for the nerves, circulation, and so
on. The details elaborate, but they do not elaborate very fast,
and they certainly do not grow into any remarkably adjustive
pattern. They are a sort of spatial, muscular, postural embodiment of the very primitive types of reverie processes that

in two of my articles [David M. Levy, "Fingersucking and Accessory
Movements in Early Infancy: An Etiologic Study," *Amer. J. Psychiatry*
(1928) 7:881–918; and "A Method of Integrating Physical and Psychiatric
Examination," *Amer. J. Psychiatry* (1929) 9:121–194]. Actually Sullivan's
reference is to conversations in which I would contribute some observations, mostly unpublished, to which he would respond when he found
them useful with his own Sullivanesque enthusiasm. The particular observations Sullivan is referring to here were derived from a study I made of the
hand movements of infants during bottle or breast feedings, and some other
activities of infancy and their later modifications. In my conversations with
Sullivan, I probably included the following examples, among others: First,
a modification of the movements of the sucking fingers which after some
years takes the form of frequent passing of a forefinger over the rim of
the upper lip. Second, a modification of an accessory movement of twirling
the hair while sucking the finger. In the case of a grown-up woman, this
took the form finally of a so-called feminine gesture—a slight pressing
movement of the hand to the hair, as though to keep a curl in place. Third,
a movement used to conceal a blemish of the mouth region, real or
assumed. This last was probably the most important one for Sullivan; it is
described in the second of the two articles I have cited. Of particular
interest in this connection is the case of a girl who, as she said, 'smiled little'
because her teeth were ugly and her sister 'smiled big' because her teeth
were pretty. In a number of other cases, the gesture of bringing fingers
to the lips was traced to an original concealing movement because of an
absent incisor or buck teeth. Sullivan was quick to perceive all the implications of these findings in terms of interpersonal relationships."

I talked about in setting up the theory of schizophrenia. And, of course, those things have never been in the self. They are no part of the self. They appear only as the self begins to sink into abeyance.

Now in between this phenomenon and the almost mad elaboration of automatic writing or of dual personality (if it ever occurs, and I guess sometimes it does) there is a great field of performances or actions which are much more a proper subject matter for psychiatric observation and thought. These are sometimes astonishingly widespread innovations—in other words, a large part of the body does something. Much more frequently, these are performances of the effectively expressive muscle-nerve combinations; they pertain to the hands, to the face, to the oral dynamism, to the eyes, and so on. In people whom we know well, we can observe, as a sort of counterpoint to their other behavior, fairly elaborate gestures and fairly elaborate interruptions of speech which go on with never the faintest sign of awareness on the part of the person. As a more refined observation, we can discover that these things occur much more frequently when the person has gotten comfortable with us and that they are only occasional, relatively speaking, in situations where the person is far from sure of how he is getting along with a stranger. That is a rather neat illustration of the relationship of dissociated systems to the self, for when the security of the individual is highly problematic, then, almost as with the rifleman concentrated for the rifle shot, a lot of the human abilities are concentrated on scrutinizing the situation and doing the right thing to insure security. But once it is no longer necessary to be particularly alert, then the rest of the personality that is denied awareness to the self goes to work and begins to do things.

Some of these things can be so glaringly meaningful that it is rather easy to see why the person who shows them is not aware of them. They mean things that the person cannot stand, that would cause the most intense anxiety because they would open him up to grave and very painful attacks from the environment. And almost in accordance with the self's capacities in the field of gaining security—that is, to the extent that the self is a very well-functioning dynamism or system of dynamisms—the expressive character, the obviousness, of the dissociative behavior becomes greater. That statement means, in essence, that the more one can rely on one's self—the more experience has taught him of his capacity to meet difficult situations and come out without any serious damage to his self-respect—the more apt he is to show quite frankly meaningful dissociated activities. It is meaningful in the sense that an intelligent observer would be able to interpret what he can see.

But to the extent that there is little certainty of security, to the extent that the self has developed in an environment that was extremely hard, in the sense of including many attacks which got through the defenses of the self and hurt, caused anxiety, and so on and so forth—to the extent that the person is easily made anxious—the dissociated behavior is apt to be fragmentary and very hard to interpret. Following this line of thought, you can quite understand why schizophrenics show in their history for a period sometimes of years before the acute onset some very small tic-like movement, a twitch, or something or other. If you pay quite a bit of attention to it, you may find that on the occasions when these people seem to be a little bit comforable—although it is very hard to be sure that they are, because they are usually rather heavily protected against giving away how uncomfortable they are— this queer little twitch does not seem to occur. If you could at such moments, without scaring them, pay a good deal of attention to them, you might discover such brutally expressive things as an erect penis; but if you look that closely, there will not be an erect penis—there will be only a little twitch of an eyelid, or something of the sort. And in situations where they feel acutely uncomfortable, feel that their security is very really menaced, this thing will be jittering away to beat the band. Thus the frequency with which these tics occur comes almost to be an index of relative security.

Tics were regarded originally, I believe, as the response to local disease of the central nervous system, the motor cortex, or something of that kind. I don't wonder at this, because the person's great alertness to the risk to which the personality is exposed, his extreme attention to threats and so on, literally suppresses any clear expressive dissociative behavior, so that this behavior is really reduced to things that seem so far from meaningful human behavior that they might well be accidents in the central nervous system. But there are two strong indications that tics are meaningful behavior, and not just accidents in the central nervous system. First, in treating patients one sometimes finds that a classical small tic will disappear after the patient has gotten to and dealt for a while with a content which is of a very repellent character to him—for instance, after a certain type of obscene counterpoint in thought has been worked out. However, I defy anybody to interpret the relation between the content and these fragments of dissociative behavior—although the psychiatrist may bamboozle the patient into accepting as meaningful some flock of words about it. The second indication is that certain very frequent tics often disappear with the ominous appearance of certain hebephrenic phenomena. The explanation of this, I now feel quite sure, is that that which was dissociated no longer needs to be dissociated, but has become an ingredient of consciousness; in other words, an almost shockingly irrelevant stream of counterpoint observations about life is then expressed in the hebephrenic phenomena.

These two things give very strong suggestion that tics are simply, you might say, the least that dissociated behavior can be reduced to when one is in great danger—that is, when the dissociated behavior is a source of extreme insecurity by its effect on others. When a psychiatrist sees a patient with a variety of these fragmentary tics, he can sometimes find in the history evidences of disastrous experiences as a result of showing clearly expressive dissociated behavior; it is obvious in such cases that these experiences in the past were so productive of extreme anxiety, even terror, that the person finally had to abandon the expressive dissociated behavior and only the fragmentary tics remain. Thus large dissociative patterns of action become disintegrated into relatively meaningless portions. For example, a person may have quite clearly proceeded —when he was not looking, so to speak, and was not worried about the people he was with—toward getting involved in a situation he did not approve of being in. Then something entraps him into a rather shocking realization that he has been moving right into one of those situations, and is in it, and has to get out. After that, he no longer moves in the direction of this involvement, but he may have tics. He may develop such compulsive things, as we often call them, as clearing the throat in a particularly loud and disconcerting manner, or stuttering, or almost any of a number of other things that must, I believe, be regarded as the intrusion into communicative performance of dissociative activity. While such activities are intended to bring about integrative situations, they are actually so incongruous to the operations of the self that they give the impression, both to the person who manifests them and to the innocent bystander, of being an interruption—of being something that breaks the situation up. Perhaps only because I am abnormally sensitive to that sort of thing and have therefore paid a great deal of attention to it, throat-clearing tics and tic-like interference with speech seem to me to be remarkably frequent solutions of the fact that major dissociative activities have gotten one into trouble. One has become, as it is ordinarily said, much more obsessional, and one then shows these recurrent disturbances of vocal communication, and so on.

I do not want to develop the topic of dissociation more fully at the moment. But I had to bring it in here to show what you might call a hierarchy of things that can happen about awareness of events. It begins with selective inattention, where the recognition is perfect but the drawing of inferences—the eduction of relations, as Spearman would say—simply does not follow. The second major step—that is, the second abstract position from which to view things—is the position where one has to go through some effortful business to avoid seeing things one doesn't want to see or having impulses one doesn't want to have. Then, in the next abstract position, lo! everything is gone, and it is a stupendous job to get the thing recalled as a real event in the person's life. And in the final abstract position, nothing happens; the patient simply hasn't any of this business of being aware of events. You know from his subsequent behavior that an event has simply sidetracked itself, for it was part of his life, even though it is not part of his known experience.

Hypochondria, Algolagnia, and the Paranoid Development

So FAR, in considering the dynamisms of living, I have kept pretty much to the order of the developmental scheme. In other words, I started out with sublimation, which is obviously the principle of a great deal of early education, and passed on to the obsessional states, which can appear and certainly are founded rather early in life. I then went on to selective inattention, which I suppose first becomes conspicuous in the juvenile era. In discussing this process I touched on all the substitutive types of reactions in which something conspicuous in the self serves, in one way or another, to keep something very unpleasant out of the self except for the group of conditions which pertain to suffering and to the paranoid development. I shall now turn to these.

Hypochondria

Since everybody complains about his health, it is very easy for us to say that there are a lot of our patients who are hypochondriacal. But that isn't quite what I mean by hypochondria. Everything in the realm of psychiatry appears in everybody sometime or other, you know, and the mere hypochondriacal preoccupation that lasts for a week, let us say, is not the same thing as the intense absorption in ill health to which I am referring here.

Hypochondriacal people are those who have a preternatural interest in their ill health and who—in terms of the interpersonal context in which I try to define things—have made the failing state of their health or some specific disease or disability the principal device for communicating with their fellows. It is as if their illness is the presenting point of their personality, and the only thing in which they still retain strong enough interest for attempts at communication.

Clearly the *self-system* in the hypochondriac has been so organized that unfavorable aspects of the information or sentience that comes in over the various afferent channels from the body are given a great deal of very pessimistic attention. Minor sensations (perhaps sensation is not the perfect word for it, but it is related to sensation) from any region of the body can be captured and treated with attention by any of us, I suppose, if we have nothing better to do. Certainly the weariness which is so often seen as a conscious content for unacceptable resentment is built up by treating some of the sentience from the body with rather elaborate attention. This business of feeling tired when one must not be aware of one's resentment is perhaps the most widely prevalent use of the hypochondriacal dynamism in ordinary life. A very striking thing about it is that the moment anything else comes along, the weariness is apt to drop off. In other words, attention is not held very firmly by it.

But the strikingly hypochondriacal person shows an intensity of preoccupation with morbidity of his body. This intensity is in direct proportion to the stress of the situation in which he finds himself. I say that in an ex cathedra fashion, but I think it is fairly easy to demonstrate with any hypochondriacal person you care to try it out on. And from it we derive the formula that this is a peculiar device for performing the self-system function—namely, maintaining security.

A great many good and bad rationalizations have been directed at explaining particular instances of this. For example, you will hear people rattle off the notion that if a certain man were not sick, then he would have to assume responsibility for his failures; but since he is sick, other people are not justified in being hostile to him, treating him unkindly, reducing his self-esteem, and so on. For all I know, this general group of rationalizations for the hypochondriacal states are valid insofar as the self-system, the security apparatus, uses the morbidity as the exclusively important device for feeling secure. Many hypochondriacal patients show, of course, other security devices besides their preoccupation with physical illness. But this is their preeminent security device, and it is always very much in evidence in a situation that causes anxiety.

So much for the self-system in the hypochondriacal state. What of *the rest of the personality?* What of the needs for satisfaction which do not ordinarily require intervention of the self-system except insofar as their satisfaction may imperil security and may require certain restraints, modifications, planning, and so on, to avoid criticism by other people? It would appear that the hypochondriacal dynamism would tend to thwart many needs for satisfaction. For example, a preoccupation with ill health and a demonstration of this preoccupation to anybody with whom one is integrated could have a rather desolating effect on the development of an integration for the satisfaction of lust. The person who is suffering terribly with his fallen kidneys or something like that would not, of course, be expected to be an excellent bed-fellow and, in fact, might easily find himself in the awkward position of feeling that if he is so sick, he ought not to have very highly developed lust. What actually happens, in my limited experience, is that the pursuit of satisfaction in an interpersonal situation does occur, perhaps no more frequently than usual, but that it is poisoned by the intrusion of hypochondriacal considerations. Thus, when this type of substitutive process, or dynamism, is called out by a person's insecurity, it would seem likely to thwart his needs for satisfaction considerably.

Correspondingly, according to our formula, we would expect a great deal of disturbance of the *sleep* function, due to the large amount of unfinished business left over from the period of surveillance by the self-system to the nocturnal period of comparative freedom, at least for implicit process. That, however, is far from necessarily the case. While a great many hypochondriacal patients, of course, report that they suffer from the most fearsome insomnia and disturbance of sleep, they can be observed to be sleeping very soundly six or seven hours a night. Sometimes their insecurity is such that they have to wake up every now and then and make considerable noise—knock the glass off the table, or something like that—for the benefit of the record of their insomnia; but still they sleep pretty well. Considering the thwarting that a good many of their needs for satisfaction get, they sleep incredibly well.

And so what are we going to do with this fact? Clearly, unlike the obsessional personality, the hypochondriacal person's peculiarities in the pursuit of security do not give him extraordinary facility for direct satisfaction of his needs; quite the contrary. The hypochondriacal person does not seem to get many satisfactions, yet he does not have disturbed sleep. How are we to account for this? It is at this point in the theory of personality that we have to lean rather heavily on the old term regression.

REGRESSION IN THE HYPOCHONDRIAC

Years and years ago the conception of regression harassed me to the point where I attempted to find out what, if anything, I did think about it, and the upshot of one of my most elaborate attempts at clearing my own mind was the following. I do believe that all the various important abstractions about living can regress. By abstractions about living, I refer to motivational systems—in other words, the needs for satisfaction compatible with the pursuit of security, the types of awareness of emotion, if you please, and the levels of symbolic operation which we call the cognitive, which are all those manifestations of symbol operations that are supposed to give us useful information about the situation confronting us, or about the future, or even about the past. All of these can, under certain circumstances, drop back and persist for some time at a chronologically earlier stage of their evolution. This reverting is truly astonishing in that as long as the regression holds sway—as long as the motivational system continues to be regressed—there is no evidence of subsequent experience after that stage of development. In other words, with the dropping-back to an earlier state of function, the subsequent elaborations that we know happened cease to manifest themselves in behavior or in implicit processes.

The regression of some of these things is very hard to describe clearly. The regression of the cognitive aspect, the implicit symbol operations, however, I have perhaps made moderately clear a little earlier, when I talked about the obsessional's preoccupation with certain autistic verbal rituals and the often terrifying symbol operations of the schizophrenic. I said, for instance, that the obsessional neurotic, in the pursuit of security, regresses in certain cognitive operations, knowing operations, to the stage of quite autistic speech. Thus the implicit activity of the obsessional contains certain terms which are not communicative, even though they may sound like words of adult speech. This might be called a very small instance of regression; and I think, in order to make the whole concept somewhat clear, that it is useful to look at it that way.

Hypochondriacal people are busily engaged in counting up all their heart ticks, or something of that kind, and telling you all about it, sometimes with every sign of being able to keep on indefinitely on the subject. And they are not having a good time in any ordinary sense; their lust is gummed up, all sorts of things are gummed up. Often their appetite—the experience of hunger and the frank satisfaction of food—is all gone by the board unutterably. That is pretty nearly impossible to explain without calling in the conception of regression. But what I want to emphasize here is not particularly the regression of cognitive processes. In their own particular way the cognitive processes of hypochondriacal people may be very acute. In other words, hypochondriacs can rattle off possible implications of symptoms and so on, using their deductive powers and remembering the curious timing of the symptoms, which nonmedical people are not apt to think of. But the cognitive aspect of the situation which is actually producing insecurity, of course—just as in our obsessional business— doesn't trouble awareness and doesn't cause anxiety. The nearest approach to an index of anxiety in these people is the extent to which they get more intensely forceful about how sick they are, what grave risks there are in their sickness, and so on. They can show the most intense anxiety, but it is always anxiety about impending physical doom, anxiety about their symptoms —not about other persons or about the social situation in which they find themselves or anything like that. Thus the hypochondriacal dynamism in a way actually blunts the utility of anxiety in very much the same way that preoccupation with numbers or something of the kind may blunt my anxiety so that I can get something done below the level of awareness.

But so far as the rest of their lives is concerned, hypochondriacs don't live, in the sense that most of us do, at least now and then. And so we simply are forced—more by the demands of my theory, it is true, than by any vast documentation I have ever belabored myself into developing—to presume that the integrative tendencies connected with these needs for satisfaction—in other words, all the behavioral patterns and refinements of sentience and so on which make satisfaction—have reverted to a much earlier level, and the experience in between has disappeared. I cannot present any reasoning as to how two or three years of life can disappear, so far as any effect is concerned, although one can be led to recall incidents from them.[1] But anyway, it happens. There is no sign of subsequent elaboration, and the thing just thoroughly regresses. The hebephrenic, of course, is the most extreme instance of all, but we will discuss that later.

What is the state of the total personality if a very considerable section of those processes concerned with the pursuit of satisfaction has regressed to a decidedly earlier state of development? The answer, of course, is to be found in what state they have reverted to. Take, for example, lust. If the lust dynamism regresses below the level of preadolescence—which I consider the earliest approach to anything meaningful in terms of this dynamism—the person would be engaging in prurient stories and obscene jokes, peering into the neighbor's windows at night, and all that sort of thing. Regression still further back we see only, I think, in the genito-urinary hypochondriac, and there it is very closely related to schizophrenia. The symptoms show, in some cases, the same degree of regression that we see in certain of the schizophrenic masturbatory activities—namely, regression to the point of reactivation of urethral components of the orgasm, and so on. They have experiences with a drop of mucus, for instance, in lieu of anything which ultimately becomes the genital dynamism.

You are not likely to find out very much about the hypo-

---

[1] *Editors' note:* Sullivan referred at this point to an earlier paper of his on regression. See "Regression: A Consideration of Reversive Mental Processes," *N.Y. State Hosp. Quart.* (1926) 11:208–217, 387–394, and 651–668. (For a later statement of Sullivan's ideas on regression, see *The Interpersonal Theory of Psychiatry;* p. 197. In general, Sullivan's ideas on regression changed very little if at all through the years.)

chondriacal person's regression in the pursuit of satisfaction from what he tells you, because as these things regress, communicability about them also regresses. But if you had competent observers, you might expect to find that their biologically conditioned needs have literally reverted to the parallels of what would be distinctly earlier conditions of these needs. And the so-called emotional life is very sharply restricted to the field of hypochondriacal preoccupation. In essence, the emotional life of the markedly hypochondriacal person ranges from a pleasant interest in one's ill health to actual and very intense anxiety about one's impending dissolution. So far as I am concerned, all the rest has certainly regressed except possibly affect.

When I say that in regression recent experience becomes as if it had never been except for rather toneless and not very useful recall, I mean that so far as tensions and so on in the total personality are concerned, this experience isn't there. It has just faded. It can all come back into action again, showing that it is in some mysterious state of memory, but its function is not shown in accumulating tensions. Thus regression to earlier types of functional activity can be completely satisfactory—it can work, in the sense that it does not pile up tensions. There is no accumulation of tension that disturbs sleep, as there is in certain cases of sublimation and in certain other states.

Algolagnia

In algolagnia, in the sense in which I use the term, it is the world rather than the body that is treated as ailing. Algolagnics are possibly the most gifted of all people at taking the joy out of life. They are the people who suffer life—who are always glad to tell you how terrible things are and who can only with great difficulty be led to show any particular interest in anything except how badly everything is going and how grim the prospects for the future are. Their absorbing preoccupation is with the suffering life has caused them.

The hypochondriacal and the algolagnic states sometimes overlap; that is, you will find people whose principal theme is their ill health, but who will at times gallop into extensive diatribes about the disastrous state of the world. On the other hand, the hypochondriac may be entirely free from any necessity to impress you, or to be impressed himself, with how ghastly the world is. There are, in fact, hypochondriacal people who really radiate all sorts of optimism about everything but themselves. The algolagnics are apt to be very much more intact than the hypochondriacs in the sense of preserving their relatively contemporary motivational systems, but that isn't saying a terrible lot, because these people are in no sense mature personalities. Algolagnia is, I believe, a distortion which begins in the juvenile era, or at least certainly appears rather early in preadolescence, and represents an inadequate fruition of the preadolescent development. Therefore, we might expect the sex life—or, let us say, the genital necessities —of these people to be definitely autogenital, or at least to be of the type where a sexual partner is used merely as a convenience because the hand is somewhat taboo, or something of that kind.

But in general there is not a particularly conspicuous element of regression in the algolagnic adaptation to life. The algolagnic process is, as I see it, more a way of handling a good deal of fear and anger—in other words, hatred—and, as such, would appear to reflect what can happen to a person who has been subjected to extremely deleterious influences from a certain point in comparatively early life. There must have been something of affection and security in the beginning, but fairly early in life things bogged down. And these people discovered that they could put others at a disadvantage by recounting how wretchedly they are being treated by the world. Other people will, insofar as they grow discomposed and embarrassed, serve the purpose; and if by any chance the algolagnic person can milk other people of not only sympathy but also money, or some convenience of that kind, then the thing takes on the attributes of being a very effective security device indeed.

The Paranoid Condition

The so-called paranoid condition requires the algolagnic, you might say, as a spring-board; but nonetheless it has a close connection with the hypochondriacal, if for no other reason than that it can clinically alternate with the hypochondriacal state. Pure paranoia is one imaginary pole and pure schizophrenia is the other; and the paranoid conditions which I am talking about at the moment are those somewhere near the pure paranoia pole, rather than states of very paranoid coloring on the schizophrenic illness. These paranoid conditions, which are said to be the prevalent psychosis of the highly intelligent, range from a very troublesome attitude in interpersonal relations—which, however, seems to get no worse over the years and possibly gets very slightly better—to very florid developments of persecutory delusions with any amount of impressive documentation and a very considerable feeling of grandeur, accompanied by certain delusional rationalizations.

The single most illuminating thing that I know about the paranoid condition is its alternation with the hypochondriacal state. While this alternation isn't frequent, it does occur. In other words, you see a few patients who are hypochondriacal when they are not paranoid, and paranoid when they are not hypochondriacal, and the paranoid state can be very marked. Thus as soon as their paranoid ideas begin to appear clearly, their health improves markedly; and as the health begins to deteriorate, paranoid ideas again fade out of the picture, so that there is a very clear alternation.

The central question in the two conditions is, What becomes of the needs for satisfaction? It is quite clear that the paranoid mechanism works beautifully for security, for how can you avoid respecting yourself if you, the very embodiment of goodness and mercy, have been persecuted and driven by surrounding enemies into a state of impotence? Very clearly there is no discredit in our social order in being the victim of persecution. Thus the feeling of worth is as well protected by the paranoid transference of blame as by anything I have ever heard of. The paranoid technique is just the simplest device for the purpose that anyone can use. Yet, remembering that we must all exist in interpersonal relations or deteriorate, it does entail some great hardships in living, for it makes any satisfaction-giving interpersonal relations very difficult. This is simply because the paranoid's security depends on being persecuted; and while it might seem that he could sort out some people as sources of persecution and other people as sources of satisfaction, it is not very safe to do this. Why? Because that is the way all of us grew up; the people who were our original sources of satisfaction were the same people who inculcated in us the need for security. And so the people who are our sources of satisfaction are the only people whom we are drawn close enough to so that they can become a menace to our security, can diminish our self-esteem, directly wound us by criticism, or something of that kind. Thus it comes about that this apparently very nifty paranoid solution makes it extremely difficult to be in a constructive integration—in the sense of a satisfaction-giving and good-promoting integration—with anybody.

So what becomes of the paranoid's needs for satisfaction? They too have to undergo regressive distortion to processes of an earlier level. While at times and in particular settings the paranoid is apparently able to act quite maturely in the pursuit of satisfactions, the setting gives a good many clues to the paranoid dynamism. For example, a number of paranoid men have, in the midst of their psychosis, managed to get out of the hospital and have then proceeded to impregnate a member of the other sex. When you look closely at this, however, the astonishing part is that the woman who is involved in this satisfaction of lust can seldom, by any stretch of the imagination, be regarded as the man's social equal. There are unmistakable evidences of a great social gap; thus the woman can be regarded as an inferior creature, not unduly invested with humanity, and therefore, perhaps, perfectly all right for genital experimentation, but scarcely a real menace to one's self-esteem. Or, if there is no great social difference in terms of the open markers of social status such as speech, clothing, schooling, and so on, then she is someone so very different from the women with whom the patient has had significant experiences in the past that we can picture a large element of autistic fantasy being mixed in with the thing and can again assume that, so far as the paranoid is concerned, she is scarcely a human being; she is more a fantasy product of his than a person who can be taken as threatening, critical, and so on.

At times the paranoid also works out a good many other things in the way of needs, usually by the self-same device of having these relations of comparative intimacy with people who are in some way at a very much lower level in the hierarchy of prestige—and prestige is one of the great securities. So here is a device by which, if you could ever find a world that has nothing in it but people who look up to you as great, you might become a savior instead of being a mental patient. And lo! that actually happens; there are paranoid worlds in which some highly intelligent paranoid is the leader and everybody else is very, very much the follower, and at a respectful distance. Surprisingly enough, there, too, a great deal is developed in the way of techniques of the special social prescriptions, and so on, for the obtaining of satisfactions of biologically conditioned needs. Thus the paranoid process gives a little further clue to the circumstances calling out regression.

If one cuts oneself off so completely from intimacies with others that, at the level of verbal communication, the only dependable topic is the wretched state of one's health, as in hypochondria, one is very much more shut out from a moderately satisfactory life than if one restricts these communicative and cognitive aspects to how wretchedly one is being abused by other people—by particular, specific other people —as in the paranoid state. The cost of maintaining a self-system in which the sentient flux from the interior of the body is the only matter that can be attended to in extenso is that most of the personality must be reduced to a much earlier state. But let us say that the person finds the simple device of transferring the blame for all his faults which have hurt his self-esteem and disturbed his feeling of security uncontrollably for years—which have made him afraid of many contacts lest someone should point the finger at these faults. If now the self-system so reorganizes itself, you might say, that it finally discovers that these faults are the other fellow's, the personality can then function fairly well. But the person must not stay long in contact with the people who once were dangerous, because they might point out these intolerable weaknesses. In other words, the self-system cannot completely disfigure reality, cannot invert itself from a device for the promotion of security to the maddest kind of a device for producing insecurity. There is no way in which that could happen. The self-system is always a device for maintaining security with our fellows and for keeping intact the illusions of them that make up our mores, social prescriptions, and so on. Thus in the paranoid, the self-system continues to function to entangle into the protective system anybody who would be critical or with whom one would be exposed to criticism. It faces society in general hostilely and with danger flags flying from all parapets. It permits relationships which are sometimes pretty

fantastic, but still may be quite physically intimate and sometimes of reasonably considerate intimacy, but only with people
who do not present much danger in the sense of reminding the
person of what really ails him.

The Dynamisms of 'Emotion'

Fear, Anger, Rage, and Hatred

As a PRELIMINARY to a central attack on dissociation, I want now to consider as dynamisms some entities which are ordinarily called emotions, and I shall begin with the dynamisms of fear, anger, rage, and hatred. I am somewhat in the dark as to which of these shows up first in the development of personality, chiefly because I do not know how much experience there is in the process of being born. Be that as it may, perhaps fear is entitled to first consideration.

FEAR

The probability is that fear consists of a very severe drop in euphoria. In this respect, it is related to anxiety, which is at the root of the development of the self-system. Anxiety, however, is a dynamism that is called out by empathy and that is a product of education and of living among significant people. Fear does not have these characteristics; it is a very widely distributed device of living organisms for purposes of self-preservation. Thus it is not so exclusively human or preternaturally social as anxiety. Perhaps fear and anxiety feel much the same. But fear, as it is ordinarily manifested, is that 'bundle' of processes called out either by the great novelty of a situation or by something in a situation that is really dangerous, or at least very unpleasant in the sense of causing pain or severe discomfort.

Fear is ordinarily mediated by some of the distance receptors; and if it is extreme, it is characterized by their increased acuity. While this last may be somewhat of an overstatement, it does tell a large part of the story. Fear causes an increasing alertness and creates changes in the internal 'economy' of the body, so that the supply of energy available for muscular action is increased. Along with this "preparatory aspect" of being afraid—as Cannon [1] has called it—go certain effects on the content of consciousness—namely, the level of consciousness is raised and bent upward, you might say, in the shape of an intense concentration on the fear-provoking situation and on the way to escape it. In some people, at least, the concentration may be such that it deletes the fear-provoking situation and all its implications except for finding the direction of escape, or any other more or less corrective movements. This may be true of everybody, although I speak with certainty only of the markedly schizoid, who ordinarily can sidetrack their feeling of the ingredients of emotion until they have carried out the action on which they are concentrating.

Although fear and anxiety must be carefully distinguished, they do, in man, come to have certain connections. Thus we find that the organization of the self-system—the device for maintaining interpersonal security—in some people includes elements which are connected with the dynamism of fear and which make fearful, or fearsome, if you please, situations that are essentially quite harmless—that is, harmless in the current living of the person. As I have said, man, like all of the higher animals, has a tendency to fear things which have a certain degree of novelty, even though that novelty may actually have nothing dangerous in it whatsoever. In other words, fear is

[1] *Editors' note:* See, for instance, W. B. Cannon, *Bodily Changes in Pain, Hunger, Fear and Rage;* New York: D. Appleton Century Co., Inc., 1929 (2nd ed.).

called out when orientation does not begin automatically following the perception of more or less external conditions. Now the self-system of man—his security device—may affect the recognition or orientation which would ordinarily follow perception, for the self-system controls awareness, and it is within awareness that we have our best acquaintance with our means of perception, our sense organs. Thus when a person has abnormal fears (and I am not talking about anxiety), what happens is that there is some interference with the recognition—which depends, of course, on recall—of an essentially harmless situation. And even though this situation recurs, it always retains an ominous novelty; the person never gets acquainted with it, and so he is always afraid of it. His inability to get acquainted with it usually pertains to some past interpersonal experience in which his security was concerned and in which there was a coloring of anxiety.

Now the reason why I harp on this rather transparently simple dynamism—which all of us are acquainted with and continue to be in spite of everything—is that in psychiatric thinking there is often the most reckless carelessness in the discrimination of fear from anxiety. I do not mind much what people *call* things if they know what they are talking about, but I do think that a patient's difficulty is often increased greatly if the psychiatrist's thinking is fully as unclear as the patient's. One reason why anxiety tends to be confused with fear is that a prerequisite for even a vestige of feeling secure is the ability to say something. So when we are anxious about something and somebody asks us about it, we are very apt to rattle off some rationalizations about what we are afraid of, just for the security value of feeling that we can say something about it. In that way, I suppose it gets to be almost second nature to feel that when people are anxious, they are afraid of something. But the fact is that anxiety, as a warning signal, implies (and here I am trying to draw a parallel with fear) that the danger is from within—that one has to do something to make sure that one's security doesn't sink suddenly as the result of the action of significant people or significant ideas.

Both fear and anxiety may be so extreme as to amount to terror. In general, when you see a person in a state of terror, the way to approach this is to determine whether the terror results from anxiety—in other words, whether the person is afraid of something erupting into awareness that looks as if it would wipe out all security—or whether he is terribly afraid of something that has 'objective reality.' If the thing has objective reality, other than the disapproval of one's fellow mortals, then the more clarity you can introduce into the formulation of what it is that is fear-provoking, the more apt the person is to improve—that is, there will be a diminution of the relatively blind tendencies that accompany extreme terror. But any attempt of that kind in the case of anxiety is, of course, beside the point and doesn't make much sense. Now in certain severe mental disturbances, a person may be both horribly insecure, suffering anxiety on very slight provocation, and also definitely afraid of attack by his fellow mortals. He feels anxiety—which may amount to the verge of panic —over what he is impelled to do to others or fears that others are impelled to do to him, because he is projecting part of his conflict of motivation; and he also misinterprets certain movements so that they can actually be defined as threatening physical violence. And if this seems extremely finespun, let me assure you that a careful discrimination between what could easily appear to be actually threatening and what is more purely projection on the part of the patient is often absolutely necessary in order to calm a terrified psychotic patient. As long as you do not discriminate, then what you have to say means nothing to him. The value of making the discrimination is this: When one becomes oriented in a situation which at first provokes fear, its capacity to call out this dynamism of fear is generally diminished, if not abolished. Thus if you help the patient to become oriented—if you encourage him to observe the fear-provoking situation more carefully and to entertain alternative hypotheses for the apparently threatening maneuvers on the part of the personal environment—he may be able to discover that the things which were apparently threatening are essentially harmless and merely novel. But if you attempt to talk away anxiety—and anxiety, by definition, means that the self-system is very seriously threatened with failure—you are just encumbering the field with meaningless jargon and destroying what little contact you may have had with the patient. That is why I harp on the importance of discriminating between fear and anxiety.

ANGER

In the minor events of life we are seldom clear on the nature of anxiety and seldom know that we are being driven by anxiety to follow the blind path which is laid down by our past experience. This fact has particular pertinence in relation to the dynamism of anger. Anger is one of the ways of handling anxiety that we learn early, at the time of the empathic linkage with significant adults before there are any particularly analytic thought processes. This way of handling anxiety is, I think, probably struck off by the first time that a significant adult makes the young child anxious by mistake —in other words, the adult is wrong. In such circumstances, the young child almost invariably, if not invariably, feels abused and angry. And when he has once experienced something which affects him as vividly as anger, he looks for it in the surrounding world and recognizes it as one of the things in his environment which has always been conducive of intense anxiety in himself—that is, which has led to this sudden and very undesirable dropping in euphoria. In this way the child learns the given pattern of being angry, the social expressions of anger, in the mild degree that parents show it toward people in late infancy. Thus anger takes on the beginnings of social conditioning. At the same time it takes on a very important justification for existence in that it spares one anxiety. The child needs only a very little random experimenting with this new discovery to find that if he gets angry, he does not suffer much anxiety. And so various degrees of anger, from what is politely called irritation up to a feeling that borders on rage, come to be the most frequent expression, so far as can be objectively detected, of situations that provoke mild insecurity, except when one is in the company of people who are so significant that it is dangerous to be angry with them or—a very much smaller group of exceptions—among people who can be so unpleasant that it is not wise to provoke them. Thus when another person seems annoyed or angry, we are most likely to approach a simple understanding of the situation if we ask ourselves whether what we did had in some way impaired his security, so that the anger was called out merely as an avoidance of the anxiety that would otherwise have been aroused.

Anger itself, as I need tell no one, is an element of the biological equipment which has much somatic machinery tangled up with it. Its purpose presumably is not to enable us to escape threatening and injurious situations, but to destroy them or drive them away. Anger does not appear, however, in threatening situations which are so novel that fear appears instead, or in situations which are so purely dangerous that it would be obviously very risky, indeed, to attack. Some of our military psychologists have sometimes speculated on whether fear can be translated into anger. If it can, I am sure I would not know how. Nor do I think that this transmutation in the very special circumstances of practically certain destruction—which is the military problem—would be particularly useful. Anxiety, which is vastly more important than fear in a great many of the operations of life, generally is translated into anger if there is time enough—in other words, if the anxiety has not become too acute. Anger blunts the feeling of personal insecurity—that is, insecurity in terms

of social values and the respect of others; but in this performance anger isn't particularly refined; it simply concentrates attention on attack and injury, on driving away the
supposedly threatening personal situation. Consequently, I
would not expect anger to be particularly useful in meeting
an intricately dangerous situation. In such a situation, I would
prefer to provide what little orientation one could as an
antidote to the fear of things which were simply too novel,
using foresight to prepare the persons concerned as to the
limits of possibility. I think that this would be an infinitely
more practical attack than an attempt to accomplish such a
mysterious transmutation as the conversion of fear into anger.

I might mention here, however, the way in which fear
might *appear* to be converted into anger. When people are
startled—and you remember that Landis [2] has worked out
many of the elaborate patterns of being startled—if they do
not feel fear, they are certainly utterly ready to feel fear;
and I surmise that in the earlier stages of being startled by any
given type of situation, one does feel fear. Being startled
includes a lot of things in the way of more or less indicative
behavior, one of which is to sort of hunch down as if to
emulate a turtle, which is, according to our standards and
our ignorance of the startle pattern, not particularly estimable.
When people have been startled by a loud and unexpected
noise, for example, they often feel quite insecure at having
been startled. That does not mean that the startle pattern is
accompanied by anxiety; but it does mean that the person's
orientation of his position with other people, immediately
after being startled, includes the anxiety pattern. The person
feels that he has been undignified—that he has been afraid,
if you please—and the culture says that one should be ashamed
of those things, however physiological and unescapable they
may be. Very often, because we are ashamed of having been

[2] C. Landis and W. A. Hunt, *The Startle Pattern*; New York: Farrar &
Rinehart, 1939.

startled and are therefore on the verge of having anxiety—
a feeling of insecurity as to the respect of others—we may feel
angry as a defense against anxiety. And so, I suppose, one
might think carelessly that this was an instance of the conversion of fear into anger. But even if that were true, the
state of being angry is not conducive to the most practical
operations for group preservation, and in many cases it is
definitely antagonistic to the proper movements for individual
preservation.

RAGE AND HATRED

If the tantrums of children can be called rage, as I surmise
they can, they must be about the earliest appearances of this
dynamism. The central core of the definition of rage is that
it is a symbolic discharge of a high degree of anger, when the
direct purpose of anger—that is, the destruction or driving
away of the endangering thing—cannot be accomplished. Thus
rage is more intricate than anger. It discharges a great deal of
energy in random activity—perhaps it is typically the sort
of situation in which a person who is very angry kicks the
furniture around. Its great significance for psychiatrists comes
from its relation to hatred, which is an extremely important
integrating tendency of very considerable complexity.

Before I plunge into that, let me say that one gradually comes
to dislike the people who provoke the minor degrees of
anxiety which one promptly meets by being annoyed or
angry, and such experiences with another person would certainly undermine a tendency to develop cooperation in something with that person. Now I regard cooperation as a rather
juvenile way of working with others because it pays—as
against collaboration, where there is a strong interest in mutual
achievement, a strong interest in the other person's achieving
as well as in one's own. Anything like recurrent insecurity
with a cooperating person would tend to discourage the maintenance of that situation, for even if the anger which appears

recurrently is a disguise or an escape from anxiety, its biological function—the preparation to drive away or destroy
the troublesome person—is amply served by merely moving
out of further contact with this person, simply developing
some minor avoidance.

But the situations that call out rage are, from my definition,
not capable of being handled in that way, for rage occurs when
anger, however great, cannot accomplish this destruction or
avoidance of the situation, but has to be sidetracked into a
relatively symbolic discharge. It must be sidetracked because
the person who calls out the rage is either of such extreme
significance or of such power that it would be extremely risky
to attack, and very harmful. Recurrences of that type of
situation are almost bizarrely different from recurrences of
the situations which call out minor insecurities, irritations, and
anger; instead of avoidance and the gradual dropping-out of
the person who provoked the anger or irritation, a rather firm
situation is often, if not invariably, integrated. When we
stumble upon a well-developed situation of this kind, we discover that we have a couple of people who are bound to each
other by the ties of hatred and whose chief interpersonal
activity may be best categorized as mutually destructive. Now
I believe it is because of these miracles of human biology that
Freud may have been provoked to discovering the death
instinct. These integrations of hatred are almost the parting
of the way for an obsessionally rational person; that is, he can't
make any sense out of his need for these integrations. If you
get nothing except frustrated anger—another way of saying
rage—from your continued relationship with a person, then
it stands to reason that that person becomes utter anathema
to you. But while this is so in your thinking, he becomes
strangely necessary in your living. This living that one con-
ducts when one is integrated with the most significant other
person in a hatred situation is unfortunate. It proceeds in
general in the direction of deterioration, unless the paranoid

process comes into service. If this process does appear, the simple reality of the situation evaporates into a very august and cosmic type of operation, which I shall come to presently.

I hope I have said enough to suggest that we really need to look to our tripartite position to make any sense of situations of hatred. Clearly such situations are not 'reasonable' from the standpoint of the self—the standpoint that we ordinarily mean when we talk about being reasonable. How then do we expect to make them fit a theoretical position which, I trust, is almost shockingly reasonable? When one studies one of these hateful integrations, one finds that certainly the only thing that both parties have any real enthusiasm for is damage to the prestige of the other. I suppose that among my countrymen at very low social levels physical violence is not uncommon; but still that is a feeble imitation of the real thing, for a hateful person really feels he has gotten somewhere only when he can hurt the other's feelings, make him feel small and humiliated. Thus, since the trick is to diminish the other person's security, and since the pursuit of security is at the very root of the evolution of the self-system, the real explanation of this peculiarly durable, destructive integration of hate must have a great deal to do with the self. And we generally discover in these situations that, in each person concerned, there is an organization of the self which includes a large element of motivation that cannot be treated by the dynamisms we have thus far discussed. In other words, it is motivation known to the self-system—that is, accessible to awareness—which is not capable of being accepted as proper, right, and natural; which cannot be sublimated, for there is no outlet for it by means of partial satisfaction that is socially approved; which cannot be handled by the relatively early magic of the obsessional neurosis; which has not caused a schizophrenic dissociation; and which cannot be dissociated in the nonschizophrenic fashion. In other words, it is something that has had so much access to the experience in which the self was born that it is part of the self—unavailingly and eternally part of the self—unless a very considerable reorganization of personality occurs.

From all of this, one expects and finds that in the relationship such a person had with early significant people, this emotion of rage was a relatively frequent part of the interpersonal processes that bore on the child. In that very early environment, rage was sufficiently conspicuous so that social sanctions were not effective against it, even though they made it awkward. In other words, when you stumble over a thing several times a day, even if society disapproves of its existence, still you know it is there. You may even expect to stumble over it the rest of your life. Thus rage has been part of the security machinery; it has been a powerful dynamism well within awareness at the early stages of the evolution of the self. And it is only in subsequent periods—perhaps in the school society of the juvenile era, sometimes not until after the child has gone through several grades of school—that the weight of social censorship and disapproval have so borne in on rage behavior, on the rage dynamism, that additional elaborations of the self-system are built to get rid of this source of insecurity within the very machinery of getting security. One might say that that in itself shows why the dynamism of rage—as well as the much more elaborate integrating system of hatred—cannot be dissociated. Rage has always been there since the self existed; so dissociating it would indeed be a piece of magic. But it becomes strongly marked with disapproval. It is made to be a misfunction of the self which causes insecurity, and as such is inhibited as best may be.

One of the neatest of all ways for a person to dispose of something in the self-system which has come to be marked as disapproved, wrong, bad, weak, or what not, but which cannot be got rid of because it has always been there, is to develop what I once called "specious ideals." This is a peculiar elaboration which is almost like a second self; in many ways it acts like a duplicate of the self-system, but it acts in a very small field only. The way it acts is exceedingly well known to all of you, but not with this elaborate setting. One becomes very sensitive to, and extraordinarily critical of, the type of behavior in others which one is constantly afraid one will show. That is the simplest device that I have seen utilized by people to dispose of some very important ingredient of the self-system relatively late in life. Thus, under strong social prohibition, this business of rage—this anger which reaches white heat because it cannot do any of the things that anger should do and which simply demands symbolic discharge in random activity—is quite often converted into an extreme sensitivity toward and intolerance of such performances by others. Many ideals follow very much this same pattern. Actually this handling of rage involves much more machinery than is involved in many ideals, but it works so suavely and yet so obviously that it provides a good clue to the more subtle and far-reaching effects of some of the ideal structures.

In his dealings with others the person goes around with special receptors, you might say, for any behavior that represents marked anger, adopts a disapproving and forbidding attitude toward such behavior, and carries away a derogatory estimation of the personality which shows it. By this serious overcomplication of life, he avoids a great many of the occasions that might otherwise unwittingly lead him into rage. In other words, if you are warned that some people are easily angered, and lift yourself to a position of greater security and prestige because they are so unworthy, then the chances of your being angered, of being exposed to the situations that would provoke you to rage, are very markedly reduced. And by very virtue of having detected the danger and warned yourself away, you feel more secure. This works very neatly.

But this secondary elaboration, which works all too well, is certain to interfere with the quiet and progressive elaboration of a constructive integration with another person. The action of this business is called out so easily that there is little chance of one's really getting deeply entangled with another person who is not particularly sensitive to anger—that is, who is not particularly apt to anger—who is secure and fairly well oriented in life, because such a person senses difficulty, trouble, and awkwardness in this unduly complex person. Thus you might say that the common run of people are always being fended off. The person who has this secondary elaboration concerning anger derogates them by his prompt disapproval of their bad temper, and therefore any close integration is avoided. But when this unfortunate encounters another person who is very like himself in this respect, but who in other respects actually has a peculiar suitability for intimacy, then the suavity with which the overcomplexity works has a doubly thwarting effect. First, it permits intimacy to be approached because it thwarts the ordinary way of avoiding it. That is, they are both so disapproving and so sensitive to the possibility of anger that that trait in both of them tends to ward off the performance that they would ordinarily derogate in another person. Under cover of this, the possibilities of real intimacy act in these people as they act in all of us; that is, as the positive constructive integrative tendency brings two people together, events occur which tend to provoke anger. We have no genuine education for tolerance—or whatever the proper term would be for what we think we mean when we talk about tolerance. In other words, we are not taught to respect personality. Most of us are taught to believe that our blood is a little bit better than that of others, or something of that kind. And so it is a rare movement toward intimacy that does not have a good many minor bumps in its early stages. Even in preadolescence, when there are far fewer handicaps than there are in current adult life, the development of intimacy is not entirely without its cares, its experimentation, its rebuffs, and one thing and another. Now in these people I am talking about, as intimacy thickens, injury—in the sense of that which calls out anger and particularly rage—also thickens. Perhaps this is the first time that one has really felt close to another person, and—as it is ordinarily rationalized—everything would be lovely if it were not for this perverse tendency of the other fellow. That works both ways, of course; and so the horrible miscarriage of human intimacy, mixed with an almost omnipotent struggle as to who will hurt the other fellow worse, rapidly comes about. So the second thwarting effect is that the possibilities of intimacy come to little; they are simply what gives hatred its integrative character. The rage, as well as the never adequate defenses against rage of the type I have described, is in the self; it is part of the security machinery for dealing with other people. Therefore it is always in the way, except when the person is asleep.

This brings me to the other points of my tripartite viewpoint, for so far I have been discussing only the self-system. In this dynamism, the self is the most important thing simply because of the natural history of the hateful person; hate was a normal ingredient of life at the earlier stages of the self-evolution and therefore requires elaborate machinery in the self to handle it when it becomes socially disapproved.

But because there are possibilities for two people such as I have described—minus their rage and their rage defenses—to collaborate together in real intimacy, one may expect the impulses which would make for simple collaboration to be represented in the rest of the personality. Thus in the rest of the personality one finds great longings for warmth and lust and love and all sorts of things that are gruesomely truncated and grimly caricatured in the waking intimacy. One sees processes which strive to diminish the constructive tensions which are unsatisfied in the waking hateful life together. The impulses which would make for simple collaboration exist in what is ordinarily called the unconscious, and manifest themselves in unwitting, unnoted behavior—sometimes in automatisms or other dissociated behavior; and in this behavior the person sometimes seems to come very close to manifesting a deep love for the other person who is always being tortured and who is torturing in turn. Any such impulses which are not manifested in dissociated behavior must be dealt with in sleep. Thus the dream processes of people who are full of hate will be found to include symbolic operations which actually have the purpose of releasing the tension of positive, constructive drive; this is one of the curious situations in which the nearest a person comes to warm human companionship is in his sleep. If in no other respect, these people are truly sad caricatures of human life. But their significance from our standpoint is somewhat greater, for it often happens that after the hateful person has encountered this sort of thing for a while, he simplifies things enormously by including certain primitive operations in his appraisal of reality and becoming paranoid. This is a very much simpler way of life than these hateful integrations in which a person seems literally to be using most of his human ingenuity to bedevil somebody who suffers but also reciprocates by bedeviling him.

Grief and Guilt

GRIEF

The dynamism of grief, like all other dynamisms of living, is a necessary part of human equipment. In normal human experience, grief is a series of processes, very unpleasant to undergo, by which the fantastic sequel to serious affectional loss is erased and the integrating tendencies which had been involved in a relationship that is now ended forever are gradually released for life—that is, for a new attachment. As such, grief is an extremely valuable and protective device.

Grief in this biologically human sense is dependent on the integrative tendency which I call love—the capacity for intimacy which first appears in preadolescence. Below the level of preadolescent development, all ties between developing personalities are fugitive in terms of the ability for closeness. The juvenile, for instance, may have a very keen awareness of what is lost, of awkwardness about a playmate's moving to another city; there may even be some feeble attempt at correspondence. But the whole thing withers very rapidly, and other people are discovered to fill the place very nicely. Nothing of that kind applies to the chum in preadolescence. The chum's death, for instance, is a major incident—literally the most important thing that has happened to the personality in the area of recollection. Such an incident is usually handled in personality by the dynamism of grief.

Let me explain from my theoretical position what I mean as to the biologically human use of grief. We are very largely a product of acculturation: our security depends on others, for our self-system is developed exclusively from communicated values which we have picked up from others; and the satisfactions of our most difficult needs—those which call for the most refined and complex behavior, extending over the longest period of time—also involve other people. For these two reasons, both from the standpoint of security and from the standpoint of satisfaction, we are peculiarly susceptible to evil consequences from the natural accidents, such as death, which destroy people who are valuable to us. And because the culture is in many ways so irrational, any attachment to anybody exposes us to another group of dangers—namely, that our incompetence in some fashion or other, our diffidence, or merely the malice of some comparatively irrelevant person—may also destroy the real effectiveness of a relationship that has come to be very important to us.

Because we have to acquire so much, we necessarily learn by rote, as it were, and accumulate our habitual operations by sublimatory processes; and consequently, when we are deprived of a valuable relationship by accident or design, we are in great danger of translating a more or less real intimacy into a wholly fantastic intimacy. We learn only slowly to separate our idealizing expectancies about people from what is justifiable expectancy. In other words, for a great many people it is extremely difficult to discover the character—the consensually valid character—of a person who is strongly liked or strongly disliked. Thus you can realize how shockingly probable it is that even two or three years of intimate life as husband and wife may leave relatively untouched a large body of illusion in each person as to the character of the mate. Very real and objectively demonstrable interaction has been unable to brush aside this great body of illusion about the other person —of what we ordinarily flippantly call wish-fulfilling fantasies. Surely, then, you can see what I mean when I speak of the danger that the death of either person in this situation will deliver the other over to life with a fantastic illusion of the person who is gone. Illusion had entered into the pre-existing relationship to a certain extent; now the reality is dropped out and the surviving person simply builds the illusion further, and goes on. The utility of grief lies in the fact that it normally erases these attachments which menace us by leaving us fixed in an illusory life.

Grief in its way represents an almost obsessional repetition of the statement, "He is lost; this is horrible; he is lost." And the iterating of the loss neutralizes the tendency to carry on the pre-existing pursuit of satisfaction and security with the purely fantastic objective. The statement that the person is gone is, as it were, an insurance against that which is chiefly necessary because of the irrational elements that are incorporated in all of us. The picture from our tripartite viewpoint that one finds in what I call normal grieving (to distinguish it from what I am going to discuss shortly) is rather as we might expect. We find in the self, readily accessible to awareness, a diminishing preoccupation with the reference that events have to the lost one. The first day after the loss, since intimacies interpenetrate so much of life, it is almost impossible not to be reminded of the loss by any little thing—even the position of the saltcellar on the table, for instance. But each time this happens, you might say, the power of that particular association to evoke the illusion of the absent one is lessened. The associations run through awareness in much the same way that the obsessional neurotic's early magical verbal formulas do. The obsessional's use of the verbal formula is possible because he never observes its real function; it just works, and that is all he looks at. In fact, he practically runs away from anyone who tries to attract his attention to what is being done. The grief dynamism is really a very practical use of this obsessional device. Thus, immediately after a loss, the position of the saltcellar may be reminiscent to you of dear John, because it was always placed half-way between you and John. But the next time you see the saltcellar, you might become a little bored; its power to evoke dear John is diminished by the very fact that you have clarified the associational link with him. And so it goes: by erasing one tie after another, and releasing the personality to move on into life and seek satisfactions by cooperation or collaboration with other people, grief protects us from making a retreat. The grieving that goes on in the self-system preoccupies us with what, so far as the total personality is concerned, is actually an erasing of all these superabundant linkages of nearly everything with the lost one. The experience is, of course, an extremely painful one, but the pain diminishes day by day; fewer and fewer things have the power to evoke this erasing process, which I insist grief is.

In the rest of the personality there are, of course, many things which do not in any sense pertain to this purpose. It is extremely difficult in this culture to have found a companion so perfect that all of one's personality was expanded and more easily fulfilled through collaboration with this person. One may assume that even in very happy married life, which I have had the good fortune to observe at great length in several instances, there are nonetheless certain needs which are not met by the mate, and there are certain operations of the mate which are conducive to insecurity. In other words, the relationship is not perfect, however unusually workable it may be. And in the period of grieving there is fairly evident a new movement of the aspects of personality which have been chronically sublimated, chronically substituted for, chronically dissociated, and chronically avoided by selective inattention. Thus aspects of personality now appear that it would have been rather hard to find any understandable evidence of during the real relationship. Now one finds automatic interest in things which would have led to no show of interest during the actual relationship. Thus at the same time that grief in the self is making tedious the once-valuable associations and so releasing one from persistent preoccupation with the object of one's loss, the rest of the personality is, so to speak, renewing its youth, looking with new hope at possibilities for the future. All of these movements show, not only that the erasing process is going on, but also that it is getting a certain encouragement from long unsatisfied needs which were not adequately met in the very satisfactory relationship. Correspondingly, even early in the period of grieving, along with all this desolation which one feels and which appears in all that one says and does, sleep can be magnificent and untroubled; and the energy of the personality is renewed for new grieving, which, however, gets less and less. And so we see in that very fact the smooth working of an exceedingly important dynamism which saves us from becoming victims of having been happy once in this culture.

MORBID GRIEVING

And now, what of the grieving that is of much greater interest to the psychiatrist? Like all the other dynamisms of living, grief can be distorted into a horrible caricature of its function by certain complex operations. It becomes dangerous and destructive to the extent that the erasing function is abandoned and grief becomes an adequate mode of life. This means that in some fashion the security of the person is involved in the maintenance of a position of loss. In a situation in which the relationship not only contributed a considerable amount of satisfaction and security in what I might call the more obvious fashion, but also contributed mightily to some morbid result in the sense of an overcomplex or neurotic way of life, there the loss entails the giving-up of this complex pattern of life, which would in turn expose the person to grievous insecurity, far more grievous than would be readily apparent. Under those circumstances, the self, of course, is not engaged in erasing processes, for the self-system is solely concerned with the maintenance of security. That is, if the loss throws one terribly open to anxiety and to the loss of one's self-respect and prestige in the community, the erasing action of the self will not appear. Instead, these associational links will become a preoccupation in many ways analogous to any other substitutive process that we have touched upon. We find that, instead of progressively losing its power to evoke tragic recollections, the saltcellar is now surrounded by a very elegant doily, or is in some other fashion enhanced and made a symbol, extravagantly fortified in its power to evoke the lost one. We also find that certain statements are being rattled off over and over, until they are gradually perfectly threadbare, and that these statements are in essence a creed: "I cannot live without John. John is with me, in spirit if not in fact." Then, if we look into the situation more closely, we discover that the relationship with John was, in an interpersonal sense, criminal.[3]

---

[3] Crime in its interpersonal significance refers to action, overt or implicit, which violates the assumed rights, the most sanctified rights, of another person. In other words, it is not a crime for me to express what comes to my mind if, for example, another psychiatrist demands that I tell him what I think about a patient I have seen in consultation with him. It is a crime, however, for me to so lose track of what I am doing with a patient

That is, the relationship was always much more important in a never-formulated way than it was in the ostensibly formulated way, and to lose this love-object means that the person would stand convicted of something—which may be any of the tawdry, unhappy performances to which we are driven in our best of all possible worlds, ranging from marriages of convenience to facilitations of death. But the point is that the self-system is now manifesting a practical utilization of the dynamism of grief for the protection of security; grief is no longer an effective and constructive instrumentality of life.

In these situations, of course, one finds conflict in the rest of the personality; the needs which had been satisfied in the real relationship are now being thwarted by the morbid use of grief. Sleep is disturbed, and operations in dreams are called out in an attempt to maintain quiet outside the self and to maintain in the self a tenuous control of things which were formerly controlled by the really substantial relationship with the other person, and which are harder to control by a purely fantastic relationship with this now dead person. Thus one discovers in morbid grief anything but a contribution to the

---

that I profoundly wound him by throwing out some verbal rattling of something that comes to my mind. That is a crime because my system of values makes unwarranted and unconstructive injury of another person justifiable under only one circumstance: namely, if that person is of no earthly importance to me and is using me as a signpost on which to hang a lot of social nuisance. Even this sort of unkindness to innocent bystanders would be a crime for some people, who are inspired by an intense conviction that man should always be kind. That is no part of my valuational equipment. But a high sense of responsibility for careless damage to patients whom I am seeing is part of my equipment, and therefore I commit a crime when I fail to live up to this strongly held valuational position in my interpersonal relations with patients.

Now that this is a crime is not proved by any amount of reasoning, of course. Yet there is a mark by which we know that it is a crime for us in our relations with others; it is to be found in what we ordinarily cheer ourselves by calling the 'emotional' aspect of the thing. I say "cheer ourselves" because no one can make sense about a good deal of life, and what we experience as emotion is one of the things that you can talk yourself to death about without communicating anything to a person who hasn't experienced it.

release of this highly acculturated creature from a now forlorn and lost entanglement with another person. Instead, the fantastic continuation of that person is resolutely used as a barrier to life—as a barrier to any change, any further progression. As I have often said, isolation from interpersonal relations is most disastrous to the human personality, and is indeed responsible for the appearance of the things which we sum up under the name of deterioration. And so morbid grief is inevitably attended by deterioration; that is, elaboration of needs for satisfaction and of behavior for the securing of those satisfactions begins to disintegrate, and becomes of an earlier type; the social sanctions begin to lose their power to refine behavior and simply drop away; and the field of interest in others shrinks. Presently one of two things befalls these people. Either they cross the line into the, to my way of thinking, very dangerous condition of depression, or they become unhappy wreckages of life by the slow deterioration process of the fantastic life with the lost alleged love-object. So morbid grief is a serious maladjustment, a very definite mental disorder which comes from the undue dependence on or the preternatural duration of the particular group of tendencies which is part of all of us and which is ordinarily adjustive.

GUILT

The mark in awareness which, barring overcomplex situations, is a safe criterion of whether we have violated something really important to our particular personality organization is the feeling of guilt. The subject of guilt is worn threadbare in psychiatric conversation, if not thought, but I have to consider it from my own theoretical position before I can feel that I have done justice to my subject.

When you hear a person talk about experiencing guilt, he may actually be talking about guilt, or he may be talking about a rationalization by which he escapes clear awareness of anxiety. Very often it is the latter, which is a nuisance, particularly if you are a psychiatrist who falls into unnoted collaboration with this confusion. A person may rattle off a great deal about his feelings of guilt when it is quite clear from any calm, objective study of his behavior that he is controlled by no elaborate and obviously highly valued ideal in the field in which he allegedly feels guilty. That simply doesn't make any sense by my definition of guilt. If a thing is not a crime, in an interpersonal sense, as demonstrated by the person's everyday behavior in full awareness, then for him to feel guilty of a particular instance of this thing is just nonsense, and such nonsense is the queer kind of sublimation with which we hound each other to death—rationalization. If the person finds something plausible that will sort of stun his own referential machines or stop them, and if it gets by with a supposedly intelligent bystander such as a psychiatrist, then there certainly are no residual problems of formulation, and he can rest there. All this happens when the person is made mildly insecure by something that would ordinarily call out anxiety, which is very unpleasant and cannot be cultivated as sport. And so he gets all wound up with a flock of moving thoughts about guilt feeling, which spare him the anxiety and the additional insecurity of perplexity as to why he feels insecure.

Statements about guilt are particularly facile to use in complicating the clear manifestation of anxiety for the reason that there is a very conspicuous component of anxiety in the truest kind of guilt. This is because we are trained fairly early to feel insecure when we fail ourselves as well as when we antagonize, distress, or disturb the significant personal environment. That is the way in which we adjust a good deal of our behavior so that we will be inoffensive and our conduct will not lead to the losses of euphoria called anxiety. And so it becomes necessary to define guilt as the peculiarly colored anxiety which attends a clearly observed violation of an important governing principle. Thus guilt is a function of behavior in central awareness; that is, it occurs in circumstances in which people know just what they are doing, or at least know what they have done an instant after having done it—and it is the only form of anxiety, I suppose, that most people ever experience in which there is such clarity. It is, for instance, a pretty far cry from the situation in which behavior of a more or less dissociated impulse arouses anxiety, so that the person simply suffers this primordial and terribly repellent experience of anxiety without any clear awareness of the dissociated impulse that called it out. But guilt is a drop in euphoria due to our not having lived up to our most important convictions of what we are good for and how we should live; and this drop in euphoria—this anxiety—is horribly unpleasant and, like all anxiety, practically always provoking in personal relations, real or fantastic.

But it gets to be the bane of a psychiatrist's life to encounter people who have not performed this intrapersonal operation of the self and the ideal system, and who never experience anxiety and cannot imagine what you are talking about if you mention it, but who gradually decide that they "must have felt a little guilty" about something or other. You find no evidence in their ordinary life that the alleged cause of guilt is a governing principle. Now for therapeutic purposes, of course, it is terribly important, again from our tripartite viewpoint, to realize that this crazy guilt, which is a rationalization of anxiety, is a security operation that complicates the inevitable use of anxiety as a warning away from a situation which produces insecurity. And the overcomplication is significant for us in that the content of the self, the readily reproducible data, will be in itself a way of avoiding the cause of insecurity. It will be beside the point. It must be traversed and gotten rid of, usually by an appeal to other instances where the person has violated this alleged principle with utter impunity and an absence of guilt. It is only after you have disintegrated the rationalization, which the alleged guilt is in such an instance, that you get anywhere near the actual cause of the underlying anxiety.

But in the case where guilt is really guilt, where the person for relatively clear reasons is justifiably and properly shaky at having fallen down on his own standards of life, there one has a much simpler therapeutic problem. And it is a problem to be handled in a quite different way—namely, by finding out what the circumstances were under which this occurred, because a strong ideal does not ordinarily rest and let things happen which violate it. Something or other has allowed the unusual to happen. Referring again to our tripartite viewpoint, we have to expect it to be found in the rest of the personality and to be anything but immediately accessible to awareness. We may also expect it to entail great anxiety in its ultimate elucidation because it is obviously a field where something in the personality collides with the most valued ideals in the self-system, and so, of course, it represents a grave threat to security.

In crazy guilt, sleep is not particularly disturbed; if sleep is disturbed, then it is because of what is being rationalized away. That is, nothing in any way related to the alleged guilt appears in the symbolic operations recalled as dreams; instead, what appears is the underlying insecurity which would otherwise be manifested as mild anxiety. But in the real guilt that I am talking about, there is a very great disturbance of the sleeping section of life, for the violation of ideals means that there are powerful impulses which are not represented in awareness and that there is pressure toward some goal in their direction which has to be toned down, possibly during sleep. The tripartite glimpse is necessary, therefore, in order to grasp such discriminations as that between real guilt and the guilt which is really only a rationalization of anxiety.

Pride and Conceit

PRIDE

I am now going to take time out to discuss one of the perhaps most subordinate of the dynamisms that I want behind us, the dynamism of pride. An examination of it is most easily approached by the usual psychiatric route—that is, when does a person suffer from the dynamism of pride? When, in other words, does this particular aspect of personality—which may be presumed to be ubiquitous, but which may be very well concealed—get to the point of being a serious handicap in life?

Sometimes a person tells me that he cannot bring himself to do some particular thing which seems to me a necessary part of a scientific attack on a problem. If he can be pushed some further, he says, "Well, I won't humiliate myself that way." And so one may take it that, in some cases, the lack of pride is felt as a particular type of low self-appraisal or humiliation, which is very different, indeed, from what a student of ethics might say is the opposite of pride, meaning humility. Pride and humility seem to have a much more poetic than actual relationship. But pride and humiliation have a very intimate relationship in everyday life, as can be observed from the way people act.

I would like to explore next the question of what is humiliating and why it is humiliating. I think that mere casual attention to what people do and say in your presence will in the course of time prove to you that almost anything can be humiliating to somebody. This means that humiliation probably is very largely a product of early acculturation. Occasionally one runs onto a person who, in spite of having pride, will strangely enough take any humiliation in the interest of some particular idea. For this reason, I think that the thing called pride, although it may be a very conspicuous aspect of personality, can scarcely be regarded as one of the great important dynamisms, in a class with jealousy and envy, for example—which

I shall discuss presently—or with the various things that I think of more as tendencies, such as sublimation.

It has seemed to me that people are always proud, in this specific psychiatric sense, of things which are not so. In other words, pride seems to be the presenting aspect of an elaborate self-deception. The organization of the self is inadequate to meet some of the recurrent needs for security; but this inadequacy would be much more poignant if the person observed it. We have seen that, under some circumstances, very extensive supplementary processes occur in the self to maintain a dissociation, so that correct recall and appropriate impulses just never appear because the exciting elements do not get to attention. In the same way, the façade which we call pride excludes from recognition this inadequacy in the self—this relative inefficiency of the self as a security device. This is why I say that one is *always* proud of something that is not so. Pride appears always for the purpose of concealing a literal insecurity which one's past experience has not permitted one to avoid or to handle in some other way. I am, you must remember, using the word pride in a restricted sense, as the name of a process; I do not mean that what one is 'proud of' in a more general sense is necessarily not there.

Perhaps I should say something here about what is *not* pride, to make my point more impressive. From what I have said about selective inattention and various other things, I think you can see how I would account for the fact that a person who almost never makes an arithmetical error, for example, can still live in a sort of chronic expectation of error and will generally check or get someone else to check his addition of a column of figures, particularly if the results are important. Clearly that person is not proud of his arithmetical ability. In fact, he is morbidly deficient in appreciating it. He distrusts something that over and over again has proved to be superior. There are a good many reasons why that may be the case. Sometimes it is as simple a situation as his having been criticized by mistake; perhaps someone else's error was at some time attributed to him, and he was told that he would simply have to get over his stupidity with numbers. Then no one ever happened to correct the mistake or to tell him, "My God, you're good at numbers." And very few of us fall into the happy circumstance of having to sit down with ourselves and say, "Now look here, am I good, bad, or average in such-and-such a field of activity?" Such judgments are not a part of the culture, and many people are never confronted with an opportunity to make them about themselves. A person can go through life with fancied inadequacies which may be explained simply by the fact that he has never done anything that had an adequate corrective influence. Usually, however, these things are the presenting signs of some of the dynamisms of difficulty, and most of the people who, without any justification, have always distrusted their ability in a given field show other evidences of obsessional substitution.

But now, with that semi-digression to clear the ground, let us imagine the following situation to illustrate my point here. Let us say that in interviewing a person to see whether he should do a certain type of work for me, I ask him, "How is your accuracy in addition and subtraction?" This person says, "I think it is pretty high. I believe I'm unusually apt to be right in that sort of thing." Now at this point I have two highly justifiable hypotheses. I may, I think with much safety, infer either that he is pretty good at adding or that he prides himself on something which is not so.

If in the subsequent weeks I find that his operations in the field of arithmetic are almost always right and that the error is far below the probable error in such operations, then I may say, "Well, this bird is good at figures and has learned that he is. He knows it." In other words, this person has had an opportunity to discover that he is really dependable when it comes to addition; so that part of his definition of himself has contributed a certain amount to his security and reduces a good many possible problems that he might have. Perhaps, along with knowing that he is unusually good, he knows that under certain circumstances this might not prove to be the case. But at any rate, he has developed a definition about himself which makes him extraordinarily secure with other people in his field, and he is not likely to have any disagreeable failures.

Now let us take the other hypothesis: What if this person who has said that he is really thoroughly good at arithmetic demonstrates in the weeks to follow that he can get a different total every time he goes over a column of figures. Then I have to say to myself, "Well, how come? What is this nonsense? This man, who obviously can't be trusted to add three and three, has gotten himself on a job where skill in addition is imperative, where that's what he's paid for. He insisted that he was well equipped for this job, and it's obvious nonsense." Well, there are again at least two possible explanations in this case. One is that there is something about the job that calls in collateral disturbing factors which ruin an otherwise average ability to add. The second is that somewhere in this person's past life great value was put on a fraud, namely: "While I am no good at addition, I must never admit that. It leaves me defenseless to a certain type of humiliation." And so the following formulation becomes an important part of his easily accessible definition of himself: "I am a person who's good at addition." But he is just unable to demonstrate that. He just is not good at addition. Now the odd thing about this is that he can fail to live up to his own description of himself again and again without any particular perturbation. But if, on the other hand, he encounters a situation in which he says, "Well, I'm good at arithmetic," the other fellow says, "I wonder," and a test is run off in which he shows up at about his usual level of competence, then he suffers terribly. He is acutely insecure, and the lengths to which he will go to restore his damaged feelings are sometimes nothing short of fantastic. How do we explain this peculiarity? Pride, you see, is based on a fictitious self-appraisal, set up to conceal something that is not adequate in the self-organization. How does it come about that it works in spite of reality's continuously providing contradictory data? And why is it that, if it is confronted with a particular type of test situation in which it fails, really remarkable insecurity is turned loose?

I have already touched on part of this story, for this is one of the many instances of the process of selective inattention. Vast numbers of negative instances are ignored; they are nuisances. And selective inattention functions smoothly enough so that this person's pride in his ability to add is not affected by the numerous instances when this ability just is not shown. The meaning is that this pride in an ability to add is an important part of the definition of the self. This is simply a special instance of the rule that in large measure the reason why we do not change, despite experience that happens to us, is that what does not change is pretty necessary, according to anything that we have in us, and therefore it is protected by selective inattention or even by rather extensive operations of some of the other dynamisms. It is as if there could be nothing else if this were lost. That generally means that this is a relatively static situation, reaching far back of the present. To understand why a person gets himself out on such a curious limb as considering himself good at addition when he really is not, we would probably have to go back to his early school days, when addition and such things were possible sources of very real pain and prestige and what not. We might venture that somehow or other this person's inability to do simple adding must have put him on the spot so awkwardly that he couldn't afford to have that vulnerability. So he did one of the many rather glaringly magical things that people can do—he altered the fact by words of power. The fact that he cannot feel comfortable with the knowledge that he is no good in arithmetic is remedied by the magical statement, "I am good at arithmetic." And because in those early days, when he was suffering from insecurity, this magical statement served the purpose, it has become one of the dependable pillars of his not very strong, not very effective self. Since this self would otherwise be vulnerable to the large amount of negative experience he encounters, it is always protected by selective inattention or some other dynamism—except when such protection cannot work. That is why the endless errors he makes are not humiliating to him, however troublesome they may be, but a specific test *is* humiliating and causes a vast to-do that a mere question of arithmetical ability can scarcely be considered to explain. Somebody says to him, "Oh yeah? Well, show it," and then he fails and he is in a bad state.

There are two unfortunate aspects of the pride dynamism, both of which I think I have gotten into this context. The first of these is that where security depends on any striking use of the pride dynamism, a great deal of selective inattention is inevitable and the person is going to be poorly acquainted with the particular aspect of reality in which this pride is centered. The second is that such a person is vulnerable to frontal attack. A situation which threatens to "show him up" breathes the same ancient breath that was connected with the original adoption of this dynamism as a part of the self. There has been little development since that time; this part of the self which operates by magical verbal power—"I am the bird who is good at mathematics"—has been rather remarkably static. Now if things are so engineered that this person cannot be inattentive to what is going to happen—and you remember that in selective inattention you have the data, but you never do anything with them—he is carried back to the time when he had to build this dynamism, when there was a great deal more insecurity connected with a mathematical failure than would probably be the case with any such failure in his more adult life. He reacts to a threat of great insecurity just as he did then, when it was a question of his ability to add two and two; and probably this insecurity interferes with what ability he has. So not only is he out on a limb, but the limb is badly rotted by the extent to which he is discomposed by this attack; and so the failure carries, for months afterwards, this deep humiliation and fierce hatred for the person who put him on the spot. And this is to be explained on the basis of the strange way in which the pride dynamism arrests critical valuation of oneself at a much more primitive level.

I have used this very simple illustration to show that when you ask a person how good he is or how he compares with other people in various activities or operations, and you get a positive answer—which may be anything from a very simple and direct statement of merit to a very emphatic statement of merit—you should have in mind the following questions: Is this statement merely factual, a valid self-appraisal? Or does it represent the operation of this queer, essentially quite young process of magically obscuring a field of chronic inadequacy from his own attention—is it, then, quite incorrect but very important for his feeling of personal security and adequacy to the demand? There is one other possibility—that the answer may reflect mere ignorance, that the reply is incorrect for the simple reason that the person doesn't have any standards by which to judge but has formed an opinion which he hopes is right, simply because he feels, as we all do, that he has to know the answer to whatever he is asked.

Within the self there is a not necessarily conspicuous, but always very real group of processes which can be called the organization of *self-respect* or the organization of *self-esteem*. The striking thing about this whole system of processes is that it can be expressed more or less adequately in communicative speech on demand. Under certain circumstances, it is possible to rattle off this system solemnly as a description of the worthy human characteristics that you have. Now this is not the whole self, but only a part of the self (if we must talk in fractions), because we always know many things that contradict almost anything that we say positively at a given moment. Thus it is not astonishing that a person may respect himself for things he does not have or may respect himself for his essentially trivial attributes rather than for certain real greatnesses that he apparently never realizes he has. All this is to be understood from the fact that the self is made up by acculturation out of what one has a chance to learn from others in the eternal struggle to be secure and free from anxiety with them.

In certain families, for example, the possession of a truly uncanny capacity for getting music out of appropriate instruments could conceivably be of no particular moment because everybody can do it. There might be some minor evaluation in terms of which members of this family take naturally to the wood winds, which to the organ, and which to the strings, but this astounding musical gift would be assumed to be in the nature of being human. It is ubiquitous in this little group, and so the possessors of this gift are not astonished by it. It is only when they are compared with other people who show little or none of it that this capacity begins to take on considerable significance.

Moreover, in some homes there seems to be a tacit parental conspiracy not to praise, not to stress the possession by the children of exceptional capacities, for fear the children will feel that they are better than other people. Consequently, we now and then run onto a person whose gifts in a particular field rather stagger us, but who is just totally unaware that there is anything remarkable in them. Generally this is the result of excessive parental caution to avoid conceit. Such parents would include recognition of one's own gifts in this conception of pride. But I think that it has to be rather sorted out of it.

A great many of us do, however, incorporate into ourselves in the juvenile era rather realistic data on where we are good and where we are bad. In the school society, where competition is rather an outstanding trait, there is a good deal of actual exploration and rather careful comparison of how one rates with other people that seem to matter. By and large, most of the things that the juvenile builds into his self as guides to where he stands in comparison with others in particular fields function pretty well. His valuations may, of course, be unduly low in some fields and unduly high in others. In certain fields the picture may be very much distorted by certain circumstances, emotional disturbances, specific taboos, and one thing and another. It is only where these valuations are strikingly and unduly high that one can observe this abnormal use of the dynamism of pride. Where they are unduly low, we know that some special circumstances account for that. But, by and large, the solid core of the self-respecting system is based on fairly well-evaluated real experience.

The peculiarities that are of psychiatric importance occur in the instances where the valuations of the self-respecting part of the self are unduly low. Generally you will find that the low appraisal of one's self does not mean that one is really not adequate for life, but that certain dynamisms of difficulty have become quite effective in the period of development; there is a chronic aching void, a chronic extreme vulnerability to anxiety, a chronic insecurity, which may have so obstructed the process of normal self-appraisal that the person never did get a very clear idea of what he was good for. Instead, he constantly suffered because he was no good at something that it was terribly important for him to be good at, and he did not throw off this suffering by any magic of pride. As a matter of fact, the operations of pride as a morbidity have to be rather restricted, for you get on the spot too easily if you are not moderately conservative in using such a device. In other words, like sublimation, pride cannot be overloaded without falling of its own weight.

CONCEIT

When you try to find out from another person what his capabilities are and what his limitations are, you will always notice that his replies to your questions are never absolutely explicit in meaning. For example, they sometimes are so autistic, the terms used deviate so strikingly from their approximate meaning in general usage, that that in itself becomes a peculiarity for the psychiatrist to notice. And among the kinds of replies which may be most illuminating is that of the person who—when you finally get to the point of wanting to know what he thinks he is good at and what he thinks he has some limitations for—is very sure that he is good at two or three things, and there it stops. But far from giving any impression that he feels an inadequacy or incompleteness, he is beaming; this very limited definition of outstanding abilities amply suffices. If you are just normal, you will engage in a discourse on this, and pretty soon rattle off the conclusion to yourself, "Well, this man is a conceited ass!" And you mean just what? You do not mean that he is not good at these things, but you do mean that his feeling of worth among men is queerly related to the integration of merits on which a healthy, easily workable, efficient feeling of worth is based.

Perhaps I can make this clear by using a personal measure. I would very much hate to fall into a position where I had to enumerate carefully the things at which I am distinctly less able than a good many of the people that I have bumped into in life. That, in my particular case, would be an almost unending performance, for two reasons. One is that my experience has brought me into at least brief contact with a rather astoundingly wide field of human performance, so that I know a great many things that some people do well. The other is that my particular life course has been such that quite dependable abilities in a few fairly narrowed fields have served all purposes necessary in the way of my self-esteem, leaving me no sense of having been denied opportunities and one thing and another. For that reason, even if I had some abilities of which I am entirely unaware, there would not have been the circumstances which would promote their continued manifestation to the point that they got fitted in as of just average, or sub-average, or super-average magnitude. Thus if I started telling you what I was good at and what I was not, I would sound like a classical instance of this conceit I am speaking of, for a few abilities that I can demonstrate seem to suffice perfectly to keep me feeling on a reasonable par with my fellows. This is an example of the effect of a life course on the extent to which one is clear on what one is good for.

But the conceited person depends for a very considerable security—in fact, a feeling of definite superiority—on being able to demonstrate average or better abilities in certain immensely overvalued traits. The conceit arises from an overvaluation of certain things; this, strangely enough, is not so different in its origin—although it is just about the reverse of the coin—from the origin of pride. Somewhere in the earlier experience of this person, demonstration of ability in this particular field was so powerful in assuaging anxiety, brought such certain relief from insecurity, that it began to take on rather magical power; it is as if the person said, "As long as I can do that, I'm all right with people." These things stand as virtues of which he is the lucky possessor, and it takes a good man to show him that he isn't as good a man. Thus conceit is built of correct appraisals of ability, given, however, preternatural importance as dependable pillars of security. Conceit, you can see, is facilitated by the culture; and insofar as it is a valid excerpt from the culture, conceit is a pretty dependable, if somewhat inefficient, process in maintaining self-esteem and a feeling of security with one's fellows.

Of course, one does encounter unhappy situations where there is extravagance, not because there is pride, and not because the person is conceited, but because he is so desperately insecure that it seems impossible to be merely factual. Now that is quite another thing. Very few of us are much impressed by the jittery assertions of competence by a person who obviously is scared to death that you will not believe him. That is so typical a manifestation of any number of insecure situations that it does not deserve a name or any particular discussion.

Now how is this business of conceit maintained? Do lots of negative instances have to be suppressed by selective inattention? Not at all. The very organization that explains conceit means that the flow of events must fit this pattern or be relatively devaluated as instances of bad taste, bad upbringing, or what not on the part of the other people. Thus it does not require anything in particular; it works. That is what I really mean when I say that it is strongly facilitated by the culture. So frontal attack in an area of conceit may get you the reputation of being a bounder, or something like that, but it does not disturb the conceited person. Even if he does not prove to be as good as the attacker in some particular field, he comes away with the feeling, "Well, I performed it wonderfully. You see, he's really better than I am, and he doesn't know enough to appreciate himself for it." It works. But that is true, of course, of anything that has as much backing as conceit can have.

Envy and Jealousy as Precipitating Factors in the Major Mental Disorders

Envy

IN OUR CONSIDERABLY irrational social order, a great many of the material and adventitious trappings of life have significance in the shape of prestige and deference from others. Thus it is quite reasonable to take the position which, I believe, was first taken by McDougall,[1] that the clothes one wears, the car one drives, the type of house one lives in, and all that sort of thing are exterior illusions of the self. They are props to an uncertain security, and they are awfully important to the person whom they serve as props. This is another way of saying that the more immediate attributes of the person's living—that is, what he can do with other people and what he can get them to do with him, or, in other words, his direct interpersonal satisfactions—are not adequate, and so, to avoid anxiety, he requires the security that comes from these other things. And whenever such a person encounters anything relating to another person which would, if it related to himself, be a material prop to his security, a material enhancement of his prestige

[1] W. McDougall, *Outline of Psychology*; New York: Scribners, 1923.

among others, then the dynamism of envy appears. Envy is an acute discomfort caused by discovering that somebody else has something that one feels one ought to have.

It is apparent that the organization of the self-system is not very successful in the person who shows envy markedly, for a person who is fairly successful in achieving security is not made acutely uncomfortable by the discovery that some other person has prestige marks or ability or something of the sort greater than his own. But in the envious person the self part of the personality just does not work adequately; it has to have more than there is. And when we attempt to discover how this inadequacy comes about, we find that it is not necessarily related to any specific type of danger in the rest of the personality—to any particular need for satisfaction that is constantly endangering the person in his relations with others. Although the envious person, viewed as a total personality picture, is lacking in many complete satisfactions in interpersonal relations, these incomplete satisfactions are but little related to the appearance of envy. There is a relation in the sense that when an envious person has achieved a strong satisfaction, he will then overlook opportunities for suffering envy —there will be no particular necessity for the morbid dynamism to appear. But still, the insecurity which leads to envy is not specifically related to any particular need for satisfaction. A very markedly envious person may, for instance, have reasonable capability for satisfying lust, and he may be well fed. His needs, therefore, are not the answer. Then what is the answer?

Returning to the self-system and looking into the history of its evolution, we find that the people who are much at the mercy of envy have learned to appraise themselves as unsatisfactory—that is, as inadequate human beings. Sometimes envious people have been taught this sense of their own inadequacy in a simple, direct, and comprehensive way. That is, in the home environment and in the succeeding school society, they have been taught that they do not rate, that they are not the people that others wish they were. They have been children who have disappointed their parents' expectations and hopes for them. Sometimes they are people who have rather small gifts, but whose parents had expected them to have larger gifts, as a result of which the smallness of their gifts was brought very keenly to their attention.

With other envious people, the lesson may have taken a different form. Instead of being taught of their inadequacy thus directly by being unsatisfactory to their parents and failing to live up to their parents' ideals, they have been given an irrational and extravagant picture of themselves as children and as very young juveniles. Then from the beginning of the school era onward, they have constantly experienced the dissatisfaction of others with their attempt to approximate these extravagant ideals that their parents gave them. In other words, they have been taught that they are more than can be demonstrated in the world. And because they are intelligent, like practically all people, the continuous failure to demonstrate how much they are worth has added itself up to a very strong, if never quite formulated, conviction that they really do not rate. Thus the history of the envious person has included the one or the other—either the parental attitude has directly demonstrated that he does not rate; or, quite the contrary, it has set for him excessively high goals which he could not attain. And as a result the envious person comes to invest with importance all sorts of things which carry prestige or approval; he needs those things, he feels, to add to what he already has to demonstrate in the world, in order to be on an even footing with others.

It is this necessity which causes the idiosyncrasies which we find in viewing the personality from the rest of our tripartite standpoint. Because there is the unusually continuous insecurity, and the need for these irrational personalized props, such as Cadillac cars and one thing and another, the pursuit of satisfactions in interpersonal intimacies is apt to be poisoned and overcomplicated by efforts to remedy the insecurities. Thus while the tendency systems which would ordinarily result in the pursuit of satisfactions are not particularly distorted, the pursuits of satisfactions are always badly complicated by this property aspect of seeking security, which can, of course, reach rather fantastically revealing lengths. For example, a boy who is attempting to get on really intimate terms with a girl may have so much to say about himself, his family, their properties, his expectations, and so on, that he gets to be regarded as a fearsome bore. The girl is put under a demand to say that everything about him—his clothes, his family, his school record, and so on and so forth—is unusually good. And so, however attractive she finds him physically, her own security is not so great that she can permit herself to be a sex-object, because she correctly guesses that, just as he brags about other things, he also will have to brag to men about his sexual conquests. His insecurity as shown in his envious attitude toward all sorts of things is a very much more prominent feature of him than are his ideals about secrecy concerning his intimate life; and, as having had intercourse with a girl is a little counter of prestige in a society which is prevailingly juvenile, he will advertise the fact. Thus the personality of the markedly envious person is apt to show many evidences of the thwarting of satisfactions; but the thwarting is a result of the ubiquitous envy operations, and therefore is somewhat different from that which occurs in some of the other dynamisms we have discussed.

Correspondingly, the sleep of these people is only occasionally of a deep and utterly restful character, because there is always a lot of unfinished business which carries over from the day, unless the day happens to be well out of the usual pattern of their lives. These exceptions occur on occasions when, by accident or design, envious people fall into a position where there just are no superior people, or people endowed with greater trappings of power and prestige than they. This is likely to occur when they are in a wholly novel environment—that is, an environment where the people who might signify are so novel that they cannot immediately be categorized. Then the envious person may be quite comfortable and give the impression of being what is ordinarily called "a natural, comfortable person to have around." On such occasions he has a wonderful time, and he gets a lot of rest at night. Thus vacations are sometimes delightful for the intensely envious person unless they are fairly prolonged. If they are long enough so that he gets over the novelty with which he has been charmed, then the need for these prestige marks becomes more and more apparent. This is partly because envy represents a deficiency in the self, and there is a corresponding alertness which the self controls, so that he alertly notes the evidences of his losing ground with strangers, and so on. At that point this thing approaches a little the paranoid dynamism that I shall come to presently.

All in all, this dynamism of envy, which is rather painfully frequent, especially in America, is a fairly poisonous ingredient of the personality. For instance, I think that envious people quite frequently die of the results of hypertension. And envious people tend in their later years to develop what might be described as a paranoid attitude. In discussing how this comes about, I should first point out that envy is very unpleasant to the person who suffers it. There are perhaps two reasons for this. In the first place, in the Christian world, lip service at least is given to an ethical norm that one shall not envy—or covet—the possessions of one's neighbor, and so envy carries heavy social disapproval. In the second place, envy is not pleasant because any formulation of it—any implicit process connected with it—necessarily starts with the point that you need something, some material thing that, unhappily, someone else has. This easily leads to the question,

Why don't you have it? And that is itself enough in some cases to provoke insecurity, for apparently the other fellow is better at assembling these material props of security than you are, which makes you even more inferior. Thus not only does the religious-cultural disapproval of envy have some tendency to make it an unworthy thing to talk about as one of your guilts, but also the intrusion of envy into a verbal context is attended by this implied further insecurity because of the unfavorable comparison of one's "getting" ability with somebody else's.

And so you must make elaborate rationalizations. These elaborate rationalizations—since they have to explain why you are inadequate and do not have something that somebody else has apparently been adequate enough to get—must have planks built into them which make the other person's having this thing a type of atrocity perpetrated against you; if there was justice, you would have it, instead of him. In other words, here is an element of the paranoid projective business. And that is rather risky, for with the paranoid business you either go whole hog or you often find yourself in extremely awkward positions with the processes within awareness.

Because it is not very satisfactory merely to think to oneself, "If he wasn't a scoundrel, he wouldn't have any more than I have," the envious person attempts to give the statement a little more verisimilitude by getting it more or less tacitly accepted by others. The only way that these bitter derogatory expressions of envy can be stated freely is by saying them of people who do not matter to the person to whom one is talking. Thus, even though you are not on particularly intimate terms with a markedly envious person, a good deal of his conversation with you takes a form which implies that you and he know that present company is excepted from the general derogation. Of course, nothing on earth is more evident to anybody than that present company is excepted only for the purpose of the communication; you are also one of these so-and-sos who, if things were fair, would be beneath his notice. And yet he is so driven by this need for props to his security that he goes through the struggle of tacitly and sometimes quite outspokenly excepting present company so that he can derogate others comfortably.

CULTURAL ASPECTS OF ENVY

The envious person's derogation of others naturally reflects the aspects of American culture that have been most disastrous to the evolution of an adequate self in these people. Here I refer to our singular dearth of good prescriptions for intimacy and accommodation to other people, coupled with our really staggering success at doing things with our natural resources —both, I sometimes think, unparalleled thus far in the history of man. The reason why I want to consider these things here is that they pertain to what little remedial effort can readily be made in dealing with the dynamism of envy.

If you look back over the relatively short history of the American commonwealth, you will notice two striking things. First, the population is the outcome of one massive wave of immigration after another. And as we all know from our own experience, the foreigner—the "boob" who has different standards, a different language, and one thing and another— is especially useful as a target for enhancing one's prestige by the somewhat treacherous route of seeing one's faults in others. Thus these successive waves of immigrants have become the targets for the hostilities that have grown up in the people who have lived here longer. One group after another, they have been regarded more or less as public enemies. And their children have grown up with the dubious asset of being the children of public enemies, regarded by their confreres who have been one generation longer in America as being anything from somewhat human—but, of course, of foreign parentage— to definitely vicious ingredients of the school society. Then, by the time they have reached maturity, they have become

American citizens and taxpayers and permanent members of the Chamber of Commerce, and so on, and by that time there is someone else coming in who is foreign, who is a threat to the security of the country and—in the last few decades— to the democratic system, which is supposed to be one of our copyrights, I gather.

Now along with all this, the dynamic by which people have progressed so rapidly in an upward direction in social status here has been the combination of the vast resources and the brilliant pioneering work that has been done in communications and transportation, together with the almost miscellaneous education of everybody in everything natural or scientific. These things have combined to increase our national per capita wealth at a rate which is unparalleled in human history, and have culminated in the perfectly stupendous development of mass production. The result is that gadgets—and even such gadgets as money—come with preternatural ease, and commerce has developed fabulously; and at the same time the cultivation of that vicious misuse of human credulity—advertising—has become one of the most lucrative of all activities in America. So the business of making things as conspicuously different from each other as possible, and grading these differences in terms of cost, has become an extremely successful way of accumulating other people's money. As a result, the material trappings with which one frantically tries to relieve one's envy—and thereby magnifies it—grow apace.

At the same time, development of understanding of the essential factors in life has been profoundly backward. The reasons for this include the very swiftness of the vertical rise of wave after wave of immigrant stock and the democratic freedom with which we tie our hands when it comes to any very long-range public welfare. The fast turnover in the lower houses of our federal and state governments in itself guarantees that we cannot carry out any very long-term educational policy, particularly if it is one which might impress the newly powerful group in each generation as endangering their new-found position.

Thus the understanding of the essentials of life and the evolution of a culture which would include the development of charming ways of human intimacy have lagged. Americans have many erroneous prescriptions and few correct orientations for human intimacy, and therefore are not apt to feel automatically secure—at the same time that they are impressed from all sides with the importance of the kind of paint they have on their houses and the number of horsepower in their cars. And so there is nothing very mysterious about why Americans are not really particularly friendly people; they can be polite and genial, as long as there is no strong movement toward intimacy. Nor is it mysterious why they are so horribly afflicted with this need for prestige marks that so often culminates in the extremely unpleasant attitude which we call envy. Thus envy is a very widely distributed dynamism of difficulty of which everybody is ashamed but which a great many people cannot avoid showing, for it rests more or less directly in the self-system.

COMPETITION AND ENVY

Perhaps I should say something here about competition, which I regard as somewhat different from envy. Competition is, I suppose, the inescapable concomitant, in the juvenile era, of leaving the exclusively home society in which one knows certain things to be true—including what one's own status is in various respects—by means of obscure, somewhat divine ordinance; that is, these things are the un-understood valuational attitudes of the parents. When one enters the school society, he encounters a group of people, each of whom also knows certain things by the same sort of obscure, somewhat divine ordinance. In the school society, where these valuational attitudes are compared, the only way in which any of them can be confirmed is by struggle—by more or less trying them out on the other fellow, on one's compeers. This testing-out can easily flow into the channel of competitive sports, which are tryouts of physical endowments coupled with mental agility; or it may appear in purely intellectual forms of competition.

Now intensely competitive adults are people who continue to live at a relatively juvenile level—that is, who live as if they always have to prove that they are better than the other fellow. More specifically, the trait which is practically pathognomic for diagnosing a continued juvenile organization of interpersonal relations, or personality, is perverted or morbid ambition. The morbidly ambitious are extremely impatient, and sometimes horribly insecure under the impatience, about the speed at which they ascend to greater social position. They may be quite free from envy, insofar as you can find anybody in this culture quite free from envy. They are out to get the other fellow down, not because they have anything in particular against him or because they need any of his prestige marks—they intend to have much better prestige marks pretty soon—but because he is in the way. Their ruthless kind of behavior is, I think one has to admit, ever so much nearer adjustment than is the gnawing, clumsily disguised suffering of envy, which can exist in people who have anything but a burning, driving ambition, and who may be, in fact, just simply shiftless. Incidentally, the classical business of the bad loser—the person who gets terribly angry in the face of defeat —is not really to be understood from the standpoint of competition, nor do I think it is adequately explained by an appeal to the dynamism of envy. To such people, any little skid in their own performance is so oppressive that one can assume that they suffer terribly from anxiety, and their anger is an example of the handling of anxiety by rage.

Jealousy

Just as the term guilt is sometimes used to mean what I consider real guilt and sometimes to mean a rationalization for something quite different, so there is a confusion in the use of the term jealousy. Sometimes it is used to mean envy; and sometimes it refers to actual jealousy, which is an exceedingly unpleasant emotional experience—perhaps the most unpleasant that man is heir to, except for anxiety itself. Thus a patient may rattle off an infinity of words about how jealous he is of somebody else's position and so on, thereby overlooking the fact that he is envious and is practically all but advertising that he himself, without pomp and circumstance, does not feel adequate as a human being. It is important for the psychiatrist not to enter into any such confusion of reference as that. It is just such confusions that sometimes result in his missing an opportunity to make a frontal attack on the profound problems of personality—namely, what holds off intimacy—and instead barking up trees about the need for prestige.[2]

If, because of the necessities of security—which, in turn, mean unfortunate early experience—one is not capable of complete intimacy with another, one may be said to be

[2] One might say, of course, that jealousy is the envy of others' capacity for intimacy. In a way, it is. But envy in any field except that of the capacity for intimacy is a relatively mild suffering, while jealousy, from all the data that have ever come to my attention, is a horribly unpleasant mental state; and so I think that the distinction is still important.

It is possible that I underrate the extent to which one can suffer envy, for I recall few instances in which I felt intensely envious. I think that possibly the capacity for missing the more extreme suffering of envy is, in my own case, an artifact of the particular juvenile era in which I lived, an era in which it was necessary to become quite expert at finding and using defensive tools. One of these tools was to provoke envy, as a minor malevolence toward troublesome people; and I suppose that provoking envy in others is one way of sparing oneself the most acute development of it.

But even in the people who suffer envy quite acutely, the suffering still doesn't seem to me to be anything compared with the misery that is experienced in jealousy.

incapable of unique satisfaction with any one person. In other words, if one has only partial intimacy with another person, there are bound to be unsatisfied components of personality, and these unsatisfied components tend to integrate relatively identical situations of intimacy with still other people. Jealousy occurs under those circumstances when two other people involved with the subject person in one of these truncated and relatively abortive intimacies manifest, or are fantasied as manifesting, greater capacity for satisfaction with each other than with the subject person. It is at those times that this devastating dynamism of jealousy takes over, and the mental state of the person concerned is abysmally unhappy. And because of the excruciating misery of the situation, supplementary processes are very apt to appear which are, in more ways than one, very closely related to the appearance of the paranoid state.

Thus jealousy is a dynamism which is complex and devastating, so far as the feeling element is concerned, and which occurs always in a context of three people. I do not say that it cannot occur in a context of larger numbers, but they will still be entangled in a three-group relationship. Jealousy is quite a different matter from envy and shows quite widely different characteristics in terms of our tripartite view of that hypothetical thing, personality. Jealousy appears in its most obvious and understandable form in the rather rare circumstance where person A, the person who is going to be jealous, is on terms of comparative intimacy both with person B and with person C. Person B and C are at first relatively unacquainted with each other. But then some unhappy event brings B and C close together, and they immediately manifest a tendency to develop a situation of intimacy. At that time the person in the central position has the poignant and horrible experience of jealousy.

Since intimacy is among us perhaps preternaturally related to sexual intimacy, it is not strange that when jealousy came to the attention of thinkers in dynamic psychiatry, it was discovered to indicate the presence of a component impulse —namely, homosexuality. I question this as being in any sense a generally correct explanation of jealousy. It is true that only under the most extraordinary circumstances would jealousy be suffered by a person who has matured without serious warp, who has matured in a series of situations rather rich in experience so that he has actually developed a fairly well-rounded personality, free from any major handicaps to obtaining satisfactions from his fellows—which means, incidentally, that he is possessed of considerable self-respect and personal security. The more adequate a person's preparation for a theoretically complete satisfaction of needs in interpersonal intimacy, the more impossible it will be for him to stand in such relation to two or more people that he will pursue the same satisfactions in each of these intimacies. This is true because very few people who have gotten on pretty well into complete development of personality escape the impression that interpersonal relations, in our cultural setting at least, increase in demands, risks, complexities, risky misses, and so on, in direct proportion to the magnitude and profundity of the needs they satisfy. So for a person who has a fairly well-developed personality and who has a wholly satisfactory lustful relation with another person, just ordinary considerations for the difficulties of life will discourage any surviving curiosity as to whether a similar intimacy with another person could not be even better. In other words, by the time one gets to the stage of collaboration with other people, one has a great respect for personality and for the problematic steps in the development of intimacy; and for this reason, a person who is rather well-matured in personality is not apt to have a series of parallel intimacies. Or if he has, they are very widely distributed in space; in other words, I can conceive of a really strikingly mature sailor literally having a wife in each one of several ports, for that is practical. But I defy you to find many rather mature people who have relations of very great and perfectly parallel intimacy with two people in the same town, for example. Thus the chances of one's being involved in this potential jealousy situation are in inverse proportion to the extent to which one has mature or adequate personal equipment.

But the reason why one should not fall into too exclusive preoccupation with sex as a means of understanding jealousy lies in the explanation of why jealousy appears when these two objects of at least somewhat intimate relations move toward each other. This is where the defect in the self, which is somewhat parallel to the defect in the case of envy, steps in; and the most general way of describing this defect is to say that the person has grown into his present position in life with a deep, however unwelcome, conviction of relative unworthiness. The setting which produces jealousy is one in which the person feels, as you could find out if you knew his most secret thoughts or heard his most profoundly self-revealing communications, that regardless of all the front he maintains, he is to some extent getting away with murder with the people whom he enjoys. In other words, he does not deserve them. They are better than he is. They have more capacity for what is going on than he has. There is a feeling of relative emptiness of value in the interpersonal field where the jealousy occurs; and it is that, combined with the coalescence of love objects, or objects of intimacy, that gives rise to the poignant emotion of jealousy. The movement of the two love objects, as I will call them, immediately awakens and brings clearly to awareness a thought process something like the following: "They can really love each other, whereas I have not really been up to that standard." All sorts of rationalizations or referential processes occur here, sometimes more or less schizophrenic in nature; and, in fact, jealousy and definite paranoid developments may frequently be singularly closely related.

Thus looking at jealousy from our tripartite viewpoint, we find the self-system so organized that, regardless of skill in meeting risks in interpersonal relations, there is a fatal defect of security in regard to the most important of all securities—namely, there is a feeling that one is not up to the level of the people in whom one is interested. At this point, you see, we move out of the exclusively sexual field into any of the fields of interpersonal needs. The person concerned feels actually inferior in some significant respect to the people with whom he has various types of cooperation or collaboration in the pursuit of satisfactions.

At the same time, there is a barrier to the development of interpersonal relations to the point of what I would call love, in which the satisfaction of the partner is at least as significant as one's own satisfaction. Therefore the jealous person, however he may value the partner, does not honor the partner as much as himself; so he can attempt to minimize his insecurity by means of additional personal entanglements with the sometimes fairly explicit idea, "Well, if this person finds out about me, I'll not be utterly without harbor—there'll be the other one." And by this very device for bolstering up his security, he opens himself to the very grave disturbance of jealousy if some of these personal entanglements tangle with each other.

The state of the personality in this situation can be of several orders of complexity. Among these is the type of barrier toward sexual intimacy with members of the other sex which gives rise to the picture of homosexual interests after the preadolescent period. Since we are the sort of people we are, and particularly since the emancipation of women has proceeded at a rather staggering pace in the comparatively recent past of the American development, it is probable that a great many people do reach chronological adulthood and set up homes without having achieved freedom for integrating love with a member of the opposite sex. A person who does not achieve this maturity is not able to achieve a relationship with another person which even approximates my definition of love; and to that extent, given the other things I have mentioned, there is every reason why jealousy should appear, under suitable circumstances, and wreak havoc upon the person who suffers it and sometimes upon all concerned.

But it is by no means exclusively in situations where there is a barrier toward full heterosexual adjustment that jealousy appears. Merely because of the difficulty of achieving heterosexual intimacy, particularly in our superficial type of living, jealousy in that connection is much the most apt to be noticed; but that is just the most frequent, rather than the exclusive, picture of jealousy.

One finds in the jealous person, as I have already suggested, none too adequate satisfaction of needs, and therefore one finds a certain amount of tension and a certain amount of use of some of the processes that I have already spoken of— sublimations, substitutions, dissociations, and so on. The gravity, you might say, of these difficult dynamisms or of the problems that they are dealing with determines the manifestations of a difficult life in the shape of uncertain sleep, sleep disturbed by terror dreams, and so on. But that part of the picture has, in a great many ways, nothing to do with the actual *incident* of jealousy. In other words, jealousy is an acute, dramatic thing, quite as acute and dramatic as the onset of schizophrenia.

In fact, symbolic operations in sleep which look like the very essence of jealousy are not necessarily attended by jealousy, but instead may be frank schizophrenic phenomena. Let us consider a man who has had, shall we say, a rather comfortable relationship with his wife, although he is probably rather self-centered and devoid of ability for real intimacy in his marriage. This man has been under increasing pressure in various ways so that he is becoming increasingly disturbed. One night he has a dream in which his wife is eloping with a colleague of his, and this dream ushers in a schizophrenic episode. Now his wife and the colleague have never been more than casual friends, and the man has no feelings of jealousy. Thus even symbolic operations in sleep which look like the very essence of jealousy are not necessarily attended by jealousy or by anything that we ordinarily connect with jealousy, such as paranoid developments, but may instead be frank schizophrenic phenomena.

I have been using this discussion of envy and jealousy as a springboard for the discussion of paranoid projection and certain of its relatives. The person who has recourse to the envy mechanism almost has to produce derogatory rationalizations about the people he envies; these rationalizations are rather necessary for the simple reason that this is an interpersonal process, and he is often in the presence of another person when he shows envy. Thus the rationalization appears, "Other people wouldn't have the things they do if things were fair"—which is the rudiment of the paranoid attitude. To the extent that this sort of thing is utilized, it precludes the development of insight; the person never gets any better, and, in fact, the thing tends to become a vicious circle which gets worse.

Jealousy acts as a precipitating factor, as one might call it, in both schizophrenic illnesses and the paranoid state. That is, it is an experience which in a number of cases progresses directly into frank schizophrenic phenomena; and it is very frequently the situation in which frankly paranoid falsifications of reality occur.

The Paranoid Dynamism

THE PARANOID dynamism is rooted in (1) an awareness of inferiority of some kind, which then necessitates (2) a transfer of blame onto others. But before I discuss these two processes, I want to make it clear that these alone constitute merely a paranoid slant on life; for a full-blown paranoid state, something else is necessary—the misinterpretation of events to constitute an explanation, usually rather transcendental in nature, of what is troublesome.

The awareness of inferiority means that one is unable to keep out of consciousness the formulation of some chronic feeling of the worst sort of insecurity, and this means that one suffers anxiety and perhaps even something worse, if jealousy is really worse than anxiety. The fear that others can disrespect a person because of something he shows means that he is always insecure in his contact with other people; and this insecurity arises, not from mysterious and somewhat disguised sources, as a great deal of our anxiety does, but from something which he knows he cannot fix. Now that represents an almost fatal deficiency of the self-system, since the self is unable to disguise or exclude a definite formulation that reads, "I am inferior. Therefore people will dislike me and I cannot be secure with them."

As might be expected, such a failure of the self-system to perform its essential functions calls out increasing effort, just as unresolved needs for satisfaction call out processes in sleep. And the efforts that are effective follow the precise pattern of the self-operations that we use in making very careful, consensually valid statements which will communicate just what we mean. That is, it is by means of refined cognitive operations that the self-system develops the group of processes that make up the paranoid dynamism; and like the sudden inspiration all of us have had as to just how to say a thing, so the paranoid dynamism, when it is finally invented, comes with all the trappings of a great insight and illumination. In many cases, as you know, the person will report, "And then I saw it all!" He shows that this was terribly important; this was a great thing. And the great thing is that finally a happy hypothesis has been received into awareness: It is not that *I* have something wrong with me, but that *he* does something to me. One is the victim, not of one's own defects, but of a devilish environment. One is not to blame; the environment is to blame. Thus we can say that the essence of the paranoid dynamism is the transference of blame.

The way by which a person can make this sad transition from unhappy sanity to the relatively more comfortable psychosis of the paranoid state is not very recondite. The self is built out of entities from the culture. It is in its very essence a working system of adjustments, compromises, and what not, that were arrived at in the days before we could work out a rigorously rational way of life. The evaluations which establish our security or insecurity have come to us very early in life by empathically experienced significant people. We cannot reach back to that time, to the origins of our security and insecurity and say, "I would be perfectly happy and entirely content if it were not for the significant people in my infancy and their evil effect on me."

But we can reach back into late childhood when, certainly, significant people blamed us at times, taking out on us their disgruntlement with their own carelessness, their own mis-

carriages, their lack of judgment, and one thing and another.
They were unfair to us; and in case we were secure enough
with them to attack their unfairness, they compounded the
felony by defending themselves, by claiming that they were
fair, and so on. While this made it a double offense, it also
gave us reassurance, for we then knew that they were very
inferior people; a person who cannot admit a fault is obviously
not as secure as he seems. Thus everyone has experienced in
the self—immediately accessible to awareness at any time—
something like this: "I wouldn't have this horrible feeling of
discomfort with others if *they* weren't there, and if I hadn't
been educated the way I've been educated by other people."
And under certain circumstances, one can think the following, which was true at times in earlier years: "And I wouldn't
have this sense of discomfort if other people didn't treat me
unfairly."

But this operation of blaming others for our feeling of discomfort is not bomb-proof; that is, it can fail when we attempt
to validate it consensually, because it includes things we do
not understand. In other words, the real causes for our discomfort—the roots of the self, the origins of the anxiety
process—date back to late infancy and early childhood and to
the empathic linkage with the significant people in those early
years, before we could possibly discriminate who was to
blame for how bad we felt. Therefore this mere intellectual,
cognitive transference of blame, by which we say, "It is not
I who am unworthy but these people who make me unworthy,"
is unstable. It can be held as a religion, and you will actually
find people who most religiously miss no opportunity to work
out a faith based on how wretchedly people treat them and
how false a light is shed on their most benevolent actions by
nasty people who misinterpret them. But while you might
describe this as quite a paranoid slant on life, it is far from a
paranoid state. This is demonstrated by the fact that if a
psychiatrist, for example, sits down with the person concerned

and really discusses an instance in which other people have apparently been misinterpreting and so on, and demonstrates that they have actually been extremely patient with the person for a good many years, this can be very awkward for the person. In other words, while this person has transferred blame for an inferiority, an inadequacy, or a defect which is poignantly undesirable, he has not achieved that feeling of power and certainty which we are likely to get when we are absolutely sure that we have the right answer, according to the present state of knowledge. The person who has only transferred blame is always at the mercy of someone who is not taken in and who starts an inquiry. He is in the same position that all of us find ourselves in at times when we discover in the moment of saying something that it is not so, or at least that we cannot prove it, which is quite an insecure situation to be in.

The Misinterpretation of Events

So the paranoid dynamism, to become full-blown, must achieve another thing: In addition to transferring blame to the evil people among whom he lives—who make him feel so uncomfortable, so inferior—the paranoid person invents a specific, rather transcendental (in the sense of thoroughly psychotic) explanation of why these people do this. It is not merely that unhappy fate has put him to live among disagreeable people, for the obvious question then would be, "Why don't you move?" Instead, there is a conspiracy, which may be a most exquisitely built-up plot, substantiated by an amount of introspective falsification that would produce stunning mystery stories and permit him to live in the lap of luxury on royalties for the rest of his life. A highly systematized paranoid state may appear under the guise of litigious paranoia, revolving around the business of courts; or, in the person who is simply shot through with insecurities in dealing with people, it may be a nightmare of practically transcendental persecution. In such cases the paranoid dynamism works because a substitute activity has finally been found that is a completely adequate occupation for the self. And that substitute activity is, in rough outline, the scrutinizing of every event that impinges on one and gains one's attention, to see how it is part of this plot to injure one, or, using the generic term, to make one feel insecure or anxious.

This, like the other substitutive activities that we have discussed, can be studied from the standpoint of what is in the self, what is elsewhere, and what is shown in the sleeping life. We find that, from the standpoint of the self, any circumstance which might be expected to provoke insecurity calls for redoubled paranoid activity. And, of course, the paranoid activity is anything but an open-faced statement that "I feel more insecure; therefore, it becomes more necessary for me to see how you have persecuted me." Instead, anything that increases or threatens to increase insecurity calls out more vigorous operation of the paranoid dynamism of misinterpreting events to show that one is all the more unutterably correct in the paranoid formula, "I'm a very important person against whom certain more or less devilish people are engaged in a destructive plot."

The type of self-operation also varies under the pressure of the circumstances provoking insecurity in this general way: the greater the insecurity, the more risk there is of schizophrenic processes appearing. Under pressure of certain types of approach, even a person in the very highly reasonable paranoid state—for example, the litigious paranoiac—may express some pretty far-fetched, practically dreamlike elements in the process of fitting events into the paranoid system. Correspondingly, in the much more common type of paranoid person—the paranoid schizophrenic—the greater the pressure, the more incomprehensibly schizophrenic will be the content that comes forth. That is both an interesting and a fairly obvious aspect of the process, since cognitive operations, which

are such an important part of the consensual validation process
—and this, in turn, is such an important part of communication—were invented and developed and are chiefly utilized for
the maintenance of security. As soon as these cognitive
processes begin to increase insecurity—which is the situation
before the paranoid system appears—they clearly are disas-
trously the wrong tool, and so the level of the mental process
sinks. It always sinks when the available tools ordinarily accessible to consciousness prove entirely inadequate, and so
more primitive types of process are used.

Certain Misconceptions about Paranoia and Homosexuality

So far, most of what I have said about paranoia has to do
with the self. I have to approach the rest of the personality
and sleep somewhat circuitously, and begin by tracing the
developmental origins of the ubiquitous and harassing insecurity that drives one into using the paranoid dynamism. For
if I immediately discuss the simple and most obvious manifestation of this insecurity—the barriers to sexual behavior in the
paranoid person—it may contribute to the possibility of your
maintaining what I believe to be an erroneous connection.
Because the paranoid processes that we encounter in our
patients are to so high a degree the results of incomplete development of personality in the preadolescent and adolescent
phases, this factor can be used to give credence to theoretical
formulations on homosexuality which I believe are misleading.
And misleading formulations are dangerous from the standpoint of therapeutic efforts based on them.

Where, in the developmental eras of personality, can one
find a source of anxiety sufficiently devastating to result in the
paranoid dynamism? If an infant has anything like an adequate
amount of encephalic tissue, he acquires the human characteristics that are usually acquired in infancy. The only people
who fail gravely in acquiring these 'fundamental' conformities

to social life are idiots. Thus we do not expect that any eternally recurrent attack on our security, such as prevails in the paranoid dynamism, has its beginnings in infancy.[1] In early childhood, the final refinements of control of the sphincters are completed, along with the acquisition of language habits. Although control of the bladder sphincter is sometimes rather at the mercy of serious interpersonal problems for years after the end of early childhood, still there are few grown people who are, for personality reasons, so incontinent that they smell of urine in public. That is ordinarily a sign of very serious deterioration, possibly a schizophrenic state. And we do not expect insecurities about language to be a sufficient cause for the recurrent intense anxiety in contact with others which calls out so grave a thing as the paranoid dynamism. In fact, one can use inadequate performances in this field, such as stuttering, to pinion the environment, to hold other people down and obstruct their movements, and so on. In the juvenile era, one again does not anticipate such recurrent causes for insecurity with others that any such massive violation of cognitive operations as the paranoid dynamism will happen. The algolagnic people, for instance, can make virtues out of juvenile inadequacies. They go about reeking statements of their incompetence; they cannot do anything particularly well; isn't it too bad, and don't you sort of pity them, and won't you give them a helping hand? Other relatively juvenile people who are slightly more secure are tickled to death to have somebody that they can be superior to, and that is a fine working arrangement in life. Thus in the juvenile era, there is nothing that would call out this terrifying hash of life that the paranoid state is.

When we move into the preadolescent era, however, we see paranoid developments. Occasionally we see a bitterly para-

[1] *Editors' note:* Sullivan agrees with Margaret A. Ribble that such extreme anxiety in infancy would produce apathy and eventually death. So it is that an infant experiencing such anxiety would not survive to adulthood. [See *The Interpersonal Theory of Psychiatry;* pp. 60–61.]

noid preadolescent, and when we look into that we begin to get a clue to the particular type of handicap that makes recourse to this dynamism necessary. I might mention here the only paranoid preadolescent that I have worked with at all intensively. This boy had had an appalling life. We sometimes talk about the profound discouragement in the pursuit of affection that culminates in schizophrenic break, and this boy's life could almost be read off from that theory. He had had someone, very early in life, who treated him like a human being—it was some distant fragment of the family who was compelled to live in this unhappy home for awhile, but finally escaped, despite her pity for this boy. Everything else that happened to him was as unfriendly and frustrating and savagely cruel as one might expect. He was a holy terror in school, until preadolescence; and then he discovered that all the available kids that he had any tendency to feel friendly toward had been so impressed with his problem character—with his lack of humanity, you might say—that they fought shy of him. He tried by serious application and much disciplinary planning to convince them that he was human, but he was unsuccessful. In this particular preadolescent society, the chumships were already pretty well structured. And so, since he had so far been exceedingly unpleasant to go to school with, it took more than his changing for a week or two to interest any of the other kids in his possibilities as a chum for one of them or as one of the gang. There was nobody in the school society sick enough to take to him naturally. And lo, he came out with a fine paranoid system. He would, for example, detail to unsuspecting kids a story of how he was really quite an important person who had been stolen from a hospital for reasons of blackmail by the person who now claimed to be his mother. And he had quite an elaborate amount of alleged data to demonstrate the truth of his story. For example, he knew that his alleged family had been blackmailing ever since he first began to notice things, because they lived better than any obvious source of income would justify.

In spite of myself, whenever I try to illustrate the beginnings of the paranoid dynamism, I have to get into the stuff that I think is rather misleading. It would be very easy, you see, to say that this boy bogged down when he thought of moving toward women because of his intense hatred of his mother, who had been extremely thwarting and cruel to him, and that therefore the real reason why he was paranoid was a homosexual conflict. But in my simple-minded world, it is a little bit difficult to talk about homosexual conflict where there is no homosexual attachment. What he had was an inescapable barrier to intimacy with man, woman, or beast—as a matter of fact, he had no pets; part of the thwarting business was that the mother would not put up with his having any animals in the house. This boy had lived as best he could as an extremely difficult juvenile, hated and feared by teachers and schoolmates and quite a gifted thorn in the home situation. Then he matured to the point of requiring intimacy with a fellow human being, and made fairly impressive efforts to get it; we can picture him as driven by the need for intimacy —just as lust will drive one when sufficiently unsatisfied— to look at practically everyone he came in contact with who was anywhere near his age as a potential friend, intimate, or chum. But he always was forced to conclude from their avoidance of him, "They would have no use for me." That is an inclusion within awareness of a recurrent statement, "I am too inferior to get what I must have." But this awareness of inferiority is so intolerable that finally he reaches the solution of making the others to blame; and the necessary support for that is the secret, the explanation of why he is so persecuted.

As I have said, this preadolescent was the youngest paranoid I have ever encountered. Very hateful juveniles may look somewhat paranoid, if you do not pay much attention to them; but the dynamism actually never appears before the preadolescent stage of personality development. It sometimes appears in early adolescence, and very commonly occurs in the mid-adolescent stage of personality development. Psychiatric statistics may seem to indicate that the numerically great majority of paranoid cases appear later; paranoid states are much more common around the ages of 25, 26 and 27 than around the ages of 16, 17, and 18. So you may think that what I say about its frequent appearance in mid-adolescence is not very plausible. But in that case, you are guilty of recklessly fixing the stages of personality development according to chronologic age, which I have tried to preach against—and I have said that each subsequent stage is harder to nail down as to its chronologic limits. Mid-adolescence, according to my definition, extends up to the patterning of genital behavior. And when we actually study any paranoid who is moderately accessible, or on whom we can get highly relevant historic data, we discover no reason to suppose that he had progressed through a patterning of sexual behavior before the appearance of the paranoid state. Quite the contrary; we find that he was defeated in establishing workable sexual habits. And this final defeat was the situation in which the paranoid development appeared.

Sometimes we find that these people have had a pretty satisfactory preadolescent experience in the sense that, although they were warped, still they moved some way toward securing human intimacy. In case they were badly warped, that experience of intimacy may have been possible to them because there were other quite badly warped fellows with whom they could establish a relationship which, although somewhat inadequate, was still much better than nothing. Or they may have had a good deal of the benefits of an intimate relationship with an older person who did not really pay much attention to what was going on. In case they were not very badly warped, they may have been fortunate enough to be quite close to a person for a time. But then they bumped into the business of comporting themselves like other young men, which too often in this culture means abandoning real happiness in favor of heterosexual prestige. When it came to the business of moving out to comfortably successful relations of an intimate nature with women, the barrier—which can be called anything from fear of women to utter respect for women—was completely effective. How completely effective it can be is nicely illustrated by the fact that the heterosexual experience of a remarkably large number of people who have schizophrenic or paranoid development consists of having sought out and purchased the use of prostitutes. Sometimes the experience is really a subtly psychotherapeutic thing because the very crudeness and complexity of their approach rouses some sympathy in the prostitute, who has had her own troubles with the heterosexual adjustment; and so these women sometimes find an opportunity to be helpful, and do some fair psychotherapy. But very few prostitutes have saved people foredoomed for paranoid-schizophrenic development, for these people can go to a prostitute only because the fact of her being a prostitute removes her from the fully human class. And, of course, when a creature who is not fully human begins to nurse and mother you, you become more or less a feral child, like Romulus being looked after by a wolf. There is no basis for prestige here; this does not lift you to the realm in which you wish to circulate. So, where the prostitute, from empathy and a similar path of misery, does incline to warm one of these poor unhappy creatures with kind consideration and so on, he practically has to leave; he cannot stand it. Some of the patients I have seen cannot approach a white prostitute because it is too hard to make her infrahuman; so they cross the line into some other race, where it is easier to feel that the partner is infrahuman. Some of them who do not have even that possibility open to them try some of the dumb beasts; but that is rather unsuccessful because of certain anatomical handicaps and because of the lecherous limitations of the dumb beasts, so that they are not at all amused by anything of this kind at the wrong time and are rather wildly, rampantly engaged in it at the right time, which scarcely fits with the experience that an unhappy adolescent is seeking.

The adolescent also encounters cultural attitudes which are derogatory toward the very things that he is doing; for example, he encounters the curse upon bestiality, which is specifically prohibited and condemned in the Bible. It gets to be that every time he sees anyone of the other sex, he rattles off this derogatory business to himself, and thinks, "That woman would have nothing to do with a person like me." And since he has recently come from the preadolescent era, when his prestige in the eyes of his own sex was what was important and gratifying, it is easy to spread this feeling that "No woman would put up with me" into a valuation which he assumes intelligent men would hold of him. This idea that "Men know that women would not put up with me, that I'm no good with women" is then likely to be followed by, "They think I'm a fairy—that I'm sexually interested in them." And by that time, since he is convinced that any woman has a derogatory estimation of him and that men now have either a realization of his shameless inferiority with women or actually regard him as inferior as a man, his consciousness in human contacts has taken on this attribute of including an intolerable awareness of defect, and the schizophrenic or the paranoid development, or, which is generally the case, the schizophrenic episode followed by paranoid development takes place.

Now this wretched business of homosexual interest has gotten itself used as a complete explanation of the paranoid process. I deplore that very deeply. It is unendingly difficult to discuss paranoid states without seeming to justify the notion of some people that homosexuality is the fundamental problem —that the paranoid business was substituted to avoid it. But if you have followed me carefully, you will see that a great deal of this is quite as adequately explained if you look to nothing but intimacy—that is, closeness, or, you might say, open-faced relationships with anybody. Because that theory is more general, less specific, less elaborated, it is the better theory until you can prove the contrary.

The exceptions, which I think are not very striking, occur only in the realm of the paranoid attitudes rather than the paranoid states—that is, the exceptions occur among people who are suspicious, who are pretty certain to find that they are being treated unfairly, and who in general have a distinctly paranoid attitude toward a great many of their human contacts. Quite a number of them are unhappy homosexuals —that is, they have continued a homosexual type of discharge of lust without being able to adjust their values so that it is satisfactory. Some, although by no means all of that group, establish son-mother relationships with an occasional woman who is sexually inhibited. This particular unhappy type of homosexual is extraordinarily attractive to several sorts of women who are practically inhibited as to the possibility of heterosexual satisfaction. But the maternal satisfactions are not taboo for the woman, and they have been sadly few for the man; and therefore there is a possible field of intimacy, which, however, is not really intimate because it is nowhere near equal. The man is in a more childish relationship than he should be, and the woman in a more maternal relationship than she should be; so there is an element of the fantastic in the thing that keeps it at a safe distance. Sometimes—often under pressure from a third person—an attempt is made in one of these situations to consummate a sexual relationship; the least disastrous outcome is that the relationship is quite promptly destroyed. In these situations, it might seem that the need for intimacy was not an adequate explanation for the paranoid development. But if you look closely at any one of those things—and they really are too painfully prevalent among the professional contacts—you will discover that there are no paranoid feelings toward the woman who is bound to a rather fantastic mother role; in other words, where there is even this heavily garbled intimacy, there is no paranoid feeling. It is the need for intimacy, coupled with the conviction, the inescapable awareness, of a fatal incapacity for that intimacy, that calls out this desolating paranoid dynamism, if I am at all correct.

The Rest [Remainder] of the Personality, and Sleep

I now want to discuss more specifically the rest of the personality and sleep in the paranoid state. We have said that the paranoid substitution of a system of persecution—along with an explanatory theory of some kind or other about why one is important enough to be the recipient of so much unfavorable attention—is a measure of a fatal defect in the organization of the self. Assuming this to mean, as we always can, that, as this person came to be, he could not maintain a feeling of self-esteem in connection with significant other people, what then does this imply as to the necessary state of the rest of his personality? I think that it is not merely exercising logic for me to say that there must be serious deficits in the satisfactions which require the cooperation of others. And, as we have said in dealing with all the other dynamisms, if that is the case, then there must be an extraordinary effort to use symbolic tools during sleep to diminish the tensions of these unsatisfied needs for satisfaction which would otherwise unhorse the self.

Thus we anticipate that before the appearance of the paranoid development, the sleep function will be rather badly disturbed, and there will also be waking evidences of a good deal of dissatisfaction, tenseness, and perhaps drive which does not seem to get itself applied any too well. We discover that somehow or other the person sets out for something but does not pursue it; it gets complicated by his diminished self-esteem in feeling that he could not get it from the particular other person concerned. For example, let us say that a heterosexual situation starts out showing many traits that are identifiable as an attempt on the part of the man to effect a sexual relationship with the woman. But the situation moves rather unpleasantly into a twilight zone where the drive toward sexual gratification is no longer so clearly the purpose of the thing; and out of this uncertain twilight it becomes a matter of his quarreling with the woman as to whether women are really any particular good or whether they are entitled to take themselves as seriously as they do about sexual choice, and so on. Looked at in retrospect, such a situation is hard to interpret. We do not know whether the man was looking for a fight or for sexual intercourse; he apparently set out for the latter and wound up having the former. Thus such a person is pretty tense in his interpersonal relationships because as soon as he starts doing the right thing with the other person, this failure of the self-function to maintain security and self-esteem appears, accompanied by all the necessarily somewhat frustrating efforts to remedy that situation. And gradually these completely garble or actually put out of the picture the positive, constructive integrating tendency that the person originally manifested. In consequence, the unsatisfied person has all sorts of dream processes and one thing and another, remembered or otherwise; and then comes the paranoid development.

One of the most significant observations I can make about the sleep of the person in the paranoid state is that, while it can be very seriously disturbed, it is by no means as bad as it was before the paranoid state put in its appearance. The patient's report may indicate that his sleep is just as badly disturbed as it ever was, but if one observes him, noting such objective clues to sleep as the lines in the face, one will find that his sleep is distinctly better. But every now and then it is definitely interrupted by dramatic dream experiences which are more or less consonant with the general persecutory beliefs. In other words, the psychotic content appears as dream processes; but since those dream processes are of a piece with the waking psychotic processes, they are identified as actually real and valid. They are not different from the waking experiences; so they are just as real and valid in the life of the patient as many another of the exquisitely complicated misinterpretations that make up his orientation in reality.

The improvement in the sleep function that comes with the paranoid development tells us a good deal. Among other things, it tells us something more of the peculiar dynamism of hate. It represents the working out of a thing which, viewed diagrammatically, is a sublimation; but it is not a sublimation in the real meaning of the term. In sublimation, the person combines an impulse which is unwelcome to the self with the pursuit of some socially worthy goal, and thereby obtains partial satisfaction. In the paranoid development, the person desires to integrate a particular type of satisfactory situation with another person; however, because this situation has always made him intolerably insecure as to the other person's esteem for him, the only way he can obtain any peace for these desires is by combining them with the pursuit of security by the hostile, derogatory method.

This pseudosublimation, which is the solution of many of the impulses that were previously frustrated, gives partial satisfaction by dint of the following sort of process—and here, of course, I am assuming that I have the prescience of God, which enables me to follow a paranoid's mental processes: Originally the paranoid thought, "I want to be close to this person for a feeling of warmth which I need because I'm lonely; but if I move toward him, he will regard me as inferior and unworthy and will deny me this warmth because he won't warm so inferior a person." This is the original pattern, which now by a slight shift of locus of the needs becomes: "That person wants me to want to be warmed by him so that he can injure me by refusing. He is a hateful enemy." But, strangely enough, a remarkable amount of time is spent in all but closeness to this person, sometimes in actual physical closeness to him, and sometimes the warmth is sought in a rather subtle way, so that it may be given. The awareness of the paranoid person, however, is that of hateful derogation of himself by the person who is giving the warmth.

Thus the paranoid person obtains partial satisfactions of integrating tendencies by way of making the attitude of the other person hateful, by projecting a hateful motivational system into the picture. This, of course, is the opposite of social acceptance, although a dangerous analogy might be drawn between the paranoid dynamism and the sublimatory reformulations of life-goals to obtain social acceptance in that both are the same kind of complication in terms of the social order. In other words, paranoids are persecuted by everybody from whom they want warmth, and therefore the particular person who happens to be involved in the paranoid situation at the moment is only a representative of society, which is very easy to generalize. This is not a true sublimation, but there is a dangerous analogy in the sense that both involve the standards of the group. In the paranoid situation, these standards are inverted into wholly unfriendly, unconstructive things. In contrast, we ordinarily try to believe that the social order is constructive and benevolent; and even if we do not fully believe that, we are not convinced, as the paranoid is, that the social order is personally hateful and destructive to us.

The paranoid's partial satisfaction of impulses can be fairly high, the only rift in the lute being that, since few other people can stand the kind of punishment that he radiates, there have to be a good many changes of objects of these integrations. No integration lasts terribly long, unless, as sometimes happens, it is with someone whose patterns of distortion have a singularly close relationship to his, and they get into one of these *folie à deux* affairs in which they can be very close, as long as their closeness is out of their awareness, in a frenzy of hating the world which is persecuting them. Under cover of that, they can be moderately comfortable; and I surmise that under those circumstances there is not very much residual problem. That is how little paranoid worlds sometimes develop, I believe.

But for the person who has not been fortunate enough to find a companion in his psychosis, we must notice, just as we did about sublimation, that the satisfaction which he obtains is not complete. And some integrating tendencies are so powerful that anything that could reasonably be called partial satisfaction is not anywhere near enough. Lust can be used as a paradigm here; in this culture it is safe to assume that lust will not be content with obscure operations which do not include recognized discharge of the genital tensions. Thus the eruptions in the sleep of the paranoid—which, as I have said, he takes as perfectly real because they are of a piece with what he has been living in his waking hours—are quite frequently gross sexual assaults, which include discharge of genital tensions, but which fit into the pattern because they are done in a hateful fashion and by enemies, for his detriment. This ingredient of the psychotic experience again is not so strange in this culture, where sex often has obviously unfriendly aspects.

Thus we may expect to find the whole personal organization of the victim of the paranoid substitutive dynamism to be characterized by complex, hateful, partial satisfaction of needs and by the maintenance of a newly high level of security by means of constant preoccupation with the attacks from a hateful environment. That not only works as a substitute operation—keeping awareness free from the truth, you might say—but also has another value, in that while most paranoid people are driven to having pretty psychotic explanatory rationalizations of their importance, still at least to receive unfavorable attention so recurrently from such a vast number of people is to get something. In the prepsychotic life, these people often have been all but perfectly clear on the fact that they always get in the way of achieving what they want.

As I have indicated earlier, I think that the whole business of the homosexual entity as an explanation is always to be looked pretty firmly in the face by psychiatrists who attempt to effect any great improvement in the mental health of the patient. One should determine whether this entity is the organization of a definite integrating tendency that satisfies a need or whether it is a complex mental disorder in which the homosexuality is present because it so perfectly fortifies some abnormal mental process, some dynamism of difficulty. Where a person has felt that life is eminently worth living only in the preadolescent stage, when he did enjoy great intimacy with another person of the same sex, irrespective of whether that great intimacy was what may be described as on the nongenital or the genital level, I am quite willing to deal with that person on the basis that he is engaged in actual direct pursuit of satisfaction from members of his own sex, or in homosexuality, as it may easily be called. But where such experience is missing from a person's life, then I think one is doing a great violence to the therapeutic principle to accept the notion that that person has anything like a simple drive to secure genital satisfaction by any type of behavior with a member of the same sex. To work on this assumption, and to attempt to deal with such a patient's 'homosexuality,' is to my way of thinking one of the most vicious miscarriages of therapeutic situations. It takes out of the culture a group of terms which, in referring to behavior, carry all the culture's evaluations of that behavior. You see, if the patient has not found great warmth and satisfaction in intimacy with a member of his own sex, but later on is told by a psychiatrist that such intimacy is what he is after—or has, by his own paranoid processes, come to feel that that is what he is after, and the psychiatrist agrees with him—then he and the psychiatrist are talking about something that is, in its ultimate essence, merely a revolting difference between him and good people. That is all. It has no meaning in terms of something that he has experienced, that he has undergone, and that therefore is a part of him. But it does have meaning as a particular type of horribly derogatory formulation. Thus, to attack a paranoid state, for example, on the basis of an attempt to understand the patient's homosexuality is an atrocious miscarriage of the therapeutic process. This is a very nifty way to make it beyond the most remote perchance that any intimacy can be established with that patient. The psychiatrist's approach means: "Abandon all hope of a feeling of personal security, and then we might be able to do something." But the developmental processes which we all have to undergo make it simply inconceivable that there is any such thing as abandoning all hope of personal security. So, of course, what the psychiatrist does is to provide the patient with a new paranoid world, in which the psychiatrist is unconsciously taking a very important part. And since he is much more patiently engaged in hateful activity than anybody the patient has previously found, the patient may attempt homicide on the psychiatrist some day. But other than that I can think of no very spectacular result except the passing of time.

So it is quite important indeed to discriminate between, first, the isophilic phase of personality development and the satisfactions that can be acquired then, and, second, the innumerable unhappy caricatures of living to which the term homosexuality is sometimes applied. The people who have gotten well into the preadolescent phase of personality development before possibilities of further growth failed, and who come to us with their life problems formulated in terms of homosexual concepts, are still somewhat near reality. But people who have not gotten as far as the preadolescent phase of personality development, and who come to us with their problems formulated in terms of homosexuality, are showing a very much more complex distortion of interpersonal relations and offer a much more treacherous basis for therapeutic relationships because they are that much less mature. Thus this discrimination has prognostic significance. It is a discrimination between what is a sort of frantic exploration on the basis of merely verbal prescriptions, as compared with regressive retreats from hopelessly difficult situations to a time in the past that was actually satisfactory, with new collisions perhaps with the culture in the process. Naturally the latter is much the simpler to attack, and the prognosis—the outcome—is much more apt to be favorable. But if, on the other hand, you combine these two into some doctrine of homosexuality as applied to factors in schizophrenia, paranoid states, or what have you, then you have missed the whole point of interpersonal psychiatry, and your results will be sufficiently mongrel so that you will never be able to feel very secure about what is what. But, on the other hand, you will never have any convincing demonstration of being completely wrong.

CHAPTER
8

Dissociative Processes [1]

I NOW WANT to take up the massive dissociative processes in personality which I have so far discussed only in part. I think I have made clear why schizophrenic thought processes are so odd, so insane, if you please, by referring to the very early stages that they represent. I have also indicated my belief that we actually do have to seize upon a conception as intrinsically repellent, perhaps, to the intellect as the concept of regression, by which recent experience becomes as if it had not occurred. I have also discussed the fact that large elements of the bodily activity system can be cut off, as it were, from clear relationship to consciousness and be given impulses which lead to activity as if of that of a subordinate or secondary personality. Along with such very massive dissociated things as automatic writing, I mentioned the horribly overcondensed and nearly purely symbolic movements which occur as tics.

[1] *Editors' note:* Sullivan later became dissatisfied with his own explanation of dissociation and posited the *not-me* as a conceptual tool for the examination of dissociative processes. In a notebook written some time after this lecture was given, he says, "To account for the phenomena of dissociation, it was necessary to add to our conceptions *that which is related to the personified self in the sense of its contradictory,* the not-me, a phase of the organization of experience personal acquaintance with which must be at best (1) marginal, unelaborated observations of particular other people—real or more or less mythological—which show this personal reference by attendant experience of awe, dread, loathing, horror (with arrest of referential process within awareness), or (2) starkly terrifying events in the deeper levels of sleep."

But what I have not done—and in fact we had to go a long way before it could be expressed very clearly—is to consider dissociation from my tripartite standpoint—namely, the self-system; the personality as a whole, with a special emphasis on that which is not accessible to awareness; and the special signs and symptoms that appear in the phase of life called sleep. In other words, I am now concerned with the actual dynamic situation, if you please, by which an important system of the personality is effectively barred from any disturbing influence on personal awareness for a period of years and perhaps for a lifetime. There is a good deal of need for clarity about this. One of the reasons why we have run into considerable risk in the development of dynamic psychiatric theory is that the frame of reference which would tell the whole story is not found; and therefore a good deal of stuff which, when it is bandied about, becomes sheer nonsense, has to be excogitated to prevent the feeling of incompleteness of theory. I think the original conception of the censor and the subsequent formulations which replaced it are pretty much that sort of thing. It is because the phenomena that we encounter are not adequately subsumed by any of these more or less allegorical formulations that I want to present something different. What I offer you is not going to be so charmingly simple as the theories I have mentioned, but the complexity does not come simply because I like complex theory.

Thus far, until we came to dissociation, the reason why many things which one would expect to be within a person's awareness are not there is that when anything might provoke their appearance, the person feels anxious; and anxiety always has an extraordinarily arresting effect on whatever was about to happen. Anxiety is more important, in a way, than the thing that called it out, and its importance, of course, is from the standpoint of personal awareness. The appearance of frank anxiety preoccupies attention. The faint beginnings of full-blown anxiety is in many people entirely sufficient cause for doing something pretty complicated, something which is certainly not the simple awareness which the particular stream of events might otherwise have resulted in.

The business of being thrust down a particular path in life by anxiety, with or without its feeble disguise of anger, generally leads to an appallingly uncomfortable life. Take, for example, a person to whom any sexual impulse, any movement of lust, is an intolerable ingredient of awareness. Presumably the only discharge of impulses which concerned lust would occur in sleep or in some other very extraordinary situation. One would expect long stretches of waking life to remain in which the person was in the throes of lust. That would mean, from our standpoint, that he was anxious, and was therefore practically incapable of that application to reality that is necessary in order to carry out complex performances, to realize goals that take more than momentary action.

It is because of the utter impracticability of life under those circumstances that I assume that this dynamism which I call dissociation is part of the equipment of the surviving human animal. It is, in contradistinction to everything else we have dealt with here, a dynamism which does not require disturbance of the contents of consciousness and which does not act as an impediment to the conduct of life in the areas where there is not dissociation. Now it is not quite as magical as that statement sounds. In other words, one is more efficient and much nearer happiness, contentment, and all those things which we allege to be the positive returns in life, abstractly considered, if one does not have any important system of personality in dissociation. The way in which a person suffers from dissociation is best discovered from a patient who is recovering from a chronic dissociated state—who has retrieved and successfully reintegrated a dissociated system of personality. When such patients have really been communicative with me, and when the relationship has been such that I could without risk ask them how things were before and after, they have told me that they could now take things easier. Life was less exhausting; it was not so intense; it did not tire them so rapidly per hour, one might say. That is the first hint we get as to how this incredibly suave process of dissociation works. It is not perfect, it is not the solution of anything. But it is a dynamism which is useful where none of the other dynamisms can be utilized, either because they fail utterly, and one is worse off than if one had not used them, or else because they require practically the abandonment of fully human living, as in the case of the paranoid dynamism, where it becomes impossible to look forward to any simple, direct satisfactions which are fully human in the sense of one's equal status, one's relationships with others, and so on.

As a preliminary to developing a tripartite approach to dissociation, I shall try to describe how a person acts who has an important system in dissociation, using an illustration which concerns lust and the traditionally important 'partial impulse.' Let us assume that a man, Mr. A, is married and leads a relatively restrained sexual life. Sex doesn't seem to have a very large place in his life. He has only occasional sexual relations with his wife and seems to get on very nicely that way, somewhat to her chagrin. He is quite capable of giving her satisfaction in a particular act, but he does not have much sexual appetite. And we will assume that he has, in dissociation, the experience of happiness which he had in definite homosexual operations when he was in the preadolescent phase; and that therefore he has what is really a definite drive toward homosexual types of integration.

Now we will suppose that the wife taxes him with his lack of interest in sexual relations with her. With no loss of security—in other words, with nothing remotely like anxiety—he says that he often wonders about that, and wonders whether it is awkward for her that he has so little appetite. Since he has thought he might be odd that way, he has actually done a certain amount of inquiry, and he finds that most men who

seem to him perfectly normal do need intercourse more frequently than would ever occur to him. He is different, but
then people do differ notoriously in this field; some of them
have intercourse every night, and some of them once a week,
and he is just a little more different and finds that once a month
does him very nicely. It just seldom occurs to him, and this
is why he is often kindly but vaguely unwilling when he is
prodded toward lustful sports.

Now you may say that the fact that he has made this inquiry
of other men is a manifestation of the homosexual component;
but there you would be wrong. It is a clear manifestation of
the very elaborate character of the dynamism of dissociation.
If circumstances were such that this man could not be perfectly
clear on how few heterosexual relations were enough for him,
then he would be in danger of anxiety; so there is in his self a
necessity to be safe in that area, and he uses the best way on
earth that any of us have for being safe in a situation which
we think may be unusual—he gets the data. He has made a
study, not because he is interested in sexual conversation with
others, but because he senses—as we all do if we are not too
gummed up by education and early experience—that if he is
perfectly clear on a thing, he is not going to be unhorsed by
it—it is part of him. So he documents the fact that lust does not
have the place in his life that it ordinarily has in most people's;
that is one of his peculiarities—nothing to be profoundly
ashamed about, although perhaps hard on his wife. But he is
able to develop certain techniques for filling the gaps that may
be left in her life. He is unusually considerate in some ways,
very thoughtful about bringing home flowers for the dining-
room table, and things like that. He is perfectly able to say,
"Well, I don't think you get everything you want from me,
and it's a pleasure to give you what I can." It is all very nice,
you see. It is quite secure; there is no exposure to risk.

Now let us suppose that by some magic we have him meet
another man, Mr. X, who has many outstanding traits of the

preadolescent partner, so that the resemblance would in any ordinary instance be utterly sufficient to provoke a vivid recall in Mr. A of the early, highly satisfactory experience. Furthermore, from all that we know about ourselves and others, we would assume that if such a person crossed one's path, that person would, if there were no obstacle anywhere in the personality, immediately be invested with emotional expectations, colored by what had been so happy in the past. There was nothing wrong with that experience from one's early life, and so immediately there is likely to be a definite feeling of warmth and liking for this person who recalls it. This, as I say, is what one would expect to happen in more ordinary circumstances which did not concern an important dissociated system.

But in the case of Mr. A—whom we have now presented with a person who is of just the type to activate powerfully an impulse which, if it worked out very simply, would lead to homosexual instances with this person—any number of astonishing things may happen. Because I want you to see what a very remarkable performance dissociation is, I shall make this an extreme instance. Mr. A scarcely notices this person. He autonomically goes through the gestures of being introduced, but treats the man almost as a nonexistent entity. He may act decently, but without taking the trouble to look at the other fellow, and so on and so forth. You see, if he deleted the person entirely, that, of course, would be a relatively psychotic performance and would be profoundly disturbing to friends of his. So, of course, something is done, but it is reduced to the very remnant of Mr. A's ordinary social manner. And for purposes of explanation, again, let us say that this is just as surprising to Mr. A as it is to anyone else. Under those circumstances, from what we know of ourselves and others, Mr. A has a strong necessity to rationalize—to arrive at a plausible explanation. And the simplest of all rationalizations is, "There's something about him that makes me think of precisely the type of person I dislike so strongly that I can barely be polite." He may put a period there, and consider it an adequate explanation. Or he may add, "He reminds me of someone. I can't think who, but I really couldn't bear his attitude."

Now let us say that we are in a position to observe Mr. A with Mr. X. We might find that Mr. A at all sorts of odd moments will be studying the profile, perhaps the whole build, of this man whom he is treating with such extreme casualness, and who, he explains, is such a problem because he is so thoroughly detested. I don't know whether you realize how much we can do with our eyes, without disturbing awareness at all, as I tried to indicate in the story of my father and the wallpaper.[2] This study of Mr. X's profile does not interfere with anything that Mr. A is doing. He is having a very interesting conversation, let us say, on the tidal currents around Dakar, and the times he makes this ritual study are probably when somebody else is making some interesting observation; he immediately comes in, showing that he has followed what was said perfectly. The activity of his eyes is no part of the content of his awareness.

Now let us assume for a moment that this activity on the part of Mr. A had nothing to do with a dissociated impulse —that the circumstances were the more commonplace ones of selective inattention. Let us also assume that I came along

---

[2] *Editors' note:* Sullivan tells the wallpaper story in Lecture 3 of this series, as an illustration of processes of 'normal' awareness: "During my father's period of being a widower, I visited him. On this occasion, we sat and talked in the room which I had always liked best in the house. In the process, I noticed that the old gentleman was getting a bit distracted. In my usual fashion I went over the context of our conversation and found nothing at all offensive to him. And so, in the margin of my mind, I grew more and more puzzled over what was clear to me as some unsatisfactory mental state in my father. Finally he said, "Well, what do you think of the wallpaper?" On hearing this question, I was able vividly to recall that in an hour and a half's conversation, I had studied every damned line at which the wallpaper came together. I had not only observed that it was new wallpaper applied since my last visit, but I had made a minute study for any poor workmanship or regrettable defects in its application. But that had in no sense disturbed my consciousness. It required this intervention by my father to attach any awareness in my mind either of the new wallpaper or of the great care with which I had been studying it."

and said to Mr. A, "Well, what do you think of his mug?" Under those circumstances, Mr. A would sort of snap into it and say, "Why, hell, it's really quite classic, isn't it?" In other words, the data would be there; they had just been utterly inattended to.

But let us now assume that Mr. A does have dissociated homosexual impulses. Then if I say to him, "What do you think of Mr. X's looks?" he takes a very hurried glance at this other man and immediately says something polite. And I can see the wheels turning as he thinks, "Certainly, he must be dumb to ask me this when he knows that I can hardly stand the looks of this man, or his presence, or anything else." In other words, Mr. A has anything but data on what he has been doing. This is the essence of dissociated behavior; it not only does not disturb awareness, but one cannot by any ordinary device discover any sign that it occurred in awareness.

Let us prolong this example and suppose that everybody is going in to dinner and that nobody has taken any trouble to arrange the guests; and lo, we are impressed to discover that Mr. A and Mr. X are seated directly across from each other at the table. If we think back a little while, we remember that Mr. A was delayed by a slipping garter or something or other so that he didn't get into the dining room until Mr. X had gone in, and then he immediately almost rudely got in himself. He didn't seem to be in any hurry to sit down, but as soon as Mr. X had sat down, Mr. A took the chair directly across the table from him. It is just the thing one would do if one wanted to continue looking at a person in order to enjoy his physical presence; yet everything in Mr. A's awareness adds up to the idea that this man makes him feel quite hostile. We may further discover that, when Mr. X talks, Mr. A has remarkable lapses, you might say, of concentration at any complex task that we might put him at; but he will have by any ordinary available method of investigation not the foggiest notion of what Mr. X's voice sounds like; or if he does, it will remind him of the voice of some very unpleasant person whose voice actually has no noticeable resemblance to Mr. X's.

Thus here is an aspect of the self-organization which frequently appears in the dissociation of the major tendencies. That is, a patient with a dissociated impulse will experience special cognitive distortions about anyone whose combination of positive values horribly moves the patient to integrate his dissociated impulse. These positively valued people are then endowed by the patient with the negative of the feelings that would accompany this integration, so that one literally, suavely, and automatically misidentifies the meaning of such a person. In other words, in order that the dissociated tendency shall never disturb awareness, shall not provoke anxiety—because if it did, one would be anxious so much of the time that one could not do things which are necessary to life—the security system has come to include very elaborate pseudo memories, revery processes, and so on, which amount to a wonderfully thorough piece of fantasy that neatly and very adequately excludes any of the ordinary ways by which one would become aware of something. You need not marvel too much that such things can be, because our erroneous explanations of things are of the same type, and you know they run very beautifully unless they happen to break down in a particularly distressful situation.

We will get clear evidence of the magnitude of the self processes concerned in maintaining dissociation only at times when the person is engaged in such a complex task that practically all of his abilities are called upon—when he is under considerable pressure from a task requiring microscopic attention, swift placing of many factors, and so on. If, under those circumstances, he encounters another person who awakens the dissociated tendency or is suitable for integration along the path of the dissociated tendency, and who makes his presence felt to any of the sense organs—by his speech, for instance—then there will be certain evidence of the dissociative processes. This evidence will appear in the fact that the presence of this person will disturb the concentration necessary for the difficult task; but, if the person notices it, it will be immediately rationalized, often by means of a pseudo recollection, which is the easiest thing in this culture that a person can build in himself to resist the capacity of interesting people to disturb awareness. Thus, if Mr. X disturbs my concentration by talking, I can be aware of this disturbance; but I would feel insecure at being disturbed without any idea of what was disturbing me, and so it is this detestable person in my past of whom Mr. X reminds me. I am sure Mr. X is a nice man, and all that, but I cannot work around his personality; I simply have to go away if I am to concentrate on anything.

Let us push our illustration to the point where the whole thing proves to be a house party, and everybody has to stay overnight. There are only half as many beds as guests, and the deferences to polite society that Mr. A has to make have the exceedingly unhappy result that he has to share a bed with Mr. X. He is so horribly embarrassed at his disliking this stranger, and so awfully anxious not to make things too difficult for the host and hostess, that, well, the simple thing is to swallow all this stupid feeling of his and act like a good guest, and so they finally wind up in bed together. Mr. X is somewhat embarrassed by the strange casualness and avoidance on the part of Mr. A which he has suffered all day—an attitude that he realizes is quite different from his own feeling that he would like Mr. A if Mr. A weren't so distant. In fact, by this time his feelings have been reasonably well wounded, and he is not much pleased with this arrangement. So he takes reasonable precautions to get undressed and in bed before the other man does, or vice versa. But as he is about to fall asleep, his companion sighs deeply and starts to apologize rather queerly, and gets up and fiddles around a little while; and Mr. X realizes that he is listening to some queer kind of cock-and-bull story about how Mr. A has never really slept with anyone before, and is just horribly angry with himself and so on, but he doesn't know whether he can get any sleep unless he gets under the bottom sheet. And so this is what he does.

What is apt to happen in the course of the night—what, in fact, has in many such instances happened—is the following: During the night Mr. A gets out from under his cotton precaution and goes around and tenderly fondles Mr. X, and then goes back to bed under his bottom sheet. There is considerable evidence of his being in a curiously foggy state of mind, which so impresses Mr. X that he does not say anything about the incident the next morning. Mr. A acts as if nothing on earth like that could conceivably have happened, and Mr. X just says to himself, "Well, this bird is a funny one." Mr. A leaves the house with a feeling that, considering that he had had to share a room with this extremely disagreeable person, he has had a remarkably good night's sleep. He feels fine, and has no trace of any information about what has happened.

Since the security machinery is theoretically pretty feeble when one is really asleep, quite often much more meaningful behavior occurs in states of light sleep than at any other time in people with major systems in dissociation. Under those circumstances, what is left of the security mechanism of the self-system will suffice to maintain consciousness at any state that does not leave any ordinarily accessible recall. We will even, for purposes of illustration, say that Mr. X taxes Mr. A with what happened during the night. If Mr. A's dissociative system is working smoothly, there will be not the remotest suggestion in his awareness that this is true. If he is really quite a secure person in his dissociated state, he does not even have to have extremely unpleasant ideas about Mr. X. The fellow has obviously had a very, very vivid dream, Mr. A will say, and he will have no doubt that this is what happened. He may think that this dream means that Mr. X is homosexual and has a homosexual interest in him, and now he understands why he disliked him so much, and so on. That will all be kept to himself, however, if he wants to avoid unpleasantness; obviously Mr. X is simply a victim of unhappy sexual twists. But if Mr. A is not so secure, if the rest of his life does not make him quite bombproof, then when Mr. X taxes him with what happened, he will be horribly angry; he will regard it as a beastly canard, and probably the situation will develop into a very unpleasant type of business. The dream explanation will still be there, but he will tell Mr. X off rather roughly. But still he is undisturbed.

Now this, I insist to you, can happen only when the material easily accessible to awareness—that is, the self—has artifacts which neatly cut off any reasonable prospect of one's noticing a tendency to become integrated in a type of situation the impulse for which is dissociated. In the self, one gets unquestionable evidence of the wear and tear of life that is brought about by the dissociated system only when there is the right sort of person around for the integration and the subject person is engaged in something that calls for all the abilities he has. Then it goes very badly; he ordinarily finds that the other person is troublesome, and goes away. Thus people with major systems in dissociation are rather often singularly at the mercy of troubles of one kind or another; a good many things annoy them dreadfully, and they go away, get out of the annoying situation, with some excellent rationalization. They have felt no anxiety in the situation, but have just found it such a nuisance that they could not get their work done. This is practically pathognomonic of dissociation. In other words, if you find yourself disturbed by another person, but by the most minute investigation convince yourself that he does not stir anxiety, then you can be quite sure that the other person is of great significance to some dissociated impulse in the personality. It shows that way because there is such an elaborate pseudo or artifact organization in the self that anxiety simply is not going to be called out by anything short of a cataclysmic collision with this other person.

In the total personality, there is the vulnerability to situations which I have suggested in the matter of concentrated effort. Life is much more difficult in that any satisfaction of the impulse in dissociation is gotten either in a very incomplete fashion or in sleep. Ordinarily the most that happens in sleep is purely symbolic, so far as other people's cooperation is concerned. And since the tendency system in dissociation must be a powerful one—for it includes an impulse that is so extremely dangerous that it must not even be permitted to stir anxiety, which is the formula that leads to dissociation—quite obviously symbolic operations with imaginary people are not going to be very deeply satisfying. Thus we expect in the total personality that there will be an extraordinary sensitivity to anything that touches upon the dissociated system.

Unobserved alertness—a rather contradictory use of words, by which I mean the sort of activity of the eyes which I have already referred to—is much more striking in a person who has a major dissociated system than in one who does not have. In other words, let me draw a contrast between a purely imaginary sort of person who has 'repressed'—a relatively futile business—the happy days of homosexual life and not dissociated the impulses at all. Let us say that he has, after preadolescence, lived in a society that is exclusively feminine for twenty years, and then he runs onto another man who just rings the bell. He becomes almost immediately the prey of violent homosexual cravings—that is, assuming he does not immediately respond positively—but he also decides that this is all very horrible. He is so completely anxious that every time the potential love object is in any way even recalled to him, he actually gets jittery, sweats, and shows every sign of intense anxiety. He is panicky at the very thought of this forgotten desire of his, which he had supposed was just gone with the wind but which now blazes up with ferocious power and simply hounds him. When he is with this potential love object, he may gaze wildly at the fly of his pants, and then he has still more anxiety, and sweats, and looks firmly out the window. He is having a terrible time with his tendency to move toward this other person, and anything like a calm study of the potential love object's profile is as impossible to him as sprouting wings would be. With the dissociated person, on the other hand, we see any amount of this sort of unnoticed, inclinationless interest in, and attention to, if you please, the potential love object.

Impulses in dissociation have lots of experience; they grow, and they grow at not so terribly different a rate or degree from that of any impulse system. What they do not get is satisfaction —simple, direct, and everyday satisfaction in proportion to their power and importance in the total personality. So we can read off from this that a person with a powerful dissociated system is an extremely risky person to put in a type of situation that will require practically everything he has, because it is quite certain that a number of his abilities, particularly those of the sensory organs—which are much easier, you might say, to use than the motor systems—and a good deal of his energy are going to be spent in this unnoticed, fairly contentless attention to an unnoticed object. And the self struggles unsuccessfully to maintain application and focal attention on the assigned task at those times. So far as the person can tell you, well, his mind wandered; he dropped into a moment of abstraction. There are several reasons for this interference with extremely demanding tasks. One of them is that the very concentration required for this complex task tends to impair the easy operations of the self devices against awareness of the dissociated system and its operations. But since it is much more vital to maintain the dissociation than to get any mere task done, the task in turn suffers under the necessity of the self-system to devaluate the object and undisturbedly to ignore something that has impinged on one. And thus there is disturbance of the concentration on the task.

We may expect either that the dream life of people with dissociated systems will be glaringly meaningful or that the dreams will be as utterly obliterated as the dreams which characterize the night terror of very early life. Let me remind you

that night terror is a situation in which a child awakens scream-
ing in abject terror; and by the time he can pay any attention
to so mild a thing as a real person and can make some efforts
at communication, he has not the foggiest trace of any idea
of what it was all about. He is probably clear on the fact that
he was unutterably shaken by a terrible experience, and he may
be still trembling, but the curtain is immovable—there is nothing left of what happened. I do not want to get into a discussion of night terror, which is not relevant at the moment, except to draw attention to this obliteration of awareness of
processes; at the same time, I might remind you of what I
have said about schizophrenia—that it occurs when the self
loses the ability to control awareness of more primitive
processes.

The person with a major system in dissociation may recall
from his sleep very vivid and blatantly meaningful dreams as
long as nothing provides a path between these dreams and his
security. As long as this situation continues, it is all very simple;
for one thing, dreams that can be remembered come a little
nearer to satisfying the tendencies concerned than do dreams
that have to be forgotten. But if, perhaps as a result of someone else's attempt at interpretation or of something read in a
book, these dreams come to interfere with the self-system's
suave function of keeping the dissociated tendency out of
awareness, then the person will cease to recall any dreams
whatsoever. He may have very disturbed sleep; his wife may
report that he groans and yells in his sleep, and he may startle
into full awareness over and over during the night; but he will
have no trace of recollection of any dream. In other words, the
self will be on the job from then on, and sleep will be maintained at a level at which primitive processes cannot intrude
into awareness. If anything does get by, the person takes time
out the instant he recovers his waking awareness to inattend
it in some manner. And afterward, new complexities are developed in the self to make it impossible to dream that sort of

thing again—the person wakes up if he starts to dream anything like it again. You might think that for a very little while after awakening, he might be vulnerable to a demand as to whether he did not dream so-and-so. But we would be unable to guess exactly what he had dreamed, and even a slight error in depicting it would permit the self to make a flat denial without disturbance of awareness. If it were just in the process of being repressed, then there might be a vague feeling that it did stir some vague memory; but even so, the person would merely wonder how his questioner ever happened to have such a fantasy. Then the function of the self to keep the tendency concerned out of awareness would go on developing, and the next time the person was simply forced to have such a dream, he would wake up the moment the thing started developing. When awareness is lifted again, the thing may run itself off at primitive levels, but it will not be a dream—there will be no record.

It is hard to tackle a thing that seems so unearthly—except when you see somebody else show it—as does the trick of dissociation. I hope I have laid enough stress on the extraordinary nature of the self-system in dissociation, the elaborate development of processes in the self, to make it clear why any frontal attack on dissociation almost always fails. Frontal attacks have long since been anticipated by all sorts of processes which immediately go into effect and which simply blunt the attack or brush it off to the side.

The Schizophrenic Dynamism:
A Tripartite View

BEFORE DISCUSSING the so-called clinical entities, it seems appropriate to consider the dynamism of schizophrenia from the tripartite view. I believe you will see as we go along that this view of schizophrenia has particular meaning in terms of therapeutic approaches. What happens to the self, the rest of personality, and sleep in schizophrenia becomes meaningful in handling the particular problems that center around communication with the patient.

Failure of the Self-System

I have defined the essence, if you please, of the schizophrenic state as a failure of the self-system to reserve attention to the types of referential process that enjoy good repute among the intelligent—in other words, a failure to restrict the contents of consciousness to the higher referential processes that can be consensually validated. But this seems, I suppose, almost extremely remote from what the young psychiatrist sees in his first schizophrenic patient; and, of course, a statement of the essential characteristic in schizophrenia is not a description of the processes which go into being schizophrenic. It is these processes that I want to consider here.

In seeking to understand the escape of attention from its

ordinary field, one has to think for a moment from the other standpoint: Under what circumstances do the earlier types of knowing processes that ordinarily go on in the unnoted areas of the mind—the ordinarily unwitting referential processes—intrude into awareness? The reason why I express the essence of the thing as loss of control of the contents of consciousness, instead of as the eruption of other things into consciousness, is that I am impressed with the effort that people can be seen to be making to control the contents of consciousness.

An illuminating instance of the way in which the schizophrenic admits into consciousness things which are ordinarily excluded might be drawn from the 'mirth' of schizophrenics. Although it is difficult, I imagine, to be mirthful when schizophrenic, what I am talking about here does look remotely like mirth. The mirth-provoking ingredients in the unhappy schizophrenic's mental state are in the general field of wisecracks, not necessarily as obscene as I had once surmised, but the sort of thing that an occasional friend or acquaintance is just too apt at.

Now the fact that some schizophrenics see something funny in various things which intrude themselves upon their attention is not, I think, to be taken as separating them from the rest of humanity. Most of us see the apropos of wisecracks, those little humorous grace-notes on thought. I presume that one way in which the juvenile protects himself from being utterly crushed by the magnitude of the cultural heritage which is being driven into him, ground into him, rubbed into him, and poured into him is by making more or less witty commentaries on a good deal of it. Such commentaries are of absolute value in one way: anything that will make one laugh diminishes tension. That can be demonstrated under the most rigorous scientific experimental situation, with no reference to subjective sensation at all. The person who is tense will, if he can be made to laugh, undergo a very rapid diminution of skeletal or visceral tension. Thus it seems to me a reasonable assumption that, along with all the other incredible capacities of human beings, we have this capacity for ridicule, for seeing things that are amusing, that make us grin or laugh, by which we save ourselves from piling up the tensions which would in various situations be extremely embarrassing, at least, and possibly disastrous. And yet many of us, in our serious concern with special aspects of life, feel that it would be a rather transparent evidence of our lack of seriousness and respect for what we are doing, or what the other fellow is doing, to give way to these impulses to relieve many tensions with wisecracks. As a result, it becomes definitely obnoxious to us to be aware of these particular slants of the cognitive or knowing process, and so they are denied access to attention. It is only in situations of no particular importance or in moments of great security and comfort with another person that we may indulge in using that particular part of our equipment; the rest of the time that sort of noticing is simply taboo—it just is not there.

Now this, of course, is not the most important thing I want to discuss. I have used it only as an illustration of the way in which the schizophrenic admits into consciousness things which the rest of us would ordinarily exclude. But this sort of thing does not drive people into panic and into all the fugues and so on that we see in the early stages of schizophrenia. What occurs then is the inclusion in attention of primitive, diffuse processes dealing with essentially rather terrifying states of nature. In such a situation, for example, I, as a person known to me, would no longer be fixed and relatively durable but, instead, would become much more like a toy boat in a real monsoon; and other people would not be the more or less truncated caricatures that I have moved uncertainly among, but would become embodiments of rather terrifying generality. And the things that become terrifying and generalized in these primitive processes are the cultural mandates—the prohibitions and prescriptions—that I have not been able to live up to, or to live with.

What we discover in the self-system of a person undergoing

schizophrenic change or schizophrenic processes, is then, in its simplest form, an extremely fear-marked puzzlement, consisting of the use of rather generalized and anything but exquisitely refined referential processes in an attempt to cope with what is essentially a failure at being human—a failure at being anything that one could respect as worth being. It is perhaps after one has somewhat got used to this that the tensions of fear and the waves of anxiety which accompany all sorts of contact with others may be relieved by the wisecracking level of cognition which I have mentioned. When attention has spread to include even that, then we see people who, we say, are in danger of a schizophrenic deterioration. Using that particular way of reducing some of their tensions is a costly thing to do because it has such a bad effect on the environment. It looks as if the schizophrenic were laughing at you, and you do not like to be reminded that you might be that humorous; and, anyway, he is too sick to be having such a good time at your expense. Thus it has the effect of separating him from what might otherwise be a slightly reassuring contact that might, in turn, go into more reassuring contact.

The Rest of the Personality

So much for a very sketchy glimpse of the self-system, the contents of consciousness, in this acute schizophrenic state. What of the rest of the personality? What goes on in the rest of the personality is the thing that is ordinarily discussed when we try to be very intellectual about schizophrenia; but, unhappily, it is very difficult to explore because all ordinary channels of communication are closed, or at least are so disordered that they are almost effectively closed. You never know whether you have something that is meaningful in the sense that it was meaningful the month before with the patient, or whether you have something that has an autistic meaning, an exact parallel of which would not be found in your own case after you had reached the age of five. In other words, you must take it for granted that the language processes of the schizophrenic are obscure. It would be recklessly optimistic to assume that a phrase or statement of a schizophrenic is simply meaningful and communicative. You must assume that it is not, even though you may later find that it is, rather than do it the other way around. If you assume, just because something sounds communicative to you, that it means what it communicates to you, that road may lead to your contributing to the aggravation of the patient's mental state, because you get meanings which he does not see were possible. When a person uses autistic language that happens to sound like ordinary speech, of course he is amazed at what his remarks provoke in others because that was not what his remarks contained, so far as he was concerned. For example, if I say, "It rained a few minutes ago"—meaning by this that I made a good many remarks a few minutes ago, the meaning of which has now completely eluded me—and you say, "Yes, I've been expecting it to rain all morning," I will be rather dazed. I will wonder what on earth you are talking about, for I had nothing in mind about the weather. And by the time I get that autistic in speech, the chances are that I am not going to look at your remark and say to myself, "Let me see, I talked about my speech awhile back, and you talked about the weather. I suppose that's some queer kind of analogical thinking on your part. Oh, yes, I see—I spoke of my speech as rain, and you took the literal meaning instead of the one I intended." Needless to say, schizophrenics do not take time out for such brilliant analyses of failures at communication. Thus I repeat: The meaning of an autistic remark is not likely to be what the words communicate to you, unless you are a very rare mortal who can guess what level is involved and return to that. And even then, because of very obscure aspects of every person's past life, it would be very difficult to arrive at the particular autistic meaning involved. Thus, getting from the patient a valid clue to anything going on outside the self-system is a very difficult task.

The Failure of Dissociation in Schizophrenia

We see in some of the essentially healthy operations of the schizophrenic something that I have never seen even remotely suggested in any other state of human beings. It is also something that I think has considerable predictive value. We see schizophrenics occasionally engaged in what up to now was dissociated behavior—doing something which, a study will show, they have done before but without, on the previous occasions, seeming to know they had done it. But now they do this thing with puzzlement, with real curiosity, with the feeling, "I ought to grasp the meaning of this thing I've just done, but it eludes me." The schizophrenic change, I believe, is quite generally due to an inability to maintain dissociation. Now in order for there to be dissociation, a rather elaborate body of processes must be built into the self to maintain it; and so when one is unable to maintain the dissociation, it does not mean that all this invention in the self totally vanishes. This invention still remains, and things that do not have simple and uncomplicated access to awareness collide with it and suffer as a result of it. Thus the schizophrenic has an unsure mental state, in which he is clearly aware of the activity of the dissociative system but unable to get the thing into clear personal focus. It is from this continued activity of an inadequate dissociating system that the profound puzzlement arises which characterizes long reaches of some schizophrenics' lives. And from the stress of being unable to maintain a system of dissociation comes the loss of control of the contents of consciousness. What ensues is that there are highly refined referential processes along with much more primitive and general referential processes, coupled with observational data which one cannot treat to anything like one's satisfaction, partly because they are primitive and deal in rather cosmic terms with things that are essentially impersonal and partly because there is interference from remaining effective parts of the self-system which were carefully organized to cut off recall of things that would imply awareness of the dissociated tendency.

Thus the schizophrenic picture is not only somewhat complicated by the large amount of autistic referential knowing operations. It is also complicated by a continuance of obstruction to recognizing a part of life which came into being to maintain the dissociation—and yet the dissociation is no longer anything like complete, but tends actually to get into behavior.

Relation of the Self-System to the Total Personality

If you will forget the patient for a moment and just try to draw in your mind a picture such as I have been talking about, I think that you will envision a person who does many things which are pretty meaningful, but then destroys your feeling that you could be right as to what these things mean by the extraordinarily incongruous character of the context. In other words, after doing something that seems meaningful to you, he then does other things which seem completely to deny the correctness of the conclusion you had arrived at a few moments earlier. Now this hypothetical person may not look very much like your schizophrenic patient at first glance, but he does look very much like what the schizophrenic notices about himself.

Thus the self-system is rather nearer in identity to the rest of personality in schizophrenia than in any of the other marked mental disorders—remembering that by a marked mental disorder I mean the point where one of these dynamisms is so extraordinarily loaded with requirements that it curiously interferes with an efficient, rather comfortable, and rather satisfactory life.

The contrast with sublimation is utter in the sense that as long as sublimation does not give way under the load put on it, the mental state is rather highly secure; self-esteem is high, no marked craving for any satisfaction is experienced within awareness, and life seems to be pretty good. The obsessional picture is, of course, the antithesis of what I have described as schizophrenic, because the obsessional is so busy going through the magical routines and thoughts that he is able to ignore the most obviously transparent performances that he may be engaged in with others. The paranoid, of course, is anything but alert to what he is doing, because it is all the result of the beastly people that he is in contact with, and he is entirely too busy with various symptoms or forebodings as to his state of health to notice what he is doing with others. But the schizophrenic has this puzzling awareness that he is doing something that he ought to recognize; sometimes he does recognize it with an excessive terror—meaning an immediate shift to more primitive types of process—and at other times he is just hounded by the fact that it ought to be clear but that some way or other it eludes him. And it seems dreadfully important because by that time he is thoroughly tired, and fatigue makes any little thing in the mind seem unduly important.

The sleep of the schizophrenic provides a strange confirmation from my tripartite viewpoint of the very things that I have indicated in describing this relationship of the total personality to the self. The sleep of schizophrenics, once dissociation has failed and the contents of consciousness have escaped from control, is apt to be profound. And that is a function of the disappearance of the very machinery that thwarts the needs for satisfaction in the rest of us. But the sleep of schizophrenics is also a different thing from the sleep that we ordinarily deal with, for when the schizophrenic is having a bad time—when he is still schizophrenic, one might say, instead of settling into one of the unfortunate outcomes—his sleep is a regressive phenomenon. Its regressive character is even indicated by the sleep picture which has preceded the eruption of schizophrenia by weeks, months, or, in some rare cases, years. I want to make that point a little better. Time and again, particularly in women —I think chiefly because of the cultural differential that they contend with—we come upon a schizophrenic dilapidation which has a rather acute onset so late in life that one might ob-

ject and say, no, the process cannot occur for the first time this
late in life; there must have been earlier episodes. And quite
often that is right. Quite often we can find the earlier episode
if we land upon the right formula—if we have paid enough
attention to the patient to know something about him, although
this is not always easy with a schizophrenic. But also we can
be wrong, in this sense: the earlier episode we are looking for
was not an episode, but it was so very closely related that it
served the purpose we think has to be served. And it explains
how a type of disaster that almost by definition, according to
my theory, must occur fairly early in life may sometimes not
occur until well in the thirties. When you effect contact with
the intimate history of markedly schizoid people, you learn
that at times which we would ordinarily say were times of
unusual stress, these people underwent for quite extended
periods a life that was more than half—sometimes nearly all
—spent in a kind of light sleep. They have literally taken to
their beds most of the time, although often they did it rather
privately and secretly. You learn also that they are quite clear
on the fact that they have not been asleep continuously during
these ten, twelve, fourteen, or sixteen hours a day of with-
drawal. And you get quite a bit of data about the particular
interruptions in the fairly long sleep binges they have gone
on; there has been some activity—they have gotten up to get
a book and read something they wanted to look up, or something like that. They will even tell you a great deal about certain dreams or fantasies that they recall from this period which
were gratifying; they lived a sort of life in Valhalla. But some
of the dream processes were not by any means as pleasant, and
some of them had extremely ugly aspects. And so here is a sort
of twilight area in which you can almost see the building-up of
the self-system's dissociative equipment. In these earlier and
milder conditions one sleeps deeply as little as possible; one
remains alert and dozes as much as possible until the establishment of a satisfactory dissociative system has been completed.

PART TWO

Therapeutic Approaches to the Patterns of Difficulty—the Clinical Entities

___

Clinical Entities as a Frame of Reference in Therapy

I HAVE BEEN asked to discuss clinical entities, but I must say at the outset that I have some reservations about discussing therapeutic approaches in terms of clinical entities. At the same time, I think that the clinical entities do have some purely pragmatic utility, if you please, as orienting points of departure for the psychiatrist. Perhaps I can make my position somewhat clearer by some brief discussion of the handicapping effect of fixed diagnoses on the psychiatrist's work.

Diagnosis Versus Prognosis in Mental Illness

As an outcome of my participation in many conferences—and good conferences—I have often been quite genuinely discouraged by the so-called formal rather than what I call factual diagnosis. In most of these conferences, an immense amount of useful, mutually profitable formulation has occurred, followed by what sometimes seems to me to be anything but scientific application of label. I have occasionally proved to my satisfaction that some of the psychiatrists who label patients cannot say what they mean by these labels; yet these same psychiatrists have no feeling of incompleteness about such labeling.[1] If

[1] *Editors' note:* In several unpublished lectures, Sullivan has also commented on the inappropriateness of personifying the disease and speaking

193

pressed, they can rattle off something that sounds rather like White's *Outlines* [2] as to what this condition indicated by the label is like. In other words, psychiatrists can often recite long definitions of schizophrenia, manic-depressive psychosis, and so on, and can often apply these labels to patients with a fairly high probability of the future justifying the labeling; but when you look at the data on this patient, the alleged basis for using the label isn't there. And that seems odd to me.

The oddness that I speak of possibly requires some further elaboration. First, even psychiatrists know a whole lot more than they run through their formulating mill; they pick up some data that just are not susceptible of formulation because they are not the ordinary data of our conscious thinking. And second—and this is the grim part of it—they also develop a very strong prejudice as to the actual meaning of some symptom or some pattern that they believe themselves to have observed; and once they have applied this label, it becomes invested with their professional prestige. So they are inclined to fight for it, and sometimes to influence the patient insidiously in the direction that the label requires the patient to move. Thus the prejudice is awkward because the psychiatrist is unknowingly looking for the things which are given importance by the prejudice and may most comfortably overlook lots of very useful and important data about a patient while waiting for these highly valued symptoms that will clinch the diagnosis. The net result, therefore, of having pretty strong diagnostic prejudices is that you can miss a lot of highly relevant information. And you can miss it rather permanently. If a psychiatrist invests a diagnosis with his prestige, it may mean, for instance,

---

of it as if it were the patient—"an obsessional" or "a schizophrenic." In this group of lectures, he has employed this device extensively himself, partly because he is talking to his colleagues in an informal setting. In his later more formal writing, edited by himself, he seems to have avoided this usage.

[2] William Alanson White, *Outlines of Psychiatry*; Washington, D.C.: Nervous and Mental Disease Publishing Co., 1935.

that he remains generally indifferent to a schizophrenic patient who, in terms of his clinical diagnosis, may be expected to deteriorate; and this may assist the patient in despairing of the outcome in such a way that he may actually deteriorate.

The culture, you see, places great emphasis on diagnosis; and after the pattern of the culture, the patient's family are very anxious to find out whether the doctor can call the illness by a label. And this gives some doctors good justification for attempting to formulate a clinical diagnosis that makes sense. That is a somewhat unwelcome activity as far as I am concerned, if only because I am very much more interested in *what can be done* than in what has happened. And the notion of what can be done is determined without particular reference to any particular clinical diagnosis. I believe that the clinical diagnosis exists more out of regard for public demand and the professional dignity of the doctor than because of its greatly simplifying effect on psychiatric problems.

A sounder approach is found, I believe, in the application of two frames of reference. The first of these is the viewing of each case in terms of the outstanding difficulties in living, the liabilities, as against the degree of ability demonstrated to meet complex situations, the assets. Now if, in studying a patient's past, the psychiatrist finds little or no convincing proof that this person has shown any capacity to meet difficult or unusually complex situations, and that he has reacted in many situations with something that we term a dynamism of difficulty, then, according to the first reference frame, the prognostic picture is dim. Of course the age of the patient is a factor in such a decision. A schizophrenic at 20 may never have had a chance to discover that he had any assets, although he may really have astonishing ones. The prognosis here would be much more favorable than for a patient somewhere in his forties, for example, who shows no evidence of any outstanding abilities in any career line, even though he seems to have had a reasonable amount of opportunity, and who has clearly used the obsessional dynamism almost steadily to handle difficult situations.

The other frame of reference is that of determining, on the basis of such information as is available from the patient, what are the grounds for therapeutic operations—what are the positive opportunities for therapeutic operations—and evaluating the possibilities of a good life after favorable change. Note that this frame of reference is simply not related to the first one; these are two entirely different types of operation with the data.

To illustrate the second frame of reference: If the psychiatrist finds that, according to any information he can uncover, the patient has never had a continuing friendly relationship with anyone, the psychiatrist has learned, insofar as he is right, that this patient is not possessed of either valid experience or parataxic surviving of experience which will readily give him 'faith' in the therapist. I use the word 'faith' because things have to start for a patient in a quite irrational way; that is, reason can come along only when the data become at least separable from the nondata. Thus one attempts to assess the gross characteristics of significant figures of the past, looking for the parataxic patterns which will undoubtedly characterize any attempt at treatment. The psychiatrist anticipates as best he can which people are bound to remain significant in the patient's future life, and even whether the significant figures who offer only the antithesis of contentment and security can be eluded. If the future situation is of an extremely discouraging character—if, in other words, the patient is hopelessly entangled with relatives who are not interested in letting him live as a person—then this must be taken account of. None of us is willing to change unless we have the hope of improving our condition; that is, recovery itself *is* increased facility for contentment and security. And if the patient and the doctor see that it will be terribly difficult to get the patient out of the entanglements that beset him, so that he can implement the increased facility for more meaningful living, then they can anticipate great difficulty in undertaking treatment.

These frames of reference, then, really constitute a study of the probable outcome from the standpoint of the tools and facilities available to the therapist and from the standpoint of the probable drive for useful results in terms of the patient's past experience.

I believe that all prognostic thinking for any intensive work with patients should certainly include these two frames of reference, for they are useful in assessing the factors which can be picked out of a reasonably good history of the patient's life—organized in terms of the developmental eras [3]—and some preliminary inquiry with the patient. If time is any objective at all, these frames of reference should be established before anything like formal psychotherapy is undertaken.

To illustrate the usefulness of this kind of thinking, let us consider the empirical fact that the schizophrenia which appears in the form of a sudden dramatic onset is usually considered to have a more favorable prognosis than the schizophrenia with more gradual onset. But in those cases of sudden onset in which satisfactory experience with significant persons in the past is totally lacking, the patient may be practically beyond redemption; he may manifest empirically trustworthy capacity for recovery to the extent of making excellent institutional recovery; but the psychiatrist is daft who expects that he can put the patient out into the world without prompt relapse.

And this leads me to touch upon another way in which this approach seems meaningful. Since all patients, I believe, manifest at one time or another various dynamisms of difficulty, the

[3] *Editors' note:* Elsewhere in this same lecture series and also in other writings, Sullivan has stressed the importance of using the developmental eras as frames of reference for organizing the patient's history. For a complete discussion of this approach in terms of clinical work, see pages 138–182 of Sullivan's *The Psychiatric Interview.*

psychiatrist can miss the shifts from one dynamism to another by a static label for the patient's behavior. This is strikingly apparent in the kind of patient I have seen so commonly in my practice: This patient is typically a fairly young person, usually under thirty; and the data on his career line show that he has had schizophrenic episodes and has been rather strikingly obsessional in between these episodes—even being a pretty classically obsessional neurotic. Such patients show up frequently in private practice; and I have even had quite a run of them in institutional practice. As I have noted before, there is really a rather close relationship between the marked obsessional distortions in living and the frank schizophrenic psychosis. In dealing with such a patient, the psychiatrist must deal with the obsessional dynamism as the principal difficulty when the patient is prevailingly obsessional in his operation. But when that same patient is definitely schizophrenic, the approaches to the obsessional picture would be terribly beside the point. And so the psychiatrist shifts his way of doing things, not on the basis of a diagnostic label, but on the basis of the presenting peculiarities of interpersonal relations. Although this lack of fixity in terms of the principal process of prevailing nuisance—the prevailing obstacle to growth and recovery—may seldom show itself so dramatically as in this sudden shift from obsessionalism to the schizophrenic picture, its less dramatic manifestations are an invariable aspect of all mankind. The hypochondriacal process may shift to a principal process which is definitely paranoid, to take another example. And the importance of keeping one's mind open to observe the presence of dynamisms other than the outstanding one is another rewarding focus for the psychiatrist in terms of time saved.

A Note on 'Mixed States'

While these dynamisms of difficulty shift at different times, I do not believe that they exist as 'mixed states,' to use the popular expression. The notion of mixed states is only a reformulation of the static Kraepelinian classification. Now I know no reason for assuming that any personality does not have available, and does not actually frequently manifest, the whole congeries of dynamisms, the extraordinary accent on one of which will give a picture of mental disorder. But I do not expect to see a person whose pattern of interpersonal difficulties will be somewhere betwixt and between. I expect, rather, to see dynamisms manifested now and then by everybody to meet particular situational stresses; and I expect the gross pattern of interpersonal relations to be rather outstandingly of a particular type. Perhaps this is just a methodological convenience of mine, and I have been inattentive to glaring exceptions to my conclusion; but I have not seen these mixed schizophrenic states that I have read about *in extenso*.

There is one other thing that I want to say on this subject. It seems quite within the realm of reason for a psychiatrist to discover in a patient whom he knows quite thoroughly that whenever a certain type of problem is the major problem of the moment, it will call out a dynamism definitely different from the dynamism that characterizes that patient's 'basic living.' Now I can make that statement somewhat more meaningful by giving a hypothetical example: Let us suppose that we have an obsessional neurotic who meets almost all the stresses of interpersonal relations by the substitutive type of operation, being obsessed with some content of consciousness. I know no reason why this obsessional neurotic might not react to a particularly domineering type of employer, let us say, by an hysterical disablement at times when the employer was particularly domineering. Under those circumstances the employer, if he were a psychiatrist, might be inclined to regard the notion that this person was an obsessional neurotic as a rather curious error of judgment, and might be inclined to pronounce the person an hysteric. But to do that, he would again have to be in the position that the good old Kraepelinian psy

chiatrists were: he could not know too much about the patient.
If he set out to document the prevailingly hysteric character
of this person's adaptations to life, then he would run into
the obsessional business, because the dynamism that gets to
characterize a sick person is like almost anything else that characterizes us in our interpersonal relations, more or less habitual.
Thus the special trimming which may be peculiarly adapted
to a particular type of problem will not be carried out consistently over a large field of living. This may be illustrated from
everyday life by our conduct when, impressed with our particular role with a stranger, we carry on quite well in living up
to that role for a while; but as the impression of strangeness
wears off, as we begin to pick up some notions about the other
fellow, we also begin to be somewhat worn out with the un-
familiar restraints that we are exercising on ourselves, and more
and more of our habitual personality or habitual type of interpersonal relation comes into play. I think there is no time when
people are so strikingly on their good behavior, as we ordinarily
put it, as in meeting important strangers. Thus I know no
reason why a quite incongruous dynamism may not be very
conspicuous in meeting a particular type of problem. But as
soon as one spreads the field of inquiry to anything like life-size
proportions, then this falls into the category of the unusual
rather than the usual pattern of living.

Clinical Entities in Terms of Therapy

Any patient will, insofar as my theory of personality is valid,
manifest toward the analyst a series of parataxic distortions
which are wholly to be understood, completely explicable, on
the basis of the past experience and the morbid experience of
this patient. These parataxic distortions reflect undigested experience of the past, things that could not be integrated into
a unitary system of motivation. Now these distortions, in my
experience, have not been very strikingly different in the main,
although the people concerned and the problems concerned

have been different. The distortions have been, let us say, the basic warp of personality, the thing that colors so much of life that it has to be dealt with if the patient is to improve. There are, of course, subsidiary parataxic distortions, representing more or less crucial experiences that have led to complications or aggravation of the basic distortion. But I am inclined to say that the major problems, at least the major presenting problems, which come up as distortions of the relationship with the therapist differ surprisingly in detail, but do not differ strikingly in the dynamisms that are concerned.[4] Why this is the case, I surmise, can be hinted at from theoretical considerations; but without going into any greatly detailed theory, let me just refer to the following considerations. The presenting problem in a patient is a disastrous experience, the first disastrous experience, if you please. It establishes a deviation from the conventional type of development which facilitates certain increments of deviation and certain diminutions of deviation; but it has no direct effect on a wholly different, a wholly unrelated type of experience. We can hypothecate a person who has a major deviation, let us say, in late childhood, and who then has a very disastrous experience in the juvenile era which strikes a previously unwarped system of the personality. Here, you see, we are overlooking the fact that these systems do not exist in utter separation from each other; they are abstractions which are useful in thinking. But even taking the liberty of talking as if they were perfectly independent and had no relationship to each other, could we imagine something happening in the juvenile era that had relatively no effect on part of the personality? Do we actually encounter such situations? I think not. I haven't seen it. In the first place,

[4] *Editors' note:* Sullivan later formulated the "one-genus postulate," which closely follows this thinking (see *The Interpersonal Theory of Psychiatry*, pp. 32–33). ". . . I have become occupied with the science, not of individual differences, but of human identities, or parallels, one might say. In other words, I try to study the degrees and patterns of things which I assume to be ubiquitously human."

it is bad thinking anyway to imagine that there are these un-related things in the person. But in the second place, the tend-ency to live and to have mental health is the thing that is affected by the initial warp; and the initial warp has the effect of leaving a person vulnerable to subsequent disasters in that field, whereas the longer he lives the less vulnerable he is to experiences in comparatively unrelated fields. So the patient that we ordinarily see has a series of disasters, following the major one, which manifest themselves as a more or less char-acteristic distortion of personality, distortion of communica-tion, distortion of observations of the other fellow, and so on. If it were not for that, I would have no particular unfriendli-ness toward the notion of clinical entities. I am quite willing, in fact, to admit their purely pragmatic utility in the field of psychiatry. They probably are useful in preparing one for what one has to do, in appraising the probable difficulties of the procedure, or even in guessing as to the future course of a patient's life.

Hysteria

I HAVE SPOKEN of the magnificence of the apparatus—the system of dynamisms, of more or less permanently running processes—which is required for the maintenance of dissociation. I have talked, you will remember, about how the dissociated personality has to prepare for almost any conceivable emergency that would startle one into becoming aware of the dissociated system and of how, as a result, one literally has to set up a whole group of special awarenesses, special alert signals, if you please. Now the clinical entity, hysteria, shows almost in caricature how that is done. Thus, although the hysteric dynamism is very much simpler than the dissociative dynamism, it is extremely illuminating for the theory of dissociation.

The hysteric might be said in principle to be a person who has a happy thought as to a way by which he can be respectable even though not living up to his standards. That way of describing the hysteric, however, is very misleading, for of course the hysteric never does have that thought. At least it is practically impossible to prove that he has had that thought. But, unlike the completely unwitting activity of sublimation and unlike the very massive and impressive dissociations which show as automatic action and so on, the hysteric can often be led, under hypnosis, to recall just the thought that was the key to how one can 'dissociate' with comparative impunity and still without anything like the elaborate apparatus of the true dissociative condition.

The collision of aspects of the personality involved in the self is also somewhat more obvious in the hysteric than in the more obscure mental conditions. In the hysteric, you see that the whole achievement of the dynamism employed is to prevent the environing people from recognizing and being able to prove the existence of the impulses which are behind the hysteric façade—or, for my purposes, which are dissociated. In the great dissociative processes, on the other hand, there is no awareness at any level of the evaluation that other people might place on the dissociated system. That is all blotted out in the readjustment within the self-system which gives security by virtue of the dissociation. In the hysteric the self-system is so sketchy that as soon as the other person hits on a fairly well-aimed guess as to what the dissociated impulse is, the whole thing shifts. In other words, one particular self-against-impulse process may be abandoned and a new one developed. Thus, hysteria is very much simpler than dissociation in its fully developed form; but it is immensely interesting as a diagram.

So, I say, all the hysteric has to do from the standpoint of dissociating his less acceptable impulses is to have a happy idea which, if true, would exempt him from 'blame.' What you see in the hysteric is thus not a high-grade conflict between ideal structures and unregenerated impulses, but just a happy idea of how to get away with something. And in the true dissociative processes there isn't the foggiest analogue of anything like that at any time.

To illustrate how the hysteric dynamism comes into operation, let us say that a man with a strong hysterical predisposition has married, perhaps for money, and that his wife, thanks to his rather dramatic and exaggerated way of doing and saying things, cannot long remain in doubt that there was a very practical consideration in this marriage and cannot completely blind herself to a certain lack of importance that she has in her husband's eyes. So she begins to get even. She may, for example, like someone I recently saw, develop a never-failing vaginismus, so that there is no more intercourse for him. And he will not ruminate on whether this vaginismus that is cutting off his satisfaction is directed against him, for the very simple reason that if you view interpersonal phenomena with that degree of objectivity, you can't use an hysterical process to get rid of your own troubles. So he won't consider that; but he will suffer terribly from privation and will go to rather extravagant lengths to overcome the vaginismus that is depriving him of satisfaction, the lengths being characterized by a certain rather theatrical attention to detail rather than deep scrutiny of his wife. But he fails again and again. Then one night, when he is worn out, and perhaps has had a precocious ejaculation in his newest adventure in practical psychotherapy, he has the idea, "My God, this thing is driving me crazy," and goes to sleep.

Now the idea, "This thing is driving me crazy," is the happy idea that I say the hysteric has. He wakes up at some early hour in the morning, probably at the time when his wife is notoriously most soundly asleep, and he has a frightful attack of some kind. It could be literally almost anything, but it will be very impressive to anyone around. His wife will be awakened, very much frightened, and will call the doctor. But before the doctor gets there, the husband, with a fine sense of dramatic values, will let her know in some indirect way that he's terribly afraid he is losing his mind. She is reduced to a really agitated state by that. So when the doctor comes, the wife is in enough distress—in part because of whatever led to her vaginismus—to wonder if she might lose her own mind, and the husband is showing a good many odd symptoms.

And the doctor probably doesn't know anything about losing minds anyway, and so he begins to wonder if he is going to lose *his* mind. But presently things quiet down.

Now let us say that the doctor in this case is a high-grade but somewhat inexperienced psychiatrist and that he sets out to get the history of the immediate situation from which this business grew. He might get an awful lot of details—details about distressing situations in the office, the terrible strain that the husband has been under from the pressure of his work—all of them within the limits of ordinary human plausibility as a basis for quite a nervous condition. And, of course, he would learn how very useful the wife has been in sort of protecting the husband from these things and in giving him as much rest and quiet as possible. But there will be no comment about anything else—no faintest suspicion of anything the least bit out of the way in the sex life. Even if our somewhat inexperienced psychiatrist, suspecting that there is possibly something a little bit off in the sex life somewhere, pushes hard in that area, he won't get any very good leads. So he will probably prescribe sedatives and a rest or a change of scene or some other damn thing, and hope for the best.

And the man's attacks will recur now and then. But even if the most experienced psychiatrist came into the case and attempted to get the recollection of this little thought, "My God, this thing is driving me crazy," he would fail unless he used some extraordinary type of investigative means, such as hypnosis.[1]

---

[1] *Editors' note:* In another lecture, not included here, Sullivan has this to say about hypnosis and psychoanalysis in terms of their relative merits: "From my experience with the use of hypnosis in the treating of hysterics, I think that each treatment increases the probability that the patient will be more disabled and more inextricably hysteric. This is not a very difficult thing to explain theoretically. The more dramatic roles that a hysteric takes onto himself, the less chance there is of finding the person and a way of life that is adjustment.

"So I think that psychoanalysis was probably the first really therapeutic tool found for hysteria that was at all established; and even in its most elementary beginnings it was an astonishingly great improvement on any-

So what do we judge from this? The verbal form that the thought takes here need not greatly concern us. It is partly slang from the linguistic culture, and it might even be a not very important distillate from popularizations of dynamic psychiatry. But whatever it is, as it occurred it was the expression of intense irritation and frustration from an entirely self-centered point of view: "My wife and her vaginismus are having a bad effect on me."

But this verbal formula becomes of great importance by reason of the fact that, as it runs through awareness, it provides what I have said is necessary—the happy idea. He has found a way that he can punish his wife for something that he is not sure is an atrocity directed against him, but that is for all practical purposes from his standpoint an atrocity. You see, he is rather too self-centered to be studying what she may be suffering. Here is a business that develops something like this: If I went insane because of this vaginismus, that would give her a bad mental state herself. Now, the man is not aware of any strongly punitive inclination toward his wife, and yet that aspect of the thing is strangely attractive. There is another element also, which he is not at all clearly aware of, namely that lust is mixed up in this thing with security operations, in the sense that his lust is somewhat tainted with questions of prestige, because he is strikingly self-centered and everything he does is of importance as such, quite in addition to its satisfaction character. So in this flippant thought, "My God, this thing is driving me crazy," quite suddenly he has a formula, which is, you might say, a very queer and inverted type of sublimation. He finds a way of satisfying unacceptable impulses in a personally satisfactory way which exempts him from social blame and which thereby approaches sublimation.

---

thing that had been done before. After psychoanalytic treatment, even if clumsy, the hysteric's personality is simpler than it was, whereas in all the other methods new and wonderful things are simply added to the pseudo living which is what hysteria is."

But the activity, if recognized, would not receive anything but social condemnation.

So he has these attacks in and out of season when the provocation is sufficient; and he remains comfortably unaware of their effect on others, partly because he doesn't pay much attention to other people anyway and partly because these are his symptoms, this is his sickness, this is something mysterious and rather awful which abruptly descended upon him at 4:00 A. M. on a particular unforgettable morning and which the doctors haven't succeeded in making much sense of.

Well, all that he has to remain resolutely incapable of recalling is the precise setting in which a related verbal formula passed across awareness; and as long as that is denied any access to awareness, the mystery of the seizures is maintained with no particular effort. The seizure itself is a special instance of all human behavior. It is directed toward the achievement of a more or less clearly foreseen goal—in this case, distinctly less clearly foreseen except for this very swift process in awareness that is now inaccessible. So, as I say, this is a sort of rudimentary caricature of the 'apparatus' in the self—the system of dynamisms in the self—that maintains major dissociations.

It is, of course, a much simpler process, for the dissociative processes have to maintain control of vast numbers of perceptions, whereas all the hysteric dynamism has to control is a particular little context of thought—that which occurs just before the dissociation. By 'forgetting' this thought or event, the hysteric is able to keep the connection between symptom and life obscure. Thus, in terms of energy, alertness, and all the various processes within the self-system, hysteria is a comparatively inexpensive way of meeting some recurrent defeat or some recurrent clash between enforced necessities for security and needs for satisfaction. All the hysteric has to do is be sure that the symptom cannot be fixed in time, and therefore there are no recallable steps by which the process became fixed. And so there is utter mystery. Here are the symptoms and here is the world, and only a tiny moment in time is omitted. And it works nicely.

Predisposing Factors in the Childhood of the Hysteric as Compared to the Schizophrenic

I next wish to consider the circumstances by which a personality becomes inclined, as it were, toward this dynamism of hysteria as a way of meeting difficulties. We can perhaps approach this best from the standpoint of the contrast between the person who uses the dynamism of hysteria and the person who uses one of the much more complex major dissociation systems.

In the person with a major dissociation, if we can fill the gap between what is manifest to him and what is not, we find a great deal of alertness, analysis, and intellectual 'success' in noticing people and in approximating a statement of his prevailing motives and so on. In other words, the interpersonal behavior of a person with a major dissociation, once we have added the two sides into a personality, has to be regarded as the behavior of a highly sensitive, highly differentiated personality. A person who does not have highly developed innate capacities cannot maintain a dissociation in this sense; he is continually falling over the dissociated impulse or the semi-dissociated impulse in integrating situations, so he is really at his own mercy. Only the remarkably alert and rather competent person is eternally warned in time and thus is able to move magically in oblivion through a painfully provocative life, you might say.

The hysteric has a rather deep contempt for other people. I mean by this that he regards other people as comparatively shadowy figures that move around, I sometimes think, as audience for his own performance. How does this show? Well, omitting the puritanical schizoid, hysterics may be said to be the greatest liars to no purpose in the whole range of human personalities. I am not talking about pathological lying. I am talking about the fact that nothing is good enough as it is.

It always undergoes improvement in the telling; the hysteric simply has to exaggerate everything a little. The language is twisted in a characteristic fashion, and everything that interests the hysteric is described in superlatives. Some hysterics, of course, are highly intelligent people, and they can give you a nice objective report of things that are official business or something like that. But when they talk about their living—their interests, their fun, their sorrows and so on—only superlative terms will suffice them. And that, in a way, is a statement of the inadequacy of reality—which is what I mean when I say that hysterics are rather contemptuous of mere events and mere people. They act as if they were accustomed to something better, and they are.

That takes us a step further back to the way the hysteric disposition gets developed. The early juvenile and late childhood eras in the hysteric are characterized by what I would call fantasies of a rather crass dramatic type. Now the markedly sensitive, shy, difficult pre-schizophrenic would perhaps engage in more fantasy than would the person who is markedly disposed to hysteria, because the schizophrenic has much more time—a lifetime to give up to fantasy. And in the fantasies of the markedly introverted person, who might easily have major dissociations of personality later, one finds that there is a constant growth in the nicety of referential detail; a myth-like daydream of last year would be just too crude to be entertained this year. Not so with the person who is developing the hysteric predisposition. A type of fantasy which sufficed in late childhood—that is, in terms of its action—may be going on five or six years later with no change except for an elaboration of the characters and perhaps a concealment of too glaring and socially unacceptable elements of the drama.

Why is there this contrast? The organization of the self in the markedly 'introverted' person is, I would say, primarily a constantly growing—a very urgently and imperatively and necessarily growing—instrument for more and more microscopic analysis with a view to more and more foresight of possible rebuffs and pains from other people. As a result, no matter how shy and how appallingly incapable of handling other people this markedly introverted person may be, he is becoming more and more capable of being forewarned so that he may have some possibility of avoiding rebuffs. The idea is to spot the rebuff in time and either protect oneself from it or leave. As a result, the most private processes within awareness undergo development to meet this need for ever-increasing scrutiny. And the daydream that stirs a little feeling of anxiety —the feeling that perhaps this is not quite the daydream that other people would think was nice—is constantly modified to make proper deferential gestures to certain standards of propriety which, this introverted person has now caught onto, are other people's values. So the fantasy constantly becomes more and more refined and more obscure about obscure primitive things.

In contrast, the person who is predisposed to hysteria and will increasingly show hysterical symptoms has no such particular necessity for elaborate caution about other people because literally, from still earlier in life, there has been a disturbance of the clarity of connection between other people and pleasure or pain. The disturbance in this region manifests itself, as I have already suggested, in the unimportance of other people to him; in a very simple sense, the hysteric is self-absorbed.

In the case of the hysteric, one usually finds, in addition to this kind of atmosphere, a self-absorbed parent or some other highly significant figure who regards the child as something of a plaything—a decoration of the parent's personality— rather than as a growing personality. The parent with this lack of respect and appreciation for the child is also an instance of the relatively self-centered personality, and will show the very thing that I have been talking about—the tendency to belittle reality extravagantly and to doctor it up. Right there the child is taught by rote and example very early in life that things are not good enough. And he learns from experience in the home to improve on things in the manner of the parent. So hysteria comes much closer to being simple contagion than most of the other distortions of living.

The self-absorbed person is not particularly hostile to others; others don't really matter enough. He can be intensely annoyed if someone goes to great trouble to rebuff him; but ordinarily he moves aside from direct rebuff. With some slight belittling of everything except what he wants to recall, and with the feeling that people have no real importance anyway except as an audience for him—someone to talk to when he is bored or someone to notice how well he does things—he doesn't need to feel particularly hostile to mankind. He is relatively invulnerable to the type of damage that an unwelcome child experiences in early childhood from parents who are not so self-absorbed—the direct, carefully focused, and terribly warping hostility to which a good many preschizophrenic children are exposed. But the easy access to others which is developed by parental respect for the appearing characteristics of the child—by a warmth, a well-aimed warmth toward the child —is not there either. Nor is there any expectation of the nice show of appreciation that many parents ask of their children. So it is in the lotus-land sort of existence surrounding the self-absorbed parent that the child readily comes to have this self-absorbed characteristic. The relatively unrefined fantasy, daydreams, and revery processes on which this characteristic depends are not, in turn, particularly refining to one's behavior and to one's skill in formulating others' behavior. And they are correspondingly less and less apt to involve one in interpersonal adjustments that are refining through pleasure or pain. Self-absorbed people tend to move in relatively superficial contact among other self-absorbed people.

Characteristic Interpersonal Relations of the Prevailingly Hysteric

What are the characteristics of the interpersonal phenomena, the observance of which justifies a strong surmise of the presence of the hysterical entity? The observable interpersonal relations of the prevailingly hysterical person are characterized by an extravagance of emotional color. Euphoria is higher than an appraisal of objective reality would seem to justify, and it alternates rather vividly with equally extravagant negative emotions. Unlike the excitement or the depression of the person who is prevailingly cyclothymic, the emotional aspects of the hysteric are highly labile. Moods come and go as fleetingly as summer showers and there is no close relationship between the prevailing mood of an hour, let us say, and what might be described as the most important personal events of that hour. The hysteric can be very angry, immensely pleased, very devoted, and very hostile in rapid succession. But if these dramatically extravagant emotions effect their purpose, that's the end of it. And I suppose that no other group of people show such amazingly sudden shifts in emotional address to other people as the very hysteric people do. This is in many ways a function of their formulated role, which is both much cruder and decidedly more spectacular than the formulated role that the rest of us try to live. The maturity of the motivational system is shown to be quite incomplete in the hysteric. The proportion of hysterics whose personality development has not progressed through preadolescence is, I surmise, quite notable. The relationship of the hysteric with other people is therefore never a relationship that amounts to love as I define it, and sometimes not even to intimacy in the sense in which I define it. Quite often there is a conspicuous predominance of the competitive motivation that has such prominence in the juvenile era, and the competition is often with members of the same sex.

Hysterics ordinarily have a rather bad time of marriage. But whether they advertise the bad side or the good side of it is a function of the particular moment in which one encounters them and, beyond that, is an index of the ease with which their morbidity is solving their problem. A markedly hysterical woman who has told her neighbors on every occasion what an idyllic home life she has, may, when encountered by one of these neighbors after a row with her husband, give an astonishingly different account of what a beast he is privately. Such a deviation from the usual account of the idyllic home life would not bother the consciousness of the hysteric particularly. She would provide herself with fairly crude loopholes, and return later to the prevailing mythology. And again, even when having a dreadful time, hysterics may for a short while be so swept by their euphoria that they give a divergent account to some neighbor; but again they provide themselves with fairly crude loopholes before returning to the conventionally unhappy state. The competition is, as it were, a competition in exaggeration. Nothing seems to irritate the prevailingly hysteric person so thoroughly as someone telling what cynical bystanders might call a better whopper. In other words, anyone who is more extravagant than the hysteric is the bane of the hysteric's life. And sometimes this competition gets the hysteric into singularly awkward positions with the calmer part of the community and leads to new hysterical symptoms to cope with the difficulties in interpersonal relations into which his competitive extravagance has led him.

The relationship with the more or less innocent bystander is more striking in the case of the hysteric than in any of the other entity types because so much goes on in words. And since language is a very important part of the culture which is built into all of us, the nonhysteric—or the not prevailingly hysteric—part of the community takes the verbal communications of the hysteric with a certain amount of seriousness and has to build up ideational processes of evaluation and dis-

counting with regard to them. Soon after the innocent bystander shows up for the first time, he is involved in a not
particularly realistic fashion in some more or less dramatic fantasy of the hysteric. So hysterics seem to inexperienced or
superficial people to be quite sociable, quite warm and out-
going. Hysterical women are particularly attractive to markedly schizoid young men as an improvement on obsessional
mothers and as the kind of people one would like to live with
for the rest of one's life. And since people who are schizoid
are relatively meek and disinclined to protest about tales thrust
upon them, a good many of them get themselves bound to
hysterics in holy wedlock. Then the schizoid husband has
something to do for quite a long time, and the hysterical wife
is no worse off than previously.

The sexual relations of the hysteric are often badly marred
by immaturity, and disorders arising from genital impulses are
so common that I think that accounts for the libido of orthodox psychoanalysis being indistinguishable from a generalized
lust. In looking for what is the trouble with the sex life, one
encounters the crudest expression of Oedipus survivals. It is in
this field that one would expect to find the woman who quite
cordially hates her mother and is all but obviously still very
devoted, very firmly attached, in fantasies to the father; and
one finds wives who frequently run off comparisons between
the husband and the father which are quite simply derogatory
of the husband. One also occasionally hears the hysterically
predisposed man make open, uncomplicated comparison between the woman he unfortunately married and his mother.
The notion of the Oedipus complex is therefore not at all difficult to maintain if one works with this type of material. As
another manifestation of that, one finds more open revolt
against the certainly prescribed role in life—that is, the sexual
role—in the hysteric than in any other group. In other words,
the hysteric woman can be a man in a homosexual relation
with an abandon which is scarcely conceivable in any other

type of human organization, and the hysterically predisposed man can act the woman with incomparable thoroughness and lack of cynicism.

Conversion Hysteria

The distinction between conversions and other hysteria is perhaps less important than one might think. The conversions are solutions of conflict by the utilization of some part of the somatic equipment—some part of the body—on very simple ideational grounds. For example, conversions are much simpler than the rather astounding way in which hypnosis may affect particularly suitable people, or the dynamics of such 'psycho-somatic' disturbances as neuro-circulatory asthenia or the peptic ulcer syndrome. The conversions are at the level of ideation which corresponds to the time when the hysterical type of disablement—the hysterical dynamism—was formed. In other words, the concepts of body structure are those of the juvenile —rather amateurish, rather young. So in this type of utilization of part of the body which occurs in the major hysterical entity, the disturbance follows this rather simple notion of body structure, and also a relatively simple notion of function. It only very rarely includes vasomotor disturbance and never, so far as I know, applies to any system as the system is actually organized physiologically.

Now, when there is this conversion, it performs a useful function; and that function occurs principally within the self-system—in other words, that is where one would look for the real meaning of it, rather than the patient's view of the meaning. There one discovers sometimes the almost juvenilely simple type of operation set up to profit from the disabling system. The patient will often tell you in the most transparent fashion: "If it were not for this malady then I could do ——" and what follows is really quite a grandiose appraisal of one's possibilities. The disability functions as a convenient tool for security operations. We know that under cover of the hysterical disorder the patient works out dramas that are rather blatantly expressive of what is in his mind, and we marvel sometimes at the prodigies of inattention by which no clue as to what is the source of the difficulty reaches his awareness. Here again, as in every aspect of hysteria, we see a peculiarly simple sort of caricature of what we encounter in the major dissociations. This aspect of hysteria—the inattention, the failure to develop referential processes, to think about details in the hysterical performance—is interesting chiefly in contrast to the refinements found in the major dissociative conditions.

Amnesia in the Hysteric

The distinction between real dissociation and an imitation of it is clearly seen in the thoroughness with which a whole course of life can be wiped out and highly desirable results be brought right into the hysteric's hands by means of amnesia. Dissociation just does not work that way. Amnesia as such is not evident in dissociation. The dissociated state is characterized by a profound disturbance of attention; but the hysteric, as was recognized very early in the history of modern psychiatry, suffers from amnesia. It is singular also that, in dissociation, any juggling of external events which would necessitate acceptance of the dissociated system by the self would probably lead to panic; in other words, this cannot be attempted. But an hysteric, under the same circumstances, abandons or shifts the symptom.

I shall illustrate this by a case on which I was called in as a consultant a few years ago. The patient, one of the many children of a steel worker, had some years before been taken under the wing of a well-to-do industrialist engineer and his wife. This couple were childless, and the patient had lived with them as practically—although not legally—an adopted son. He was then seventeen or eighteen years old.

The condition on which I was called in had come about following a minor accident in some sport event at school. As a result of the accident, he was clearly unconscious for two or three minutes; but there was no blood from the nose and no post-concussion headache. His foster mother was summoned and she took him home and called an internist. Almost immediately the patient developed a tremendous amnesia. He could not by any device be persuaded that he was in truth the child of this large family, didn't recognize the members of it, had no idea what his name was, and just couldn't remember large chunks of recent events. After a few days of this, the internist called me in on the case.

In seeing the patient, it was impossible to avoid the foster mother, and from her I learned a wealth of detail about a long, long relationship in which she had been decidedly the Lady Bountiful to this family and had gradually taken over their most attractive child. She pictured the foster father as being rather unsympathetic to this boy and particularly unsympathetic to his new mental disorder. There was enough obscurity and uncertainty in his wife's communication about the husband that I was glad to have a chance to interview him. He had made a good deal of money, and he had a fairly strong interest in the more frivolous aspects of life. His wife, in contrast, was something of a benefactress, and was busy with meetings and serious public affairs. The husband thought that she was in love with the boy, and he told me quite openly and not amiably— "I think she's gone on him." But he did not think that his wife had shown her interest in the boy clearly enough so that the boy knew about it—a surmise which seemed somewhat questionable to me.

I saw the boy himself quite a number of times, and he was very genial, very ingratiating in his manner. I traced out the limits of his amnesia, and they were wonderful. There wasn't anything that provided a convenient lead to the course of events that had led to his being practically adopted. I applied almost all the pressure I could to make anything in this tight system yield, with absolutely no results—only lots of transference in beautiful imitation of the psychoanalytic real thing. And, as usual, my problem was, Is there an element of schizophrenia in this thing? I had to dismiss this possibility, however, because of the patient's uniform suavity in defeating me and in leaving a large element of suffering, and so on, sort of free-floating. In other words, he handled the situation beautifully. Schizophrenics just aren't that way. They may be terribly able at analyzing, but they are rather wooden and clumsy or unduly tense in performance. This boy wasn't.

So finally I decided to arrange a piece of awkwardness for this patient that would make his disorder very expensive to maintain. The husband was willing to cooperate. And he was able to press his wife—because of his justifiable grievance about her devotion, I think—into fitting into the following plan: Since the boy had lost all recollection of the skills which he had acquired while living with her, he was left with the prospect of returning to a machine shop as an apprentice. So that was arranged—we turned on the economic and social heat. And lo! the boy had a miraculous recovery, late enough at night to wake up the whole household. He went shouting through the house his joy at having recovered his memory. Shortly after that he went away to school, and my latest report indicates that there has been no recurrence of the amnesia.

Treatment of Hysteria by Making the Symptoms Unpleasant

Many of the older forms of therapy with hysteria, in which the patient was permitted a role, were delightful, especially if the role was easy to get onto; but they failed to cure. Whenever the doctor began to get downhearted, the particular symptom which was oppressive at the moment would be cured, but unhappily with some residuals or some new symptoms. So the thing went on indefinitely at a fairly high level of entertainment for both the patient and the doctor. But during World War I the hysterical dynamism got a very severe jolt, when some not too profoundly philanthropic or, I think, profoundly clever psychiatrists discovered that hysterical disabilities can be dispelled by making them very unpleasant. That works. They started turning high voltage sporadic current on these poor unfortunates. Well, I am afraid that sporadic electricity permits only one role, namely, to know that it is extremely disagreeable. And some of our psychiatric colleagues vied with each other, with wonderful results, in figuring out what new forms of nuisance could be perpetrated on hysterics. On the basis of this general war experience, hysteria has for some time fallen off as a subject of much interest. But there are now, in a new and even more desolatingly disturbing and threatening world war, the terrifying necessities which drive people to whatever dynamisms they have at their disposal. And hysteria may thus again be a subject worth giving some thought to.

A View of Hysteria in Terms of the Pragmatic Utility of Clinical Entities

Surely, if one puts a patient into some abstract category, such as hysteria, it is much better to do this with a view to what it determines in one's actions as a therapist than merely for peace of mind or for some obscure reference to outcome. Here we need some fairly reasonable schematization of the psychiatrist's work to guide us. And the work of the psychiatrist can, for my purposes, be schematized by the following questions which I shall attempt to answer in terms of the clinical entity of hysteria.

(1) *What can you learn from the patient, and what difficulties, facilitations, and safeguards are relevant in that connection? What must you seek through collateral channels or by dint of interpretation of obscure comments from the patient?*

The psychiatrist can feel perfectly certain that he will hear very little from the hysteric which is not merely an exaggeration of the conventional cliches of interpersonal currency.

Thus, in contradistinction to the schizophrenic, whose speech is notoriously apt to include utterly uncommunicative autistic terms—private words—there is no special problem about the language of the hysteric. It can be taken for granted that what hysterics say means simply what almost anybody would mean if he said it. It is perhaps for this very reason that hysteria has such a curiously parental role to modern dynamic psychiatry. What hysterics said *could be* translated without any very careful assay of just what they meant. On the other hand, there is a good deal about the hysteric life that is represented most conspicuously by its omission from communication; that is, if one listens with reasonable attention to the communications of the patient, certain gaps in what one expects to be the experiences of average human life become conspicuous. This, again, does not require any intense scrutiny, but rather continued alertness. In connection with these missing elements of average life, one may expect certain fairly characteristic difficulties if one inquires. And these difficulties are to me rather startling in the simplicity of the so-called defense which the patient interposes. Again this lack of refined discrimination which suggests the fraudulent comes in, and one wonders whether the patient is perhaps lying or kidding, or whether he is actually as out of touch with that detail of life as the context shows. The fact is the latter. In the dramatic world in which hysterics play their roles, things are like somewhat undistinguished fiction, and there can be these gaps that are just a bit incredible. One has always to have in mind that hysteria is a very wonderful achievement in the sense that as long as it can be gotten by with, you might say, it solves rather serious conflicts with singularly little apparatus. Even though it looks as if the hysteric is kidding himself, he isn't. The symptom must be thought of as fairly simple in comparison with the symptoms found in other illnesses. So it is that the psychiatrist should approach the patient with certain realizations as to the pattern of communication. First, you must tone down in your own mind the extravagances of the patient, trying to think what is probable or what was probably observable by an innocent bystander, in terms of the events that the patient is reporting. Second: you must attend, without excitement or chagrin, to the curious gaps in personality that the hysteric's experiences, as reflected in his communications, show. And third: you must realize that any attempt to close these gaps is going to be countered by something that can be frankly provoking. It looks as if the patient is simply lying, evasive, without benefit of any respect for your personality.

The hysteric patient will be able to give an objectively valid statement of his attacks or of the way that the symptoms interfere with his life only after some quite novel relationships are set up—perhaps in an intensive psychoanalysis with powerful transference, or hypnosis, or something of that kind. This comes about, again, not because there is any intention to deceive, but because of the rather rudimentary character of the self-organization by which hysteria is maintained, making it impossible for the hysteric to have data of that kind. Such information about himself would make the maintenance of the disorder impossible, and so of course it cannot be obtained by any ordinary method. Thus it becomes important for the psychiatrist to look to collateral information.

In general the collateral information requires pumping. That is, the really understandable, unwittingly purposive affects of hysteric performances are shown only to those who will overlook the comparatively rudimentary nature of the hysteric personality. On the other hand, a person who questions the hysteric critically, who is obviously skeptical about the hysteric's *bona fides*, or anything of that kind, produces in the hysteric a mixture of the conventional hysterical business plus more or less random dramatizations, which is not particularly helpful data. So it is that any informant who has actually been there—who has suffered, if you please, the suffering of the patient—is unable to give the psychiatrist a penetrating analysis of what goes on. But nonetheless he will have the facts, and the psychiatrist can get through to them if he can avoid scaring up the informant's anxiety. That is, the informant who has really useful information will react badly to what is so hard for the psychiatrist to avoid, namely, giving some clear impression that the symptom is purposeful.

(2) *What extraordinary phenomena are to be expected from the patient? And to what extent is one to look to the dream life, and so on, for useful and usable data? Now, secondarily to this, What maneuvers will the patient engage in as parataxic evasions of therapeutic situations?*

Since the self of the hysteric is able to maintain security without a great deal of apparatus, it is to be expected that he may dream with relatively little disguise. Therefore, once the proper guarantees have appeared in the relationship of physician and patient, the dreams of the hysteric will provide significant material for the psychoanalytic procedure. From the standpoint of theory, there is no risk associated with the use of dreams in hysteria, in contrast to certain other conditions in which any encouragement of dream processes may, by disturbing the self, be disastrous both to the patient and to the treatment. The hysteric can, in case of need, make a very considerable shift in the field of symptomatology or in the nature of the disordered episodes in order to elude rejection by a critical person. Thus he is in no danger of a grave disturbance of the self. I would be greatly astonished to learn that any type of therapeutic intervention could precipitate panic in an hysteric. True, clumsiness and even many things that are not clumsy may precipitate lots of apparent anxiety. How much anxiety, it is always hard to say because part of the hysteric's structure is that if one has some anxiety, he might just as well have a great deal of it.

One expects almost any psychiatric approach to be productive of significant material in the hysteric. But the danger again is that the really significant material may be so conventionally reported that, although you get the inference you should get about it, this inference is of much stronger, greater significance than the reported material. And in one field, where the line between sleep and waking is less sharply drawn, one may have highly significant material that has only an obscure relevance and that requires interpretation the same as the dream does to become simply valid facts of personality. That is the realm of the personal mythology, if you please, or the preferred fantasies of the patient. It is not uncommon—in fact, this has been projected into all psychology, I think, out of some hysterics—to find in these patients carefully preserved continued stories from the earlier years, somewhat different from anything else I know of in psychology. We know that in the early juvenile era persons who by accident are rather isolated fill in the need for compeers with imaginary playmates, and that some of them carry on with the same imaginary playmates through long-continued courses of imaginary events. Well, this is inherent in the structure of human personality and guarantees nothing as to the outcome of the person from the standpoint of clinical entities. But the continued stories that the hysteric has carried on in spare moments, possibly at night in bed, involve real people—actual playmates and so on; and they have gone on well into the juvenile era and are reproduced apropos of alleged simple associations to dreams, or something of that kind, *as valid recollections from the past*. So the psychiatrist can find himself facing for weeks details from the patient about something which finally, with luck, is resolved into a continued story from the juvenile era.

In these continued stories—once one has caught on, which may take an awfully long time—one has no difficulty in separating the fictitious from the real. And the interesting thing from my own very limited experience is that the people who were, you might say, plucked from real contexts and used in continued stories apparently do not have to be particularly significant people in the real life history of the hysteric; they just happen to suit, in looks or something else, his particular necessity. A lot of effort addressed to solving that problem has convinced me that the actual people who had been borrowed and made over in fiction by the hysteric had been rather incidental in the development of his personality, however deceptively it might appear to be otherwise.

From this ease of dramatization, which characterizes not only the waking life—I mean, the behavior—and the revery processes in formative years but also the development of symptoms and so on, there has come about the notion that one very valuable armament of the physician is to have the patient make up a story or run off an imaginary situation. This notion appeared years ago under "the fantasy method of psychoanalysis," in which there is, I believe, very much more unconscious humor than was ever intended. But that is another characteristic of the patient, as you could infer from what I have said about the appearance of the symptom in my imaginary case. Properly motivated, the hysteric can produce rather sketchy, very dramatic daydreams at any stage in life, and these daydreams are ostensibly of use in therapy because they are almost transparent. But their transparency still probably doesn't make them particularly useful, for the fact remains that hysterics have stayed under treatment, even with fairly well-known psychoanalysts, for years and years and years.

Now what special problems can one anticipate? To me, the major problem of therapy with the hysteric is the extreme ease with which the therapist can make errors in judgment. As long as the psychiatrist comments to the patient on material which is not significant to the patient, there is an excellent opportunity for an elaborate cooperation which, aside from a certain lack of warmth, goes splendidly. And that reduces me to the verge of infant rage because I have to question *everything* minutely, and the game doesn't seem to be worth the candle. But I have learned from others that the same thing happens with them. Given an interpretation before there is sufficient data for a good interpretation, the patient is off with the physician on a course that is thrilling but unproductive. It finally pales out; there doesn't seem to be anything at the end of it. But by then one is so far from where one took this tangential departure that it is a long time getting back.

The very simplicity of the hysteric's language and experience is baffling in that everything means just what you would expect it to mean—only, of course, much of it doesn't, because much of it is just verbal. Much of it has been picked up bodily, you might say, from other people's experience and from stories and so on which hit the flair for dramatic presentation and may actually have been run off as reveries, as continued stories, in reasonably adult years. So for all you know you may be analyzing somebody else's experience for a while, and of course that isn't profitable. The comparative transparency of the dreams makes them, I think, very important in the psychotherapy of the hysteric. It is as if they were less susceptible to manipulation and therefore do actually function as something of a safeguard in the therapy. I should suppose that if the dreams show no reasonable relevance to what is being discussed in the so-called free associations, the chances are that the free associations are just filling up time; they are a magnificent ride on which the patient and doctor are taking each other. And for that reason I am rather inclined to think that the one place in psychiatry where considerable recourse to dreams is highly advantageous is with the hysteric patient.

Although the hysteric's flow of words may provide hazards for therapy, his freedom from entrapment in autistic language is his particular facilitation for therapy. The bane of working with schizophrenics and the greatest risk, the most recondite nuisance, I think, in working with obsessionals, is probably the fact that their experience has made some words mean things so far from anything that your experience has made them mean that you will fall into supposedly communicative interchange without talking about the same thing at all. It is almost necessary in the early stages with the schizophrenic to presume that you don't understand a thing the patient says. Gradually, of course, as you begin to find the limits of the more frequently used autistic terms, all that great caution and questioning of course becomes dispensable. Now this difficulty is probably at its lowest intensity with hysterics. The hysteric's language is apt to be fairly near the dictionary language.

The other facilitation in the hysteric is the fact that the psychiatrist can get at what simply can't be, which is a rather tremendously useful achievement. When you can tell a patient that in your experience things just don't work that way, and you are *right*, the patient has heard indirectly that psychiatry is really a reliable slant on life—a bit of news which cheers the patient especially when he is spending fifteen dollars an hour. Insofar as the dynamism with which one is dealing seems to be pretty definitely hysteric—which is not necessarily always the case even with the most outstandingly hysteric person—then if the thing goes way out of what a consensus of one's suburban neighbors would regard as human and reasonable, the psychiatrist is entitled to great skepticism about the patient's interpretation, often with considerable impression on the patient. That is just rather out of the patient's line. And skepticism about unusual explanations is almost bombproof, just so it is not as fraudulent an attitude on the part of the psychiatrist as many of the performances of the hysteric seem to be to the innocent bystander. In a good many patients—notoriously again, the obsessional who is apt to become schizophrenic—before the psychiatrist says what can't be, he wants to be quite sure that he understands what the patient has been telling him. Sometimes he will reach very bright ideas about what couldn't have been the case, only to discover that the patient was trying to tell him quite a different story which he just didn't follow. That, I should say, is no problem in dealing with persons properly classified under the clinical entity, hysteria.

(3) *What major changes are to be had in mind, and what is the most promising way of getting at them? In other words,*

what are to be regarded as the necessary achievements for great improvement? Note that here I am avoiding the term "cure," since I do not think it applies in the realm of personality.

The presence of the hysteric dynamism as the outstanding way of meeting difficulties in living seems to me to imply that the patient has missed a good deal of life which should have been undergone if he was to have a well-rounded personality with a rather impressively good prospect for the future. Because hysterics learn so early to get out of awkwardnesses and difficulties with a minimum of elaborate process, life has been just as they sound: singularly, extravagantly simple. And so, even if one could brush aside the pathogenic or pathologic mechanisms, one would have persons who are not at all well-suited to complex interpersonal environment. There they just haven't had the experience; they have missed out on an education that many other people have undergone. And under no circumstance could the therapist anticipate that such persons would become as intently observant, subtly discriminating, and perhaps analytically gifted as many a schizoid who has never had any psychotherapy. All the opportunities have been missed, you see; there hasn't been this development. So the therapeutic expectation has to be restricted—in the sense that one doesn't expect the hysteric to become a great student of human personality or something of that kind. The thing, therefore, that the psychiatrist would attach to the entity, hysteria, is that, insofar as the patient tends to seek his livelihood in a realm in which very acute discrimination and careful juggling of alternative hypotheses are necessary for outstanding success—that is a morbid movement which is to be choked off as best one can. And insofar as the patient tends to move, in the therapeutic process, toward a livelihood in which his relation with others is somewhat diagramatically simple, that is perfectly consonant with a movement toward mental health.

CHAPTER

12

Obsessionalism

I TRUST I have made clear how words—verbal propositions—come very early in a person's life to have rather astonishing power to handle some of the situations that are attended by anxiety. Now, if there were no correction of this faith in the power of the right remark, then perhaps the typical development would be the psychopathic personality who feels that if the right thing is said, everything has been done. But most people learn, soon after having been greatly impressed with the power of verbal propositions, that this power is a function of the person who hears the verbal proposition, that a thing perfectly useful with mother does not click so well with father, and that some things which are quite effective with both mother and father lead to anxiety when tried on the maiden aunt who has had some experience in educating children and sees that little Willie is becoming a rationalizer.

The type of situation which leads to this more complicated grasp on the utility of verbal propositions is rather roughly after the following pattern. The child finds himself in a variety of situations, all of which may be said to have in common that they are violations—that is, they collide with something that the child should know better about, should have learned. In these situations the child uses a verbal proposition, picked up from the speech around him, of course, which, although it works, does not work satisfactorily. That is, the parent is sufficiently affected so that the verbal proposition does prevent the descent of all the anxiety or punishment that would otherwise attend the violation; but the parent is at the same time affected rather unhappily, so that there is no boost in the child's euphoria, and there is even a little anxiety. It is as if the verbal proposition were powerful, but not quite powerful enough. Earlier, saying that you were sorry for stealing baby's bottle worked all right. But in these later appeals to verbal propositions, while you don't get spanked, still the significant adult is not too well pleased with the way things come out, although he doesn't know what to do about it; and so a generally mildly unpleasant situation continues. In fact, these verbal propositions that are not too successful and yet do not fail outright are verbal propositions that complicate the simple living of the parents.

To use an extreme caricature, let us say that little Willie has—accidentally, of course—dropped from an upstairs window a very ripe tomato on his mother, who is down on the ground outside hanging up some clothes to dry, and she is incensed and sputters. Little Willie, who certainly becomes somewhat of a genius at prevarication for the purposes of my illustration, says, "Oh, mother, I was so delighted to see you that my hand let go." Well, what will mother do then? Being hit with an overripe tomato is awfully hard to associate with the feeling of delight at seeing her. The situation is not resolved; he doesn't get thrashed, and she doesn't get satisfied, and his euphoria is not what it might have been—unless it is privately greatly elevated by her being hit with the tomato, which is irrelevant to my story.

Now, let us turn from this caricature to what actually happens in some homes: No matter what aggression anyone perpetrates on another—no matter what outrages the parents perpetrate on each other, or the elder siblings perpetrate on each other, on the parents, or on little Willie—there is always some worthy principle lying about to which appeal is made. And the fact that an appeal to an entirely contradictory principle was made 15 minutes earlier does not seem to disturb anybody. The members of a group like that might be called by unfeeling neighbors 'damned hypocrites.' Here is a situation where it has been found that it is better to have this limited verbal magic than the only other thing one could have—an awful lot of fairly open hostility and dislike and hatred.

In a good many homes of that sort, love was perhaps the only thing that was of no importance in establishing the marriage; convenience and all sorts of other things entered in. If one of the partners originally didn't have this business of appealing to ancient ethical principles to excuse all sorts of selfish, domineering, and self-seeking performances, he or she had learned it from the other before little Willie came along. So little Willie is denied the high educative value of learning that what works with mother is no good with father. He learns that a great many things do not quite work with anybody, and yet they are better than nothing; he is surrounded with them from birth, you might say, so quite clearly they are a part of the universe and he has to learn them. He does not have the high educative effect of sharp failure with verbal magic, which would impress upon him how important the hearer is in verbal operations; instead he has an unclear feeling that nothing works very well in this verbal field, or if things do occasionally work very well, they may not the next time. To the extent that verbal magical operations are better than nothing, he actually is inhibited from developing some of the most valuable aspects of verbal implicit operations. In particular, he is liable to bog down in any serious interpersonal problem in his developmental course by, as it were, concentrating on this half-satisfactory verbal magical business—the stuff that does not really save him from anxiety or boost his euphoria greatly but that does arrest severe anxiety and ward off punishment.

Perhaps I have not said enough about how the ethical tags that sort of embarrass one's parents in early childhood and inhibit more devastating punishment get to be 'interiorized'—to become the obsessional verbal magic used to allay anxiety, to ward off the feelings of guilt and shame which represent the critical evaluation in the self, and which can eventuate in such things as a queer kind of overconscientiousness. This may sound a good deal like 'introjection'—a term I have always boggled at. The self grows by learning techniques for, shall I say, removing threats of anxiety from the significant people. Actually, you cannot remove the threats, but at least you can anticipate them; you find a way of picking your way among the significant people so that you do not feel insecure very often. To do that, you have to have memory. And what is memory? Memory is a fragment of the real situation. If the person is a pretty good analyst—that is, if he has a pretty high intelligence quotient, so-called—then he remembers, in connection with the act that brought anxiety, the really relevant elements of the significant other person concerned. Then on future occasions when the person is about to move in the direction of the same sort of act, this recollection appears in the form of a feeling of unpleasant anticipation, which, in turn, comes to be called by the name of guilt, or shame, or what have you—all these names are simply tags. So if you wish, you can talk about the significant person having been introjected and becoming the superego, but I think you are apt to have mental indigestion.

When I have, often enough, turned a nut in the motor of my car the wrong way and put myself to an enormous amount of trouble retrieving the bolt which has fallen out and gotten under the car, then I get to where I recollect that the damn thing goes on clockwise. From then on, I turn it on clockwise instead of putting myself to a 50 per cent chance of having to do a lot of extra work because I can't remember which way to turn it when it is just beginning to take hold.

Recollections about significant people work in somewhat the same way, except that because they are so utterly of the very essence of avoiding insecurity, they naturally manifest themselves in this vast dynamism that we call the self. Sometimes in the fantasies of patients one comes across diagrammatic fragments, you might call them, of a significant person from many years before—the significant person is still there, and still acts in the fashion that was originally relevant. This sort of thing is a caricature, in a way, of the manner in which the surviving imprints of a past situation may act very suavely in interfering with an impulse.

If this process occurs outside awareness—in other words, where neither the person concerned nor anyone else would know about it—then we find that we have described something very significantly like sublimation. Thus the question may arise, what is the difference between sublimation and the obsessional operation? I think that the type of operations which we see as obstructions of impulse by what may be called "conscience," "self-criticism," or something of the kind, are of the same genre as sublimation, but differ from sublimation in that they are clumsy, uncomfortable, mildly disturbing performances. Sublimation is wonderful, if it is not overloaded; the obsessional operation, however, is never completely successful —there is always some insecurity. Aside from the fact that the situation which provoked the obsessional operation was one of insecurity, the very business of turning the energy into the obsessional dynamism consists in giving oneself a very mild jolt, a reminder that 'that doesn't work *because*,' which in turn means that you do not feel quite so secure as you did a moment before. But sublimation, where it works, is not only entirely satisfactory from the standpoint of the mental state of the sublimator; it also is generically very closely related to our successful social learning. Most of the social heritage that gets to be ours is acquired by something which, so far as I can see, is indistinguishable from sublimation—which can be, if you must get mechanical in your thinking, described as long-circuiting the impulses into socially approved paths of discharge. But the long-circuiting is not done within awareness; if it is, what you get is not sublimation at all. It is, instead, an obsessional state, if you get anything that works fairly well; otherwise it is simply a state of very severe anxiety.

Obsessional Neurosis as a Miscarriage of the Verbal Security Operations of Childhood

In describing the beginnings of the obsessional process, I have been trying to give you a rather abstract statement of what I believe to be the first principle in understanding the obsessional states. Prevailingly obsessional people are perhaps too easily dismissed as having recourse to verbal magic. Everyone has recourse to verbal magic occasionally, but some of us are lucky enough to learn the function of the other fellow in our magical feats, and so we confine our verbal magical effects to situations where they seem to be needed. As a result, we may become quite skillful at implicit operations with words which are the basis of successful communication of novel and complex states. The person who is prevailingly obsessional may be rather poor at verbal implicit operations that are an adequate basis for communication in the most troublesome, most difficult field of communication—namely, trying to get oneself across to someone or to get clear on somebody else. He is apt to meet all baffling interpersonal difficulties with a stream of verbal implicit process which has very little relevance and which is a continuation, as a security device, of this not very satisfactory business that characterized the home. It is almost as if the child had learned that you have to have certain things in your mind before you do certain other things —you have to be perfectly ready to spring this hokum if anything backfires. So getting the hokum ready first is just ordinary good sense. And later on, when he gets rather badly baffled in his progression toward adulthood, the hokum takes over, you might say, whenever the bafflement would greatly reduce what security there is—in other words, whenever the bafflement would lead to an acute feeling of anxiety and insufficiency and so on.

The translation from the early, more or less caricatured, picture that I have given you to the full-blown thing is always a matter of very rich detail, which will prove to be there if the psychiatrist has the time and the opportunity to work with it. In other words, I think that the relevance of this consideration I have been discussing can be found in each case, although the niceties by which particular obsessional contents come to be important are as numerous as those contents themselves. Almost anything conceivable can determine that an obsessional person thinks so-and-so under such-and-such circumstances—I am speaking of the content of his thought. The notion that, by thinking this, he magically achieves security is extravagant. He does not. Obsessional people are definitely insecure. But any obsessional neurotic whom you can get to talk at all will tell you that he would feel ever so much less secure without the obsessional content; and that is so even when, instead of merely verbal implicit operations which can be expressed, whole rituals of activity are concerned. Such operations do not give any omnipotence at all, but they do prevent intense insecurity.

As I have already said, this is a business wholly of the self. It has to do with interpersonal security; it has nothing to do with the satisfaction of the impulses that do not require the intervention of the self, and it complicates them only insofar as they may have been made sources of insecurity, as sex usually has. Nearly everybody is made more or less insecure about his lust in the process of getting socialized, and so, in an obsessional neurotic, the field of lust is almost always badly complicated by obsessional ritualistic things. But that does not produce impotence or frigidity, by any means, and it does not, for that matter, seem to have very much effect on how much lust is in experience. It is the field of security which is concerned; and so, in a prevailingly sexual situation, the obsessional person provides a lot of nuisance for the other person in connection with his security needs, but is relatively free so far as the actual genital cooperation is concerned. The satisfactions of obsessional neurotics—the elaboration of dynamisms for the securing of satisfactions—are often almost painfully simple; obsessional neurotics are quite direct in some things that most of us have to develop complexities about. Their security with other people is—you might almost say, by definition of their early home situation—scarcely ever likely to be perfect. They are never very secure, and they have little of anything to give them the idea that such a thing is possible. In other words, their acquaintance with the milder degrees of anxiety is immense. But aside from the fact that anybody, from the newsboy to the mayor of the city, can be a nuisance to them—and, I might add, vice versa—they go about eating and sleeping and drinking and having sexual intercourse with sometimes rather crude directness.

Now, since I am trying to talk about clinical entities, I suppose I ought to talk about when one is justified clinically in saying that a given patient is a case of obsessional neurosis, instead of talking about people of prevailingly obsessional personality, as I am much more apt to do. If one is to find a criterion, it has to be in the realm where the great disturbance is—the security in relations with others. It will be the expression of the degree to which interpersonal relations are attended by these milder grades of anxiety that call out the obsessional content. I would say that a person may perhaps best be described as prevailingly obsessional who does not impress ordinarily intelligent, reasonably observant people he comes in contact with as being at all odd or queer or anything of the sort, but who shows, with the people he is *chronically* integrated with, a definitely obsessional stickiness. But a person who gets into this obsessional stickiness with *anybody* who attempts to have any type of even slightly meaningful contact with him is an obsessional neurotic. In other words, a person can probably be called an obsessional neurotic if he cannot enter into any actually meaningful relations with a stranger without obtruding into an otherwise presumably informative, communicative situation the sort of thing which I think, perhaps, is best described as the stickiness which is caused by obsessional preoccupation.

Now what is this stickiness? A prototype of the general type of nuisance I am speaking of is the stutterer, who makes use of verbal behavior—or misbehavior—not for communication but for defiance and domination. The stutterer, perhaps because you have been so reckless as to ask a question, sets out to answer it, and the most conspicuous thing—to me, at least —that happens thereafter is that time passes with the most shocking disregard of either his life or yours. A tremendous amount of effort is made and, along with this effort, in case you try to go away or to help out, almost a compulsion is exercised on you to stick around until finally you have your information—if you can live that long. Thus people with speech disorders are quite adhesive, once you have been reckless enough to apply yourself to them. An almost identical process occurs with the obsessional.

There are times when obsessionals are fully as maddening as any stutterer, for the value of time seems scarcely to be within their grasp unless a matter that has life or death importance to them is concerned. For example, let us say that you have some very important person on the other end of the telephone line waiting for a certain piece of information, which you have to get out of your obsessional secretary. If you can prevent yourself from having a stroke first, you will have the information by the time she gets through talking. But there is simply no way of hurrying it; and if you try to hurry it, you convert her into a mass of jitters which closes off everything. So there is no way you can win in a frontal attack on obsessional obstruction. And the reason is not so recondite when you think of it from the standpoint of the self and the enemy without—that is, acute anxiety. Acute anxiety, which is what you can precipitate by sufficiently adroit brutality, is much worse than the tension that the secretary suffers in you just as much as you suffer it in yourself, you might say. But that is the life of the obsessional in a great many contacts with other people. He isn't happy; he isn't secure; he is really so obviously at the mercy of one thing or another that he is definitely a little anxious. And the more anxious he gets, the more he resorts to the obsessional magical verbal symbolic operations in lieu of simple communicative propositions, which seem always to be dangerous compared with the other.

The Source of Anxiety in the Obsessional Neurotic

Now, what is the danger that these people are warding off? They are warding off and will eternally be warding off—until they are cured, if they are fortunate—a type of inadequate self-function which their self, you might say, began with and will forever stay with unless given help. *The obsessional neurotic has never had the satisfaction of outstanding success in interpersonal relations.* I think that much of the difficulty, even for psychiatrists, in dealing with obsessional processes arises from the incapability of grasping that fact. It is not an obvious fact, for the obsessional neurotic is not, for example, unutterably jittery, intensely anxious, and obviously a creature of profound inferiority feelings, nor is he blown up with paranoid grandeur as a mask for his feeling of unworthiness. His self-system has functioned to avoid a great deal of severe anxiety that he knows from experience he could suffer, and, as it were, to maintain a low level of well-being or, to put it another way, a very mild state of anxiety which is a background to some very vivid satisfactions. In other words, his self-function is rather poor; but poor as it may be, it is still an extremely valuable self-function. By and large, only people who are involved as necessary to the satisfactions of an obsessional neurotic can unhorse him. That is, the obsessional experiences severe anxiety only when the other person involved is of real significance, occasionally because of anticipated satisfactions, but more generally because of past satisfactions with that person.

For example, a person who is quite important to the obsessional neurotic as a source of satisfaction—let us say, the perfect genital mate—may begin to find fault with the obsessional, not in the genital field, but in much less dramatic but more time-consuming areas of the relationship. That conveys a threat—it is in itself a source of insecurity. Any intelligent person is apt to think, "Well, if I don't do something about this, I'll lose this perfect mate." But that is not the way the obsessional handles his insecurity. And so, as the mate—the wife, let us say—starts to wonder why, in order to enjoy twenty minutes out of twenty-four hours, she has to be sort of wrapped up in sticky flypaper several hours a day, then the obsessionalism gets thicker. That is, this tendency to question—which is clearly addressed against the self of the obsessional—can be experienced by him only as a singular wrongheadedness on the wife's part. Instead of calling out valuable, useful analytic and synthetic operations as to the real situation, it calls out these frustrating, because magical, performances.

I suppose that when you get two rather obsessional people together, whichever one consults the psychiatrist first will put it in nearly these words: "Well, the longer we go on together, the more crotchety and difficult so-and-so is getting." And the crotchety and difficult part proves to be that, as they grow insecure about their relationship, they get to pestering each other more and more in what sometimes seems to be a never-ending effort to, in some obscure fashion, get the other person down. And yet the one does not want to get the other down in order to lift himself by standing on the other's fallen body or anything like that; instead, each one wants to overcome the other's power to produce anxiety—to make the other fellow impotent to produce anxiety. Incidentally, to make the mate sexually impotent would be a dreadful misfortune to an obsessional neurotic, and it is that very dreadful misfortune that sometimes does encompass him and brings him to the psychiatrist; the wonderfully satisfactory mate, after more and more obscure dissatisfaction, becomes impotent. In some ways I think that that is a simple therapeutic movement on the part of the mate because, once he is impotent, it would seem that perhaps the principal significance would be gone out of the relationship so that he could presently escape without causing more than a ripple on the surface of things. But it doesn't work out that simply. It takes some pretty clear referential process to be through with such a relationship, and the obsessional neurotic is not capable of very clear referential operations about personal relations. Moreover, the self-operation by obsessional dynamics is essentially weak. The obsessional neurotic does not actually achieve omnipotence by the use of certain words, as some really virtuous people do when they say, "It is God's will"—and you know that anything you might have to offer in reply has become less relevant than the other side of the moon. Or another type of person may say, "My conscience dictates . . ." and that is final. Those things are not obsessional, you see; they work. But while the obsessional operation works, it does not work very well; it is no guaranteed buckler. Even if it never fails, it never produces euphoria; there is always the low-grade anxiety which in one sense is a statement of the inadequate self-function and in another sense is an inevitable consequence of the whole evolution of the self.

Thus, under therapy, the obsessional neurotic actually goes through the motions of operations that look as if he is getting absolutely panicky at the prospect of having something formulated clearly in the realm of his personal problems. But since one might be misled by certain implications of this statement, let me put it in another way. As the motivational pattern becomes more and more difficult to disguise by security operations, it takes on an aspect of novelty and crosses the line into the region of fear. This is true regardless of what the motivational pattern is about—whether it is something which anybody would be ashamed to discover in himself or whether it is something that is unworthy in only the most obscure way or even actually quite estimable. As I have already said, there is a degree of novelty that frightens all living creatures, although the limit varies from person to person and from species to species. And so, as the set of the therapeutic situation gets such that almost clear referential processes appear in the consciousness of the obsessional neurotic, and the doctor is about ready to make the fatal statement which the obsessional cannot forget or obscure any more because it is clear, the state of the patient is very bad. And I have often suspected that it is far more a state of fear than of anxiety. Sometimes the patient shows quite frankly a tendency to engage in random activity —almost circus movements of starting to get up and then lying down on the couch, and so on. Now these movements are not used to fight off an interpretation, however cleverly the patient will do things which make it difficult for you to say what you are attempting to say. Instead, they are designed simply to arrest process; and insofar as you happen to be part of the process, you may say they are in opposition to you—an attempt to prevent your doing something. What occasions the movements is a pretty deep type of mental state which we all experience if we hit anything that is strange enough to reach the threshold of fear. But when this business is over, the obsessional may see a lucid, really adequate formulation of something that is valid about him and his interpersonal relations —and that is improvement. To that extent, he has moved out of a realm of obsessional operation into clarity, and to that extent progress has actually been accomplished. To that extent his interpersonal relations become less complicated and less uniformly, if obscurely, frustrating to his partner.

Therapeutic Problems Posed By
Obsessional Miscommunication

The obsessional process can, if it is applied to enough of life, produce something that sounds very reasonable if one doesn't try to find out what is really being said and what it refers to in terms of obsessional operations. In illustration, I shall consider some fragments from a patient's history as reported to me. This man is clearly a person of very considerable gifts, and does rather well when he is not mentally disturbed. As I heard the development of the case, it occurred to me that the thing which is called his mental disorder is an intense restlessness which occasionally simply takes him over and drives him around in circles so that he is, at times, almost reduced to wringing his hands. But the thing that seems to stand out is that from quite early in life this man has fixed everything by a mild, rather inconspicuous use of the obsessional process. Even his social rituals have become somewhat obsessive, and also somewhat good. He is a good husband and father. He has a perfectly wonderful domestic life—as uneventful, as featureless as a drop of mercury—which gives the impression of really remarkable normality, both to the patient and to the person who hears it. There is scarcely a thing he says that does not sound all right. According to his report, he and his wife are very happy in the sexual relationship, and their interests more or less overlap. There is a curious grace note of rather striking promiscuity at times on his part, but it doesn't mean anything—everybody does it among his friends, and one simply has to fit in so as not to look different.

The thing that struck me in all this was that things had gone so simply that it could not be so. It was like a juvenile fantasy —a fantasy of a badly harassed juvenile who has finally pictured a nice quiet life for himself. And apparently this man has a nice quiet life except for the recurrent eruptions of his intense restlessness, which is so marked that it has disturbed various psychiatrists, who have made various diagnoses and attempted various treatments.

The outstanding thing about this man is the thoroughness with which he has substituted, over a vast field, somewhat meaningless thinking about life in the sense of definitely not simply communicative thinking. And it sounds very good if you do not look closely at it. Most vulnerable, I think, in his own picture of his life is the richness of the relationship of the husband and wife. This part of the picture seems utterly incredible to me, for I have heard nothing, except the patient's bare statement, which suggests this. In fact, there is evidence that they have quite separate fields of interests, and I surmise that the wife's interest is practically reduced to the children. Sex, of course, traditionally reflects all personality problems, but I doubt that anything is to be gained in this case by attacking this; the episodes of promiscuity are not episodes in the mental sense, I think, but are responses to environmental facility. And I do not think there is going to be anything of psychiatric significance to be found in studying the genital relationship of husband and wife.

But what I am getting at is that the obsessional's verbal operations, however autistic his words may be, can give a highly plausible effect.

And particularly, in struggling with the treatment of the obsessional neurotic, you are ground down by the fact that you never get anything quite right; and that becomes more and more conspicuous as you close in on a really correct interpretation of some persistent trouble in the patient's life. The case I always use to illustrate this was a woman patient of mine. She and another woman, both of them markedly obsessional, lived together. My patient had been cuffed around frightfully by a socially preeminent mother; in this, her history was quite different from that of the other woman, who had, in fact, been exploited by a socially inferior mother. As a result, there was a very striking difference in what you might describe as the hostile operations these two women engaged in. The first one, my patient, who had been walked on by her mother for many, many years, would get her feelings hurt and go off, the tears just beginning to run down her cheeks. That was about the most devastating thing she did. The other one, on the other hand, would say mercilessly cutting things that were terribly hard to forgive for weeks afterwards. But although there was this striking difference, the type of operation they both used toward significant people and toward each other was prevailingly obsessional. The fact that the companion was also obsessional finally became clear to me, and it also became apparent that the data I heard could most plausibly be interpreted as showing that these women were engaged in what was, in some ways, a microcosmic drama of a very spectacular kind. It was a battle for prestige between the two of them, conducted by the indirect, substitutive methods of the obsessional pursuit of security.

The point I want to make is what happened whenever my patient and I approached clarity about her situation. Any little context I attempted to pick up proved to be somewhat "misunderstood" by me. Incidentally, I frequently deal with very small contexts, for unless I am certain that the patient's attention span will hold what I am trying to get him to look at, I may expect to be defeated. So I pick up little things that are very revealing and work them to death. But in this case, whenever I attempted to pick up some little thing, it soon developed that I had not quite understood it. There were always additional details which hadn't been mentioned before, which made it very difficult to be clear on what I was trying to illustrate. My contexts never stuck together long enough. And it wasn't that my patient had earlier failed to say something which now, when she added it, gave an entirely different color to the picture. Not at all. It was just that as soon as I mentioned that I thought we could look at this particular context, my patient would add a new clause to the thing which made it much harder to be quite clear on just what I was attempting to talk about. There was no great change in the meaning of the thing; the reality had not been distorted at all by the omission of this clause; but it was just that an additional consideration was crowded in at the most awkward point so that the clarity of the whole thing disappeared. It was as a result of such experiences that I developed the statement I used to make to obsessionals, "Now we let the fog in." This patient and I had a very rough time in reaching a consensus about the possibility that there was a struggle going on between the other girl and her in which each was trying to force respect from the other.

Now the way in which part of this dilemma was resolved is no credit to me particularly. In actuality, the patient's unconscious and an accidental happening outgeneraled her finally—I couldn't. One very hot summer day she got out of my office without bursting into tears or anything, got resolutely into her car and, as she frequently did, nearly ran over a few traffic policemen. That was her outdoor sport; the more disturbed she was when she left me, the more menace she was to the traffic cops; she never did run one down, but she gave a number of them shocks. As she drove toward the apartment hotel where she lived, she got to thinking about the guests that would be at their place and about how hot it was and how nice it would be up on the roof garden—she was almost certain that that was where the guests would be. She decided that she would come in very quietly, rush into the apartment and take them up some nice cold drinks as she went to greet them. But as she dashed into the apartment, she discovered her companion walking toward the kitchen door, bent on an apparently similar errand. In her hurry to get to the kitchen first, the patient collided with her companion in the very doorway. Since my patient was a woman of some bulk, I can imagine the horse-power exerted in this encounter. They glared at each other and then burst out laughing—an unprecedented event in this relationship. Now I can only suggest that our long struggle with the problem had some slight connection with the particular settling of the event—but the event itself was unpredictable and fortuitous. It does take something like that, after a long preliminary acquaintance between therapist and patient, for the obsessional neurotic to drop some of the complex operations which are as frustrating to him as to anybody else—except that he is so used to frustration that it doesn't disturb him as much.

Another patient wanders into my mind—a sad and curious case of a woman 45 years old, who was seen by her physician in a very disturbed state, according to report, and was referred by him to a psychiatrist colleague of mine to be tided over the emergency. However, the emergency really seemed to be one of the most chronic features of her life. She was of a fairly successful professional family, with a curiously incongruous but very successful mother who had spent a good deal of her life as an invalid, but who had maintained a very active interest in the music world and one thing and another even during her invalidism. The patient had made an extremely successful marriage at the age of 25. Five years later, she became greatly enamored of another man—a musician who was an alcoholic—and it was a fairly open business, as a result of which the husband divorced her and got custody of the children. She went to Mexico and found another alcoholic and, not long after that, still another alcoholic. This last one wasn't really very alcoholic and actually was a very good architect, and presently they were married. Fifteen years later, under a certain amount of needling from her, he got a big contract in China; and he couldn't take her with him, so that was the emergency that my colleague was to tide her over.

My colleague had not the faintest thought of there being anything obsessional in the business of her marriages, but the thing that had struck him was that he could not keep the woman on any topic that *he* felt needed exploring. She always knew what she wanted to talk about, and to anything that he tried to bring up, she would say, "Yes, of course, but . . ." and be right back on her problem. And that, in its way, is a manifestation of what may be simply the obsessional business again. The obsessional is secure as long as he is engaged in some explicit or implicit verbal operation which is apparently communicative, but is actually uncommunicative because it is somewhat too autistic. Thrusts from the environment which attempt to interest him in some other aspect of reality are de-natured as quickly as possible, and he is back on his preoccupation. And the listener may be quite completely misled as to what is really being discussed.

I have mentioned these cases to suggest some of the manifestations of this obsessional business. In discussing the beginning of obsessional distortion, I spoke of the very highly autistic type of operation in which one has a little ethical tag which seems to be wonderfully effective at blocking or frustrating everything—both others and oneself, but others a little more than oneself, so that one has a feeling of a certain power in the thing. And there are other obsessional operations which look like awfully well-directed, well-adjusted seeking of advice, depicting of a problem for study, and so on, which are actually uncommunicative and in fact chiefly purposed to maintain such security as there is. But despite the great number of manifestations, the uniform characteristic is that while the obsessional operation sounds pretty good, it actually does not communicate—or rather, it miscommunicates, misinforms, and misdirects attention.

I think that the nosological distinction, if you must have one, between the markedly obsessional personality and the seriously disturbed obsessional neurotic—the person who would unquestionably be diagnosed by reasonably competent psychiatrists as an obsessional—lies mainly in the success of the obsessional processes. If these processes are rather successful, so that the person very rarely encounters acute and severe anxiety, then he is an obsessional personality.[1] But if, on the other hand, they have been much less successful, then the person's security at best is so tenuous that he is awfully busy, all the time when he is in significant interpersonal contacts, going through his rituals to protect it. He doesn't have time to adjust these rituals to all the nuances that come very easily to the obsessional personality; instead, he becomes very rigid in his adherence to certain magic formulae which may sound as if they referred to something, only you cannot find out what. By translation, as it were, these obsessional formulae can be reduced to a ritualistic type of behavior so that actually the communicative possibility, you might say, becomes nil. Inquiring of the person about his compulsive rituals proves rather futile, for he cannot tell you anything about them. All that usually appears in the consciousness of the person who has a compulsive ritual is simply that he does it because he feels better when he does it; if he doesn't do it, then he gets nervous. Not doing it disturbs his mind and so on, and so he does it for peace of mind. And it is hard to get any further with him.

Thus with a patient who makes prevailing use of obsessional

[1] Incidentally, some fairly useful traits are almost necessarily associated with insecurities that begin as early as the obsessional processes do and that are never either more crippling or more remedial than they are. For example, obsessional people frequently develop considerable skill at technical operations of a good deal of complexity and a good deal of economic value—skills which perhaps a person who had no such insecurities and who found other people wholly delightful or even moderately delightful would not have been interested enough in to develop. Thus obsessional people are quite often useful to have around. At least they can be if only you are able, in some way or other, to get them to function without engaging in their security operations with you in and out of season.

processes there is a certain prognostic and prospective element in noticing the extent to which these processes fit fairly readily into the given context of quasi-communication or the extent to which they are autistic and blankly uncommunicative. The more profoundly autistic and uncommunicative they are, the more extreme will be the difficulty of unraveling them. Thus one has to be guarded in one's optimism about the outcome in treating the so-called compulsive neurotic—the person who has a great many rituals that have to be gone through rigidly in the course of a day.

For a long time, one of the outstanding diagnoses in this field was mysophobia, the fear of dirt. But, and this is the joker, quite often the people alleged to suffer mysophobia had no conscious experience of mysophobia. The person with mysophobia had to wash his hands in and out of season. Sure, he would agree with you that he may have gotten germs on them or something. But, actually, what was terribly present in his mental state was nothing about germs; it was *the hands must be washed*. And all the reference to a fear of dirt and so on may have been historically true in every case, but it was far from the obvious mental state in some of these people.

And even if it is a fear of dirt that underlies this compulsion of washing the hands, the patient may no longer know that that is the case; and the psychiatrist is faced with the problem: How do you begin? The fact that some piece of gross behavior seems extremely meaningful to you does not mean that it is easy to start unraveling the personality by dealing with it. The patient may politely agree with you about the meaning that you read into it, but it is nevertheless quite possible that you are wrong. And even if your interpretation is right, there will still be a few details that you cannot possibly guess, and they are likely to be the very details which would make the relevance of your correct interpretation clear to the patient. As long as you do not have those, the patient can continue quite secure and unchanged. Thus details make a great deal of difference in whether a patient does recall an experience you feel certain must have been there. And so, whether I am dealing with obsessional neurotics or any other patients, when I feel it necessary to investigate something of this sort, I may say, "Well, this sounds to me very much as if you had had somewhat the following experience at some time." And then I repeat my picture of the experience two or three times and finally say, "Now I know that that isn't what you've had, but it is something like that, and maybe that will in some fashion facilitate recall."

THE OBSESSIONAL'S DOUBTS AS UNPRODUCTIVE AREAS FOR THERAPEUTIC INVESTIGATION

So far I have not given any attention to doubt, but it deserves some consideration because it is the outstanding feature of many people's unhappiness that brings them to psychiatrists. Its importance as a problem does not hit me as forcibly as it might for two reasons: first, because the doubters, when they actually have been reckless enough to commit themselves to treatment, soon cease to manifest doubt but instead manifest more classical obsessional processes; and, second, because I am very much impressed with the alertness and, you might say, the skill with which typically obsessional people delete certainty. Since certainty is a menace to them, it seems rather strange that the symptom they allegedly suffer from in many cases is dreadful indecision and doubt. I think that the obsessional neurotic prefers to be uncertain about a great many things because the static character of the obsessional neurosis is largely maintained by unclearness about anything that is so oppressively evident that he cannot treat it with selective inattention. Moreover, in some cases where doubts and indecisions are alleged to be the problem, it has seemed to me as if the patient had, at some time or other, hit upon the fact that a tremendous amount of misery about doubts is one of the most completely baffling things the environment can encounter.

The obsessional, in effect, asks the other people in his environment to solve his doubts—to advise him. And presenting other people with an opportunity to advise works very neatly. This is so because Americans, being among the world's most insecure people so far as close approaches to intimacy are concerned, are also the most ready to advise without a moment's hesitation; for if you start handing out advice, you don't have to get any closer—you immediately begin disposing of the situation rapidly. Thus it is almost as if the obsessional puts most of the work of his neurosis on the environment. All he has to do is to maintain the most unhappy inability to become convinced, and other people just rattle on with no effort on his part—which strikes me as economical. I think I have come to this conclusion, which may be just a satirical misinterpretation of this morbid doubt business, because people who have come to me for morbid doubts have quite soon gotten into struggles of the classical obsessional kind with me. Every now and then, as I listen to this headache of considerations that cancel each other out and leave everything just wobbly, I ask, at what is calculated to be a quite disconcerting time, "Well, why the enormous harassment about it? What difference does it make which is right?" On such occasions it sometimes becomes plain that these doubts are transparently bunk—they are not of any particularly great importance in the context in which they have been produced. What has happened is that the patient has simply been careless. In fact, you will discover that every obsessional, if you watch him closely in a familiar situation, can become awfully careless. I think the thing is so exhausting and so monotonous that he gets careless from fatigue. Thus on such occasions as the one I have described, he has been too careless to have a really valid doubt. And that is very disconcerting, for the whole thing has miscarried and he has wasted his time and mine on piffle. That is very hard on him; his prestige is shattered, and he is intensely insecure.

Thus I think that we do not learn much about what may

otherwise be going on by regarding the doubts as a preoccupation—as an obsessional process in itself. I believe that it is a matter of seeing around the doubts to what the patient is doing, and then giving the doubting operation a few jolts on some occasion when it is running a bit wildly—that is, when it is rather clearly not suited to the situation or to me as a significant person. When I do this, the other business appears and takes the place of the doubting business—the wanting to be clear, you might say, the wanting to be correct, which is, I guess, the best statement the person himself could make of it; and the patient and I are then dealing with the classic obsessional business. From that sort of experience, I have come to think that doubting becomes a vivid part of the picture merely because it calls out so much work from the environment. It simply keeps other people busy so that they are not apt to attack the obsessional very much. Possibly—and this is a quite tentative formulation—it sometimes has the added merit that the other people make damn fools of themselves trying to help the obsessional with his doubts, and therefore his security is a little better.

Perhaps I should digress from the subject of obsessional doubts and mention another element of the larger picture—namely, what we see in the way of real, abiding uncertainties in people. These can be awfully harassing things—sometimes, I think, about as painful mental states as one can chronically have. But they are never expressed in frank doubts and so on. In a typical instance of this, it only gradually occurs to you that a particular patient must be eternally wondering whether he is "a boy or a girl"—where, in the masculinity-femininity distribution, he really belongs. Or perhaps his uncertainty is —as we often hear in classic theory—"Can I be loved? Can anybody love me? Am I not essentially unlovable?" But in such an instance, you hear no rattling off of doubts of the typical harassing, obsessional kind. The patient cannot confront these things clearly, even though he is always preoccupied with them. You fall over the thing in all sorts of subtle, indirect attempts which the patient is making at investigating his problem—and the characteristic of all these attempts is that the approach does not present the problem so clearly that the poor bird has to be aware of what is bothering him. He can't stand it, and yet he can't drop it because it has become involved in the whole structure of the future. Until this is settled, there is no peace, there is no happiness; there is always doubt —real doubt—and there is uncertainty, insecurity, sometimes suspicion, and always caution about what people mean and what their actions mean, and so on. Let us say that in treating one of those people, you finally, as a result of good luck and plenty of alertness, close in on a really probable hypothesis of what lots of little details refer to, and you say, for instance, "Look, are you unclear as to whether you are mostly a man or a woman?" The patient is likely to look at you as if at last somebody had opened the gates of paradise for a moment, and to say, "Yes, I think I have always been worried about that."

But this is a great contrast to what will happen if you close in on a probable hypothesis with an obsessional neurotic. As soon as you start anything of that sort, the obsessional practically gets up from the couch and throws it at you—he does almost anything to stop you from talking. He is warned immediately when there is a shift in you that means you finally have this thing so that he cannot escape it. He certainly makes it difficult for you to get it said, and when he has nonetheless heard it, there is anything but this great feeling of relief. There is usually anger, but there is also marked benefit. If he has really grown to feel fairly secure with the therapist, he is apt to say for weeks afterwards, "Oh this—that's my damn whatnot that you made me see," with diminishing anger and with increasing admiration for the fact that you have helped him to understand something. Incidentally, when I talk about closing in on a probable hypothesis, this does not mean, in my universe, that the psychiatrist is a detective sneaking around under the

Tarnhelm picking up clues. I am referring to interpersonal operations which gradually demarcate a field which is appearing to both participants. With the obsessional neurotic, the nearer you get to this significant field, the more excursions and circus movements there are on the part of the patient. But the other type of patient—the patient who actually has these horrible, usually almost contentless doubts which he cannot stand to state clearly—is vastly relieved by your interpretation. When you say the right thing and carefully gather together illustrative manifestations in which he has participated, it suddenly jells into utter conviction, and he feels, "Of course this is what has been harassing me all this time!" And then you have a problem which can be treated by the ordinary method of seeking roots for the uncertainty in the past.

I have never, however, been fortunate enough to track down a single historic root of any of the obsessional doubts—or at least I have never been able to track down anything that I could conceive of as being meaningful to the patient, and I just do not believe that you can do things that are utterly irrelevant to the patient; he simply will not take it. In other words, real doubts—the kind of grinding uncertainties that poison many a life—refer to highly significant and unintegrated experiences that cast great uncertainty on something which seems to be essential, whereas the particular thoughts and considerations that get themselves made into problems for the obsessional are merely little tools that he picks up as he goes along. I think that tracking them to their source would really be perfectionist investigation; and anyway it couldn't be done—the patient wouldn't cooperate. Thus I do not have any sympathy with ultra-refined interpretations of the particular verbal content of the obsessional or the particular behavioristic pattern of a ritualistic gesture, and so on. Sure, it means something; sure, it is autistic—which means that you cannot see the meaning very readily—and what of it? It is not used to communicate; it is used to obstruct, to protect. And therefore why should one presume that it is relevant to attack it on the basis of seeking its original meaning? I do not see that there is any necessary evolution from an originally meaningful context.

Tic-like movements and automatisms, on the other hand, represent necessary action to maintain a dissociated system. It may be very difficult indeed to get an automatism to unfold into what it stands for, but it does stand for something, and something very important. But even though an automatism has a significant meaning, I do not believe that an attack on its origins is necessarily the easiest way to get at what you are after; for I have sometimes found, in treating obsessional schizoid people who had automatisms, that as we cleared up certain of the patient's problems, the origin of the automatism would become clear, quite without my ever thinking that it was happening. Or at least the origin would become clear to the patient; he would report wonderful and sometimes immature types of thinking which were to him an adequate explanation of the automatism, even though they were not very meaningful to another person. In other words, such things as automatisms are built by types of implicit activity that are pretty young, so far as our ordinary acquaintance with them is concerned.

This is rather like what once happened with one of my patients who was part of the time rather definitely schizophrenic. Among the things which were a nuisance to him, and which I heard about at intervals for years, was the feeling that something—not a fluid, not a stream, but something—went down his leg into the earth. It was essential that, when this happened, his foot should be in contact with the ground or the pavement or something else that stood for earth. Thus the arrival somewhere of whatever it was that went down his leg seemed to be a part of this nuisance. We worked up a lot of obscure business about his mother's relations with him and his brother, which could have been beautifully interpreted as her attempt to castrate her boys, but I do not know what difference such a statement would have made to the patient. He puttered around in very early material about the mother's getting her boys tucked into bed, and—in some fashion never quite clearly recalled—communicating to them that their hands might well be distributed so that they were a reasonable distance from the genitals. It was all very hard to recall and pretty subtle; but it was awfully meaningful. Then he startled me one day by saying, "Well, you know, I think I have at last come to understand this obscure thing that I've told you, about something going down my leg." And I think he did. I didn't understand it; nor did I ever hear anything that clearly explained it to me.

The Obsessional Neurosis and Schizophrenia

The grave complication which can occur in an obsessional neurosis is that it may progress into schizophrenia. I think that there is a fairly easy transition from the one state to the other. Although it is not by any means a usual progression, it does happen occasionally rather late in life. For instance, years ago I had as a patient an internist who had been an obsessional neurotic for some 12 or 13 years, and who was getting worse— that is, more tied up with the rituals and compulsions that complicated his living. Finally he got to the point where his office began to be extraordinarily untidy and his practice declined. He couldn't keep himself clean, and his office and equipment were obviously getting no sanitary attention. Then he was admitted to the hospital, still under the diagnosis of obsessional neurosis; but by then it was not awfully hard to scare up frankly schizophrenic content, and he progressed into a deep dilapidation.

I am reminded of another patient who had what would be diagnosed psychoanalytically as a compulsion neurosis—an obsessional state with much ritualization of behavior. The outstanding feature of his fear was that he would be contaminated by encountering feces. His behavior quite early in his hospital stay came to be marked by his frequently getting into the men's toilet in any way that he could, and alternating between washing the skin off his hands and standing under an exposed soil pipe—in other words, standing where there was the greatest possible opportunity, if there was any leakage, for him to be contaminated with fecal matter. That patient had become quite obviously schizophrenic, and he moved swiftly into the hebephrenic category. Not long after, an acute miliary tuberculosis set in and he died with startling speed.

Thus schizophrenia does, at least occasionally, appear as a complication in the obsessional neurosis. The question might then be raised whether the obsessional neurosis which progresses into a grave schizophrenia is a typical and true obsessional neurosis. My own observations, based on a rather keen interest in schizophrenia and a somewhat more superficial interest in the obsessional neurosis, suggest that there is no particular difference between the obsessional neurosis which progresses into schizophrenia and the one that does not. I have not seen anything that distinguished such patients as the two I have mentioned, before they progressed into schizophrenia, from other pretty severe obsessional neurotics who did not show such progression, and who in some instances actually improved.

Whether a progression toward schizophrenia seems likely has an important bearing on my attitude toward suicide in the obsessional. Fear of committing suicide is sometimes one of the really impressive fears or phobias in the presenting picture of an obsessional neurotic. As soon as I have convinced myself that there is a pretty stable obsessional state rather than an indefinite obsessional schizoid condition, it is my practice to treat this fear very roughly—to just assume that there is practically no danger. This is partly a derivative of my feeling that to take such a thing seriously is a collaboration in the psychosis, you might say, and that it is never very profitable to give it much respect. In other words, it is to be taken as an obsessional content which I am very willing to have all the facts about but which I do not need to have repeated very often. But there are striking exceptions to this general approach, and they are all in the field of schizophrenia.

I recall one case, which to me was outstanding, of an obsessional who showed great fear of committing suicide. The patient was a civil engineer who had become more and more obsessional until finally he had to do all of his work on the second floor of his house. His wife had to bring his meals to him there and had to take his work to his office, get the approval of the people who dealt with it, and bring it back. She was in turn a cook, a messenger, an office-assistant, and whatnot. All this, contrived with the unlimited attention to detail that an obsessional is capable of, was put on the basis of his fear that if he got on a stairway he would be overwhelmingly compelled to fling himself over and thereby kill himself. Finally he was brought to the hospital. Some final aggravation made his wife's burden impossible, and she just could not carry it any longer. To that extent he made a mistake, of course, since it resulted in his coming to the mental hospital. I saw him for a while in order to try to figure out what it was all about. By that time I had become rather definitely suspicious that there was a middle ground between what I was interested in—schizophrenia—and what I was at that stage uninterested in—obsessionalism. But although I spent some time with him, I elicited nothing even remotely suggestive of anything but classical obsessional processes. It was true, however, that he had somewhat more glaringly large returns than most patients show. In other words, he had eliminated almost everything that was disagreeable to him, except possibly his wife, by the intensification of his fear of throwing himself over the stairs. Thus he succeeded in keeping himself on the second floor, which was the really pleasant part of his house, where he actually liked to work. And so the secondary gains in this instance were pretty high. As I have said before, an obsessional neurotic does not have a good time, but he could have a much worse time.

This man convinced me that he was a pretty classical obsessional. I was not particularly skillful with obsessionals in those days, if I ever did become so with them. He simply began to pulverize me, as I think obsessionals may be inclined to do with everybody; and I didn't fool myself very long into thinking we were getting anywhere. Eventually I staged some scenes so that he got fairly well out on a limb, and then I told him, "I am transferring you to the second floor now, and issuing orders that you will not be served a tray. And so, I don't know; maybe you will die by flinging yourself over the stairs; I doubt it. Maybe you will starve to death; I doubt that too. But we'll have to see." Not very long after that he was discharged as much improved—I should say, with no material increase in his insight, except that I think I did succeed in getting him to see that there was a transparent level of profit he was deriving from his neurosis that that particular environment would not put up with. I seem to recall that his wife divorced him two or three years later, so apparently she followed somewhat the same pattern as did the hospital.

In this case—which I do not cite as an instance of particularly good treatment—strong pressure in the direction of the obsessional's fear of suicide, far from precipitating self-destruction, led to a recasting of the obsessional problem. I think that that would be the case rather generally where a fairly stable obsessional state exists—not that one can take the chances on the outside that one can sometimes take in a mental hospital with an adequate staff of attendants, nurses, and so on. But the progression toward schizophrenia certainly did not occur in this patient.

There are some patients, several of whom I have seen for a long period in intensive therapy, who fairly clearly show a shift back and forth between obsessional and schizophrenic processes. The theoretical importance of these people seems to me to be enormous. For instance, there are people who sound just like obsessional neurotics—who, I think, are obsessional neurotics—but whose history, as one drags it out of them, includes blanks which are not merely the result of the extreme caution which some obsessional personalities show. Perhaps I had better say something about this extreme caution first, in order to distinguish it from the blanks I am talking about. Very often it is rather exhausting to find out what has happened to an obsessional neurotic because everything has to be told just *right*. Dangers of misstatement, and so on, of the most recondite and subtle kinds seem to hound the poor patient, so that it may take an hour to get a fairly simple statement made, such as, "Well, I think the girl has lost interest in me, because the last time I was invited to her house she had gone out by the time I got there." (Of course my private suspicion is that that doesn't prove very much; she may have waited an hour and a half while he was struggling with his rituals, and decided that it was too much for anyone to put up with.) In making a statement of that kind, which reflects severely on his status, the obsessional neurotic has to be awfully careful as to just how things are said, so it takes quite a long time.

But when I talk about blanks in a patient's account of something, I do not mean that the patient uses extreme care about how a thing should be said and what the other person will think about it, but that he says at some point, with amazing frankness, that he isn't clear on what happened. And when you ask, "Well, can you recall any of the events?" he is very apt, again unlike the usual obsessional neurotic, to say some astonishing thing such as, "Well, I don't know, but some way or other the sun was mixed up in it," which, as I do not need to tell you, sounds pretty schizophrenic. In other words, such a patient is in some border region; when he is discussing schizophrenic episodes of the past, he talks like a schizophrenic; and when he is discussing other things, he talks like an obsessional neurotic. In getting his history you have all the travail that you have with a typical obsessional neurotic, except that now and then you hear something like, "Well, I don't know what happened; I know I had a terrible time," which is quite direct for an obsessional neurotic. If you ask, "Well, can you recall any detail about it?" the detail you hear may be pretty startling, and it is given quite directly, without cautions and protections.

I have not been able to discover wherein the obsessional phases of these people differ in any way from the obsessional neurosis. But I have found that when it was schizophrenic phenomenology and not obsessional processes that unhorsed a patient, the history of such a patient's life includes warning events. He experienced those events at times when he was very much less secure, very much nearer panic, than he ordinarily is when he is simply suffering his obsessional necessities. I think that the patient who much of the time shows evidences of the obsessional dynamism is, in fact, suffering the obsessional dynamism; but that, even though it is the outstanding morbid accent of his life process, under certain circumstances it may not be enough.

I think that I can illustrate this by a patient of mine in whom I clearly observed the shift, under stress, from obsessional processes to schizophrenic phenomenology. First I saw it almost happen, thanks to a very serious mistake of my own, and a little later I saw it actually happen as a result of certain other circumstances. This young man's mother had married, not the man she loved, for he was one of her brothers, but instead an extremely ambitious man whose harsh centering on himself and his career was apparent from very early in his life. Before very long she too became extraordinarily ambitious, concerned with the business of being his wife and consolidating a social career for herself, which was facilitated by his successes. She bore him four children in fairly close succession, and a fifth after quite a long interval and a very disastrous event. This event concerned the eldest daughter who was the only person for whom the father had any real feeling—the other children knew him only as a man who would sometimes be annoyed because they were talking to each other and would cuff them into silence. This eldest daughter was fatally injured in an automobile accident during the father's absence from home. The father rushed back home immediately, but the girl was dead when he arrived. The father's behavior reduced the mother to a state of agitated depression which persisted for a year or so. In the latter stages of this depressed period she bore the fifth child, a son—the only one of the family that was not an emotional wreck when I knew them. He became normal and extroverted, ignored the rest of the family, and was so different from them that they couldn't find any way to get him down. I judge that the mother was so paralyzed by the hangover of her depression that she just could not get him into harness as she had the rest of her children.

My patient was the most brilliant of the older surviving children, and he was the quintessence of obsessional neuroticism. Everything on earth had to be handled very carefully and cautiously, and it took an interminable amount of time to do anything. You can picture the satisfaction he was getting from studying mathematics. But he was in a profound emotional jam with one of his professors, which I couldn't get any clue to until finally I learned something about his father. This professor had the same intensely arrogant, contemptuous manner that the father had always shown, and the boy was just tied up into knots when he went to that class; he couldn't hear the professor, and he couldn't answer any questions.

I learned that there were two rather striking things in the boy's history. The first of these was some sort of difficulty of bowel function which had appeared one summer when he was traveling in Europe. He had become such a problem in the home that a young instructor at the university had suggested that the boy travel with him in Europe that summer. This suggestion was accepted. But after a short time, he began getting more and more incredibly entangled in obsessional business, and finally got so preoccupied with some problem of the bowel function that even the instructor realized that they didn't seem to be doing well together. So the instructor went on ahead, whereupon the boy's symptoms cleared up somewhat and he was finally able to join the other fellow at the port of embarkation for the return trip. I heard this difficulty with the bowels referred to a great many times. But I soon realized that I had not the foggiest notion of what the boy was talking about and that there was no immediate prospect of my finding out; it was one of those things that could not be told.

The second striking thing in the history concerned a difficult roommate he had had at the university as an undergraduate. The situation with this fellow had been perfectly awful; it got worse and worse, and at that point I did actually get the detail that the sun seemed to be involved in some way or other in this thing. As he could tell it under pressure from me, it sounded as if he had to be outdoors in the sun a great deal in order to improve his vitamin D supply, or something like that. But there would be obvious indications that he knew better—that he was aware that the explanation about his health and vitamin D was merely a rationalization that he could use most of the time, and that he knew there were really lunatic fringes to this business about the sun. Sometimes he was simply mute, and couldn't make any attempt at conversation.

In our work, it finally became evident that the mother had in some fashion constituted herself an inescapable restriction on the genital function very early in his life. It was fairly easy to fix the time, since he recalled that it was when he was still sleeping with his brother in some sort of cradle. In some fashion, what with arranging their hands under the sheets and so on, the mother got herself identified as a very serious threat to the perineal region.

As I have said, I made a nearly fatal mistake at one time in the treatment; I simply did not realize what an extremely important thing he had said in a very gentle way, and for a while it was touch and go as to whether he would pass into a lurid paranoid state at once. He didn't, and we puttered along and, I guess, ultimately repaired the mistake. Then one summer, when the boy was no longer in treatment with me, the father died suddenly, and the mother came so near to blowing up with joy that the boy was precipitated into a schizophrenic episode.

The son came back to me in this schizophrenic state, so I had plenty of opportunity to see how curiously processes can shift. After some very obscure operations concerning how great a danger it was to work with me—which, taken at face value, practically meant that by coming back to me he was abandoning every hope he had ever had of getting well—we got back, presently, out of the complex schizophrenic symbolism to the pretty typical obsessional caution that had always characterized him. This case, in which I saw the thing happen, and some other cases in which I know that it has happened, make me say that the person who has put principal dependence on obsessional processes will, under great stress which the obsessional dynamism is not able to handle, develop schizophrenic phenomenology. I am not sure, however, whether I should make this statement apply to *any* person who has put major dependence on obsessional processes or only to *some* of these people.

Therapy with the Obsessional

The indication for management of the obsessional patient is, of course, *just don't apply too much pressure in the area where he can't stand it.* The immediate question then is, What is that area? The answer is to be approached by recalling our general statement that the obsessional processes are devices for providing an uncomfortable approach to security. Thus I should say that one does not strike *directly* at the self-esteem of an

obsessional neurotic, although I have had no unfavorable results from agreeing with obsessional neurotics when they documented how low their self-esteem was. In other words, you do
not turn all of your ingenuity, if you have quite a lot of it, to
beating them to it and showing them up before they are equal
to showing themselves up. You cannot hurry their insight very
much, but that doesn't mean that they are not pursuing insight.
They are no exception to the rule that patients, once they get
the faintest glimmer of hope, are principally engaged in trying
to get well.

In dealing with the obsessional neurotic, the psychiatrist
must recognize that until the interpretation of a particular life
situation has become almost self-evident, there is no use in
offering any interpretation to an intensely obsessional person.
Otherwise, what will happen is the following: The psychiatrist hears the patient tell him about some very difficult situation he is involved in, and what it means in the sense of what
the patient is doing, and what probable returns he is getting
out of it, and what strains he is being subjected to in it. The
psychiatrist helpfully reflects to the patient what he has heard
—whereupon he finds that he is wrong. He will probably then
want to find out why he is wrong—either because he doesn't
want to make the same mistake again or because he wants to
show that he wasn't wrong at all. And this turns out to be a
month's digression; things go around in circles until the psychiatrist feels quite dizzy. Finally the slow progress is again
resumed.

Thus the psychiatrist must learn to wait until the interpretation of the particular life situation is almost self-evident and
must, at the same time, observe carefully what is going on.
Of course, when he has annoyed the patient, all that is going
on is that the psychiatrist is being pulverized, usually rather
unpleasantly. But otherwise, if the psychiatrist doesn't get in
the patient's way, and doesn't prod the patient in some sensitive region, what is happening is that the context is being run

again and again and again through the mill; and each time it is a little clearer than it was the time before. That is the way in which obsessional personalities seem to heal themselves. They run through their security operations over and over and over—but not entirely without the rest of the personality achieving something in the process, for each time the context gets a little clearer. Occasionally, just about the time when you feel certain that you can now make an interpretation of some durable difficulty of the patient's—some chronically unpleasant entanglement with another person, for instance, which he never seems able to solve by any simple procedure—the patient beats you to it. Something happens that brings the interpretation by brute force; it cannot be overlooked any longer. Even though he doesn't beat you to the interpretation, if he is quite ready for it when you make it, he will probably, with rather severe anxiety, give some faint indication of agreement, and soon afterwards say, "Well, why in the world did it take you so long?" or words to that effect. This is the type of approach to the hurdle, and falling over it, that seems to constitute the therapy of the obsessional neurosis.

Of course this can happen only if your prestige is not involved in the interpretation—in other words, if you are not attacking the patient by making your interpretation, but are merely propounding the riddle, "Well, now, actually doesn't this picture which you depict mean so-and-so? What else can it mean? I can't find any other hypothesis that accounts for the course of events." Because obsessional neurotics have been insecure and used to a rather hypocritically insecure environment from very, very early life, they are past masters at detecting blind spots in the analyst. They don't mention them, but their operations begin to involve this area, and if the analyst hurts them, disturbs their self-esteem a little, he is apt to find himself involved in something that has a little tendency to obsess *him*. It looks quite malicious, for obsessionals are the people, I sometimes think, who twist the knives in wounds. But when you apply the term malicious to a person, you imply that he knows what he is doing; and God pity the obsessional neurotic who would get such little benefit from the obsessional dynamism that he would realize that he was being malicious. On the other hand, these patients have no difficulty in seeing the truth in statements, almost always made to them by people involved with them, to the effect that they are terribly difficult to live with, that they are just awful as companions, and so on and so forth. Since they see the truth of such statements—which is part of the expense of maintaining what security they have—they are apt to take time out in therapy and in life for excursions into self-pity, excursions which are all the more spectacular in that they are also intensely obsessional. Whereas certain types of inadequate personalities and certain hysterics, it seems to me, never enjoy anything as much as a good cry over their woes, the obsessional neurotic who cries, cries from rage, and his self-pitying performances invariably are thoroughly designed to crucify somebody else. Thus there is a lot of what can easily be interpreted as hostility, because this is an attempt to maintain an uncertain security which has to go on practically all the time when anybody who is significant is around. And when you are trying to maintain a feeling of security, with the constant marginal feeling that the other person doesn't respect you, well, you are not apt to be loving, you see; it *is* a rather hostile performance, so far as the other person is concerned. But to interpret the obsessional neurosis as a mask for hatred is, I think, just dreadful hokum—the cart has been put on top of the horse there; it's not either in front or behind, it's just mixed.

The recitations of the obsessional neurotic about the past gradually come to reflect rather singular brutality toward the patient by a significant person, usually a parent. If this rather brutal recital includes some thin disguise which the parent wore, I think that you may always accept the account as being reasonably close to the truth. In other words, in a very considerable number of cases these patients have been subjected to really severe cruelty by a parent, but always the parent had a little mask to conceal the sheer brutality of what was going on. The type of atrocity which had been perpetrated on many obsessionals just did not seem probable to me when I first began working with them, but I encountered it so often that I gradually began to see what had happened. These people really know that their parents were not happy and that one of the parents, at least, was savagely cruel to them. But what has always been baffling is this constant thin veneer of convention and sweetness and light. The bafflement of the child took the form of wondering whether mother, for example, was really cruel to him or whether she was really sweetness and light and it was just his own cursed perversity that made her seem so cruel. The relevant part of treatment consists in coming to see that all the conventional sweetness and light was just a veneer; in the process of study, what was mask and what was motive gets itself somewhat clear.

This insight is often attended by bitter grieving, in which one of several things may be the case. In general, the grieving is over the many opportunities for possible happiness that were wasted because the patient was so puzzled as to whether he was right or wrong about the savage interference of the significant parent. This is true grief. It is the final emancipation from a lost object of desire which has been festering, as it were, in the personality from childhood onward. But just as grieving can in other situations become a disease instead of being a very useful dynamism, so also morbid grieving can appear in the course of psychotherapy of an obsessional—and perhaps in the ordinary process of obsessional life, if the person hits on too strong a reminder of a highly pathogenic early situation. I surmise that the so-called reactive depression of the obsessional is that sort of thing. And to the extent that grieving becomes a pattern of life in itself, I suppose it may become a type of atrocity to the environment.

So far as suicide in such a situation is concerned, if the environment just gets up and leaves—won't have any—I assume the self-destruction is not likely to occur. Thus when I have encountered vigorous threats of suicide in retaliation for my brutality to obsessional neurotics, I have usually taken these threats as merely an invitation to real brutality. For instance, I have asked such patients to do it somewhere, if possible, where it won't put me to great awkwardness in getting somebody to remove the results. I should add, however, that in one instance where I told a patient something of this sort, the results did not contribute to my low blood pressure, for although the topic of killing herself to get even with me disappeared promptly from her productions, for a time I heard things which did suggest to me that she had given busses a reasonable chance to hit her. She didn't go out of her way to get under them, but she certainly gave them a reasonable chance. Thus it came within gunshot of being a situation which one might describe—if one was intensely given to symbolic language—by saying that the death instinct came near getting unmanageable. I have said that when some of the atrocious disappointment of childhood and the juvenile era is revived, it may be accompanied by grief—which either may serve at last to emancipate the person from the lost but still desired objects or may become an operation in itself. When a person is attached to unreal love objects and denies the possibility of anything actually available ever equaling these objects or making up for them, I can conceive that he might feel, "What difference does it make whether I kill myself or not?" Perhaps it seems reasonable for him to join the unreal character of the love object. This may have been the origin of my patient's actions. But I do not think that it is usually the origin of statements about suicide made by obsessional neurotics.

One of the complications frequently associated with obsessional personalities is a subdiaphragmatic disturbance of the viscera. Sometimes such disturbances are sources of outstanding disability in obsessional neurotics. An improvement in the visceral symptoms of tension, frustration, and so on may precede a noticeable change in the predominance of obsessional implicit processes, but neither is apt to be cleared up without improvement in the other aspect of the difficulty. One such patient of mine had had a nearly fatal gastric hemorrhage and a great deal of trouble with constipation, which improved after I carried her through to insight into an utterly impossible struggle that she was engaged in as the major aspect of her obsessional neurosis. Both she and I knew that there was another extremely difficult entanglement to be resolved, but for various reasons I felt that I had done my bit on the first—the one that was really apt to kill her by gastric hemorrhage—and that she could work the other out with someone else, which she at least attempted. I have not heard how it turned out. In this case, the business of constipation, which was almost immemorial, was entirely relieved by clearing up an extremely difficult life situation, which was of much more recent origin than the constipation. How much the viscera suffer from the obsessional neurosis, and how much the environment and the patient suffer from it, is not too simply predictable. I have never felt entitled to torture patients by the month to find out something that interested me but was of no special moment to them —if only because I do not think that anything can be learned by doing it. And so I never made any attempt to discover why, in the case of this particular patient, clearing up her greatest interpersonal problem had such a phenomenal effect on her somatic health, even though a very severe problem undoubtedly remained.

In certain moods I would say that anything on earth can be relevant to the obsessional neurosis. Obsessionals have a genius for getting all sorts of things involved in their situations, but only for the purpose of befogging troublesomely inescapable insecurities. A good many of their satisfactions are pursued with almost blatantly simple directness. And quite often this simple directness is something which they cannot control, for that is all the development they ever had to make in that field. They are not as well socialized in the areas of certain of their needs for satisfaction as some of us are. Now and then they encounter somebody who points out what crude creatures they are in that area, and they cannot do anything about it. That is a real attack on the points where they are tender—on their prestige, their feeling of status. Under those circumstances, they will reach around for practically anything on earth and become harassed about it. It is just like the squid: a cloud of confusing details pours out in which everything becomes somewhat nebulous. That is much better, however, than the anxiety experienced at the threat to their rather feebly supported prestige. It is really too bad when the doctor collaborates in that and starts working diligently on a lot of stuff that is of as much real importance as the other side of the moon would be. I think that if one could really keep one's eye on the ball with these people, they would not necessarily be such remarkably slow therapeutic prospects. But it takes a high degree of alertness to sort out quickly what is relevant and what is merely convenient fog. I have invented, with very telling effect on my obsessional patients, a description of their way of life as the flypaper technique. That is, when the obsessional gets into an insecure situation with a significant person— where there is anger or a difference of opinion or something of the sort—the other fellow has just about the same experience as a cat does who has stepped on a sheet of flypaper. Every move made by this other fellow gets him stuck up somewhere else, so that finally all he can do is just glare. He may experience what the obsessional is doing as shifting the topic, misunderstanding everything, imputing the most astounding meanings and the lowest motives to him, and what not. All this simply means that in therapy you do not quarrel with an obsessional neurotic unless you want to have a lot of your time converted to as near nothing as the human being can convert time. What the obsessional is doing is a special instance of the befogging procedure that I mentioned before, except that now instead of picking up all sorts of irrelevant and immaterial extraneous details, he is picking up all the irrelevant and immaterial internal details, you might say, that he can find or suspect in the antagonist. As the antagonist, you realize that in a very remote and incredibly unrelated sense these accusations do, however, have some vague relevance; that's why they stick. So you rapidly become quite entangled; and that leads to such an increasingly foggy argument that within 15 minutes nobody knows what it was all about, but everybody is furious and frustrated. It is really not a great help to a therapist to have been involved in that special kind of entanglement.

Consultation on the Case of an Obsessional

In the course of this series of lectures, Sullivan would occasionally be asked by one of his colleagues to comment on a case which had proved difficult. These were not long formal case presentations for the most part, but were concerned with particular problems in the course of therapy. We have included three such consultations, one here and two more at the end of Chapter 15. All three of these comments on particular case-problems were made at least a year later than the period of the other lectures included in this book.

Sullivan: The problem I have been asked to comment on concerns the management of a strikingly obsessional male patient. In summary, this patient after about six months in therapy is apparently willing to manifest a consensus with the physician to the effect that he is showing a good deal of malevolence toward the environment, but he shows a striking dearth of any particular feeling about it. The malevolence seems focused primarily on the patient's mother. The patient's wife is pictured by him as having married him for, among other reasons, the purpose of helping him with his problems. She is a rather secondary target of the malevolence.

In almost all of my work with obsessionals the patient has started out with one or the other of two goals that he tries to achieve with me. The crude goal is to show that he is being treated quite badly by significant people; the other, and rather more forbidding goal as a therapeutic problem, is to show that everyone is as nice as can be to him, but still things seem to go badly—mysteriously the patient's feelings are hurt, and one thing and another. The first of these goals seems to apply to this case, and I will discuss it. By accepting a patient's notion of this rather ubiquitous malevolence toward him, I have been able at times in less than six months to get a pretty clear picture of his engaging in actions that are anything but friendly, placating, or tender toward these significant people.

I maintain that to have a clear grasp on the extraordinary extent to which the patient is malevolent in dealing with significant others, there must already be established the fact—it should be a fact for therapeutic purposes at this stage at least —that the significant others are malevolent toward the patient. I take it that this is more or less what has gone on so far in the case that has been presented. And further, the patient's mother is the target figure in much of his productions. When the mother is the target with one of these people, I really expect an awfully bad time in the sense of a most unrewarding passing of hours. I much prefer that the target be someone who is not traditionally related to the patient, in the hope that in the relatively insignificant more current situation, trends will be seen that will provide an excellent springboard to the relation with the significant mother. Now in this situation the mother is clearly in focus; but the patient *is* fairly productive of difficulties with his wife, and that, I would feel, is a rather promising area to investigate. I would expect that he had married a thoroughly difficult woman. She married him more or less to cure or at least alleviate his misery. Well, I should say she has a very healthy interest in trouble, and I would not be at all surprised to discover that she is also strikingly obsessional in personality organization. Doubtless she has had some discouraging experience to date in helping him. He, on the other hand, would suffer a great deal from her very kindly inconsiderateness. In her efforts to help him, to encourage him, and so on, she doubtless treads every now and then on his sensitive feelings. Yes, I should think he had a current difficulty that would be very rich. Let us consider it as the focus of therapeutic endeavor, and later on I will return to a situation where the patient provides nothing but the mother as a target.

It is a rare experience to find a markedly obsessional person in a really tender, considerate, and constructive environment. Obsessionals are pretty hard for comparatively comfortable and easygoing persons to get awfully enthusiastic about as a prospect of happiness, and such persons, I think, tend to veer off from them. So the obsessional, in my experience, shows a marked tendency to get involved in a situation that can be described very crudely as prevailingly hateful. I think that is a risky view to offer a patient, although I often use it for orienting my own investigation. A very gross strategy which seems to work is to discover how the important and helpful person in the patient's life miscarries in effort. The strategy sets out with a very bland observation on my part that certain things are not working too well and one might be able to discover what the other person—for our purposes, let us say the wife—does which seems to get in the way, however helpfully intended. And entanglements are usually revealed which approximate what I call the flypaper pattern, in which the situations as they develop between the two go from bad to worse.

The situation will be revealed as something like this: These people are like everyone else—that is, lousy with good intentions—so one of them—let us say, the wife—in attempting to be helpful about the husband's particularly weak-spined reaction to some imposition placed on him in his work situation, for example, hurts his feelings. She is distressed at this unexpected and unintended injury to him and attempts to explain that she didn't mean to imply that he had no backbone, but just that he was so unusually diffident about his interest. And he comes back at that with the remark that apparently diffidence is something that she doesn't value very highly because she herself doesn't show any. And then she feels that that isn't quite true, for she has very often been diffident about her own needs and deferred to his; in fact she is doing almost nothing else. He may then, feeling that he is sufficiently entangled, practically weep with frustration at how little he can appreciate what a marvelous wife he has. Whereupon, she will play her cards to this effect: Oh, she doesn't think she's a perfect wife, just nearly so. Then his move will be to say that she's far too good for him; look at how she has put up with such-and-such, "such-and-such" being things which actually she has *not* put up with, you see. That won't seem quite cricket to her, and she'll be a little defensive. And so it goes, getting thicker and thicker, and the one certainty of these exchanges is that both parties will be quite disturbed by them.

As I say, I try to get this revealed to me by the somewhat guarded communication of the patient. The way that I ask for it is really very simple but does have a somewhat defective effect as well as the appropriate one. I say to the patient that I want to know what happened, who said what next, and so on and so forth. As the patient is reporting, he is apt to get the idea that I am trying to discover just what kind of a polite she-devil he is living with; but the brute fact is that I am trying to get data that are somewhere near what actually happened. I know I may often hear what the other fellow said. I also will hear a great deal of what my patient said, except that it will usually leave out some quite important data—not in any sense deliberately; it will just happen that a number of the things that show how the melee became more and more inextricably unprofitable will appear in his account of the other person's contribution but not in that of his own. I never expect to get an accurate account of one of these unpleasant flypaper operations early in my relation with a patient; but when I have some notion of what went on, I may depict it in rough outline for the patient to hear it. Whether I do this or not depends upon whether he is likely to have some such general outline available himself. Sometimes, where it has taken an awful lot of work for him to complete the tale, it is almost too much to suppose that he has been able—what with all the caution and obsessional detail—to have very much of a general pattern left. So I take the trouble of reporting what I have heard, but I do not voice my suppositions of the patient's contributions to the melee. My report often functions usefully because, however true it may be that the obsessional substitutions are usually precautions against showing malevolence, there is nothing rash and careless about an obsessional, and he will see something. He will see that my picture, even though it reflects quite faithfully, if briefly, just what I have heard, is obviously not right. (What is wrong with it, I believe, is essentially that it puts a much better complexion on the patient's participation than the facts would warrant.) But anyway the patient is distressed at what an unfavorable impression I must have of the other person. My response to him then is that I want to know all about that. I do not quite agree that my impression is such an unfavorable one; it is the impression I got from the story; I have not formulated the story as condemnation of the other person; rather I have just said what I have heard. This doesn't suit the patient, and he sets about to fix the story up. In this process of reformulation I take singularly small part except to ask questions when I simply do not understand something. As he fixes up his story, I may get a few clues to his part in the flypaper operation; and if such a clue shows up, I am apt to mention it.

Just how I note its existence depends very largely on what I think of my opposition—the self-system. I may, for example, comment that I am quite sure that *that* was not mentioned the

first time. Or possibly, I will just *notice* the additions and say
that I think perhaps I am getting a little clearer about what
the difficulty may be. My choice of comment here depends, as
I say, on my evaluation of the opposition to me. The simple
measure of that opposition is the extent to which the patient has
to show obsessional processes in attempting to prevent my
drawing unfavorable views of him in the interchange with
the other person. Where he gives a great deal of attention to
my supposed impression with all this, I realize that I am in the
presence of a very strong opposition in the sense that the patient is quite frequently and quite noticeably anxious—or as
nearly anxious as obsessionals ordinarily get—about what is
going on in *me* in response to his story. Under those circumstances I am certainly *not* going to give any sign early in the
relationship that I doubt the completeness of the story told me;
so I go easy indeed in warning him that I am trying to catch
onto what really goes on in these flypaper entanglements.
When, however, the patient does not pay a great deal of attention to what I may think, then I figure that he has a good
deal of confidence in the obsessional substitutions and therefore is not unusually disturbed in communicating with me. In
that situation, I will ask questions that come near requesting
what I would really like to know.

So, if I am lucky, in the course of time something will be
reported from one of these entanglements that is succinct
enough and unguarded enough so that I can say, "Oh and then
you said so-and-so? That was kind, wasn't it?" (This is, of
course, an ironic statement because what he had said was quite
*un*kind.) Then I simply have to sit tight till the fireworks
quiet down; and by that time, incidentally, the patient has
usually gotten around to the point of wondering what was so
unkind about it. You see the point has hit very hard, but it
gets somewhat attenuated in his operations with me that follow on my saying it. Whereupon I repeat the story and say,
"Now *I* don't see how that could do other than hurt the feelings

of your wife, do *you?*" Well, that is as far as I ever hope to get in that session. I suppose only one out of the thirty or forty obsessionals I have worked with has said, "No, I don't. I think it was unkind." Most obsessionals will only say something vague that implies that I might have something there. That is about as close as they get to agreeing with me. Nonetheless, I know the operation has worked. The patients have seen that, however much they suffered from the start of this, they certainly got in quite a crack at the opponent. One gradually accumulates two or three instances in which the patient discovers that, far from his being utterly long-suffering and hopelessly misunderstood and just not up to the standards of the other person, he has taken extremely shrewd blows at the self-esteem of the other person. After these have been accumulated, I feel that I am really getting somewhere near to doing some therapy. I can then tackle the problem of finding out how these melees start. And so the next time that I hear of a difficulty with the patient's protagonist, I am apt to begin, "Ah, well, just let's get this entirely straight from the start. Just exactly when did you get home, and how had things been going at the office?" I want the patient to sketch in a little background for the occasion first; then I want the point at which the two met; and then the point when something happened. At this last point these patients always want to go on to a world of detail, but this time we don't go on. When I hear of the offense to the patient—*offense* is *my* word, for the patient never says it that way—then I say, referring to the remark of the wife, "Well, what did you make of that?" The patient almost invariably does not make anything of that; he asks, "What do you mean?" I say, "Well, come now, can you recall when this remark was made to you?" He usually says that, to be quite frank with me, he cannot remember. I say, "Well, this is how something began. Now I gather a lot followed it, but this is really the start of it, and I think that that remark would have called out some feeling. Three or four different things have occurred to me as possible meanings of it. What occurred to you? What did you think your wife meant by this remark?"

By sort of hounding the patient, I can usually extract a statement which interprets the wife's remark in a fashion that is hard on the self-esteem of the patient. And then I say, "Oh yes, well, that was one of the ideas I had. Tell me, what on earth do you suppose brought that out?" Again the patient wants to tell me all that has happened, and I say, "No, no, I want to get clear at the start and then I'll be happy to hear the details. Now *you* have been through all this, and you may have some clues. Have you any clue to what your wife was driving at by taking this crack at you when you came in?" Once more I have to fight off spending the rest of the hour on the report of subsequent events before finding out what the patient really thinks the wife was trying to do by this remark. What she said will turn out to be something quite unfriendly. It may seem very helpful but in reality it implies, for example, that he failed entirely in his efforts to get a raise or something like that. It will be something that made him anxious, you see—that is, disturbed his self-esteem. When I have worn this thing to a very high polish so that there are no shadows—no doubts that the wife said so-and-so and that that brought to his mind the idea that she thought so-and-so, which was not particularly friendly—then I say, "Ah yes, well it sounds very reasonable to me. Now go on, if you will, with what you can recall of the account." The considerable joker about now going on with the rest of the story is that every now and then the account, far from taking hours as the first one did, is greatly condensed. According to my lines, this shows that the patient, having gotten to the original wound in the thing, does not see very much sense now in repeating the vast waste of time that originally was consumed in showing no hurt feelings but nevertheless retaliating—all of which of course is entirely unwitting.

Having documented that on a few occasions the patient has

not been particularly kind to the troublesome companion and having documented that on a few occasions the companion has started trouble with very shrewd punctures in the tender areas of the patient, I am then in a position to comment on the amazing amount of resentment that must pile up in *him* from these rather inconsiderate performances of the companion. Then, after having been given a running complicated opinion on that, I next comment on how much resentment there must pile up *only* as a result of his shrewd, if somewhat delayed blows. This is of course harder to agree to, but we can usually get to that point. And then I can wonder aloud, "How come there is so much obscure dissatisfaction in the relationship?" And, before the deluge, I pose another question such as, "What positive aspects are there in the relationship?" I might say to this patient, for instance, "How is your wife really of very definitely constructive value to you?" That is a tougher one to get at. What I am really looking for is just what I ask for: What are the constructive values in this situation? In many instances, such patients report practically daily warfare with a marriage partner; yet real assets may appear in the picture of the companion, and it is fairly easy to infer from this that there are assets in the patient which are appreciated by the companion. But despite what is a justifiable basis for the relationship, a good deal of warping, humiliating, and attacking goes on in and out of company.

Then I can propound a little: "What on earth can be behind this? It looks to me as if both of you must be carrying on in the long phase things that belong somewhere in the past, not with each other. Let us see where in the world these patterns begin of presuming that the other fellow is taking a slice when he is saying something that is approximately complimentary. Where did that begin?" Only after this inordinately long build-up do I expect a reasonably rapid revealing of the role of the significant parent—the mother, in our type of society. By dint of discovering how the patient suffered from the mother's kindly and constructive efforts on his behalf, I can finally say, as if by accident: "God, was there anything that you did of which your mother unqualifiedly approved?" This is the last thought that the patient ever hoped to hear expressed. There is a considerable struggle to get rid of it now that it has been expressed, but I anticipate then that within a few weeks it will be agreed that the patient cannot recall any unqualified, unexpected approval from his mother. Only after this am I in a position to wonder what his emotional attitude toward his mother really could have been in view of this continuous indirect derogation and expression of dissatisfaction. How could he have helped hating mother?

Although I have taken an awful lot of time in outlining what I believe to be the way to save time with the obsessional, let me mention a further problem in this regard when the target is the mother. I once had a patient from the edges of psychiatry, a patient who had suffered a good many analyzed people. She announced very early in the work with me that her trouble descended directly, unalterably from very, very early in life and was the work of an exceedingly hateful mother who never had any use for her. I have forgotten all the details—whether she was unwanted in pregnancy, or should have been a boy, or what not—anyway I had the hateful mother to contend with. There was no difficulty about documenting the hateful character of the mother. It was dragged in as a ubiquitous explanation of everything. The target figure was right in front of my nose, I saw nothing else; there was no way of getting around it. That the mother had been hateful, ye gods, how well I knew by the end of six months! But then, apropos of some clue a little too elusive for the patient to see it in advance, I did get to what had kept her alive, which had been the vast mystery. It happened to be an old woman who did sewing for the whole family; she worked in an attic room in the house, and the little girl liked to go up and talk with her when she came, which was quite often. This old woman, who was somewhat in the role of a servant, showered the little girl with tenderness. The patient's father had long since been practically a human effigy except at his place of business. He was completely under his wife's thumb and not permitted in any sense to interfere with her very modern and reasonable education of the children. So he was a nonentity. But the tenderness in the picture—ushered in with a flood of tears in the patient's therapy—showed up with the uncovering of this nice old seamstress, who interestingly enough had developed a perfectly polite arsenal to use against the mother. (Some superior domestics, you know, amass a good many weapons of aggression to get their work done.) She would reduce the mother to a rage, whereupon the mother would back around and go downstairs and let the old woman do her work as she pleased. That made a vast impression on the daughter. In many ways this seamstress was the contrast which I needed.

Once this had happened, I was able to begin work, to start with her difficulties in current life, and really discover what, out of this dreadful contact with her mother, had been destructive. Before, just everything was wrong; it always had been; it was all mother's evil work; and that was the end of it. Mother was dead, so there wasn't very much to be done about her. But when we could finally get away from the utterly desolate childhood—which, incidentally, I think is physiologically probably impossible—we could really tackle current events and discover how this patient had trouble with living; then we could get somewhere.

This long strategy that I have sketched out is probably about the only way that will *relatively* promptly get the patient to deal with something besides words. Additionally, it provides a method of accidentally curtailing the obsessional's long accounts. When I say accidentally, I am not trying to be funny or take the fault out on the patient. These patients unwittingly leave a few details out of the accounts with the skill that shows what I think is so extremely striking—they have really great gifts of foresight. They foresee with singular clarity things that are going to make them anxious. These things are often treated with selective inattention and come up missing in an account which shows no gap, but just goes right on as if nothing had happened there. Similarly—chiefly, I think from this high development of protective foresight—obsessional patients are absorbingly interested in anything that will probably make both the psychiatrist and the patient miss the point. Not that obsessional patients have an actual motivation to murder time or to avoid getting well, but they have all had such desolate experience in early life that they do not mind being misunderstood. What they live in fear of is being understood, being revealed as what they fear a maximum of clarity would show them to be—that is, unregenerately bad. Now, they do not *think* they are bad, they fear it. In fact, you can get almost any of them to give you quite a dissertation on certain aspects of their decency. But that is not awfully wise to do; it is very much better to have them show you the decency of their protagonists.

The Manic-Depressive Psychosis

I HAVE FOUND it convenient to divide the major psychoses into two categories: those states called manic-depressive, although I am not sure how properly; and those seriously disturbed mental states that fall somewhere between the imaginary conceptions of pure paranoia and pure schizophrenia. There are in addition a number of mongrel and contaminated clinical entities —the mongrel group perhaps being the involutional illnesses, and the contaminated group including infection, exhaustion, drug deliriums, alcoholic psychoses, and so on.

I can offer very little of theoretic importance on the manic-depressive psychosis, for even in a case where the circumstances were exceptionally promising, I did not get to first base in being able to deduce anything from the experience that was any good to me in terms of making a theoretical formulation. That particular experience, which occurred many years ago, was with the disturbed daughter of a society woman. At the time I saw the patient, she had quieted down to what might be described as a hypomanic state. She was well above normal key, in the sense that it would be extremely difficult to find anybody who could talk as fast as she did, but the hypomanic picture otherwise was not terribly impressive. Her mood was not elated; in fact, at times she looked extremely unhappy when she was galloping across obviously very painful data. She was not highly distractible; and in one sense it might even be said that she was not distractible at all, for she would keep to material that was relevant to her life situation, which is certainly not characteristic of distractibility. But while she kept to relevant things, she showed a residual feature of the hypomanic state in that she moved with great speed over the surface of them and never dipped down; there was no depth to the development of any topic. Thus she unhesitatingly expressed hatred for her mother, based on fear of her mother's evil effects on her; and in our interviews she brought out a great deal of historic data regarding this hatred, including a vast documentation of the reasonableness of her attitude. But the striking thing was that, while I got wonderfully adequate insight into the type of deviltry she had grown up with, not the slightest trace of any benefit resulted from this, so far as I know. She never slowed down, and she never gave anything a chance to sneak by the self, one might say. She merely provided these glimpses of an extremely unhappy life, with an appropriate facial expression of the emotion; that is, the more unpleasant the business, the more apt she was to look sad and harassed and sometimes to shed tears.

Altogether, it was the strangest kind of a hypomanic picture, and I still can hardly believe that a manic-depressive could behave as this girl did. Yet she showed no marked schizophrenic phenomenology, even to a person who was looking for it and knew more or less what he was looking for; and although many years have passed, she has not since then developed a schizophrenic illness—I have taken the trouble to keep a little track of her. She has had some ups and downs that required care on occasion, and in general gives a fairly convincing picture of being cyclothymic. Thus her subsequent history supports the notion that here was a very curious fragment of something that can happen in a manic-depressive personality.

Manic Excitements: Some Impressions, Hypotheses, and Problems

Ordinarily, the picture one encounters in excitements is either the classic one or varies from the classic picture only slightly. In the classic picture, the person is full of energy and extravagantly euphoric. The physical activity is outstanding; and it has one queer characteristic—the large joint movements are facilitated so that the elbow may be moved when one would ordinarily move the wrist, or the shoulder be moved when one would ordinarily move the elbow. This is not conspicuous enough to be pathognomonic, and yet when one looks for it, one finds that it is quite frequent. The content is, I think, best apprehended as a manifestation of a constant necessity to have something going on in awareness, but since whatever is going on in awareness seems to get troublesome almost at once, there is a necessity to keep moving, as it were, from one thing to another. Thus part of the physical behavior may consist of the eyes literally darting around looking for things for the person to talk about. The most amazing ingenuity is shown in maintaining this distractibility, such as using clang associations to something heard in the environment; almost anything that can come in by any of the sensory channels is grist for the mill. I have repeatedly had the inescapable feeling that the hypomanic keeps busy moving from one thing to another lest he experience a drop in euphoria. Although I have never been able to prove this conclusively, it seems to me that there is some hint of the validity of the hypothesis in something which can be frequently observed in the hypomanic state: in spite of the fact that the patient claims to feel wonderful and there is the usual clatter of swiftly moving subjects of thought, in some instances he is obviously not so euphoric; in fact, he may be clearly anxious or even a little panicky. I had one exceptional patient of this kind many years ago; and it seems to me now that the evidence was there for such a hypothesis, had I known enough to make the proper investigation at the time. In this particular case, I did recurrently observe to the patient that he was obviously very jittery about something or other even though he said he felt so wonderful. This insistence of mine had a powerful impelling effect on him; I felt that there was no doubt in his mind of the accuracy of my surmise that one thought about a great many things because there was a continuous menace that something very unpleasant would occupy awareness if one didn't. But he continued to stay on the surface in what he said, and he did not say anything that would really convince me of the validity of the hypothesis. Now, whether this hypothesis is correct, I do not know. It is plausible, and it would make manic-depressive states grow out of a good many things that we see in psychiatry.

Depending to some extent on my own euphoria, I suppose, I have varied between two notions about manic-depressive states. One notion is that the central theme of manic excitement—the distractibility, the flight of ideas—is to be considered as strongly conditioned by life situational factors. The other notion is that it is to be regarded as primarily a disturbance of metabolism or something of that kind. Actually, there has to be some disturbance of the commonplace biophysicochemical existence of the person for him to maintain the enormous expenditure of energy, for this would ordinarily reduce one to utter inactivity in comparatively short order. The sustained expenditure of energy by some of these patients is one of the most mystifying and astonishing things I know about in psychiatry. Schizophrenics can perform miracles of valor, but I assure you they pay for it; the manic apparently does not. While we know some drugs that stimulate the anterior horns, and others that seem to stimulate the motor areas and so on, nothing like the manic expenditure of energy can be produced by the use of such agents. With such drugs there is not only an effect but later an aftermath of the effect, something related to what we might call exhaustion. But that does not appear in the manics. They rattle along incredibly.

Another point which might be noted is that, under some circumstances, drug deliriums show suggestions of the hypomanic type of excitement. I surmise that if we knew more about delirifacient drugs, and did not feel necessarily restrained in our pharmacodynamic research, we might find a way of testing out the tendency, for example, of a young person to have a manic-depressive illness. This does not sound like the way I ordinarily tackle mental problems; it represents the influence of my feeling that the manic-depressive psychosis cannot be explained without a good deal of attention to obscure, intricate complexes of factors in the bodily organization.

Another problem that I have been much interested in but know nothing about is the element of duration in relation to onset. People can go into a lurid manic state quite swiftly. But there is no such thing—at least I have not seen any such thing—as really abrupt onset, such as happens when a person who is having a devilish bad time in life, which is rather well concealed, suddenly realizes that automobiles are following him. In other words, here is an almost instantaneous rupture of an unhappy variant of normality, with the appearance of frank schizophrenic phenomenology. In such cases a paranoid state often shows the rupture of what seems to be an approximation of mental health; that is, such people seem to go along in their unhappy way, mulling things over and grinding their teeth from time to time, when *suddenly* they see it all and there they are, with full-fledged persecutory ideas. But in the manic, the state grows by accretion so that the change is from a barely perceptible beginning to a very perceptible state. Thus the appearance of the excitement is not *sudden*, even though the excitement may mount very rapidly in the course of, say, 24 hours, with a person passing from an irritable, uncomfortable type of active existence to a psychotic excitement. In other words, it is difficult to say just when a person becomes excited. And this growth by accretion is part of the argument in favor of somatological factors being involved in the manic-depressive. Looking at the other side of the picture for the moment, depression, I believe, deepens in much the same way. But that is not nearly as easy to see because quite often the person's depression impresses the innocent bystander as being related to a particular event, and deepens from there on, perhaps.

Although the attempt to formulate the manic state in personality terms has not proved as profitable as it might, one can say that there is a great deal of obvious hostility in quite a number of these excitements. In some others, we do not see hostility; but when we study *what is done* as part of the manic hyperactivity, it does represent a long string of violations and so on. For example, I might mention the most amiable manic that I have ever known, who happened to be a wealthy woman. Her family would know that she had had an attack when she would drive down the main city street at 60 miles an hour and wave to the traffic cop, who was so flabbergasted that he didn't even whistle at her. So far as her family was concerned, that meant that she was well up, and it was time for the mental hospital. She was an amazingly genial and amiable woman and I have never seen her in any other condition. She could crack superficial jokes by the hour. Many manics engage in a malicious sort of gibing, but this did not appear in her content. Yet when one looked at *what* she did when she got excited, one could see that she simply violated all sorts of standards, *although she did it gayly.* Thus hostility may, perhaps, show only in the pattern of activity. But, as I have said, it often shows quite frankly in the content, and the drive in the hostility is sometimes most impressive. For example, I recall a patient in the third illness that I had seen him in and in the fifth or sixth that the hospital had undergone, who at the height of his excitement could not resist the impulse to strike the night supervisor, a man twice his age, white-haired, and in general a pretty kindly person. This was a clear instance of the ungovernable necessity for destructiveness and injury to others which appears in some patients at the height of their excitement and which is, I believe, part of the picture, even if masked. (Incidentally, I would like to communicate to you something of how I feel about the menace in a situation like the one I have just described; I am simply not at all amiable about violence.)

The discharge of other motivational systems or integrating tendencies is much less strikingly consistent to me. For example, there are people who, as they become excited, have a great expansion of their lust and engage in really manic sexual relations. But there are others who become excited only after they have become simply impotent; and lust, while it may color their thoughts, does not express itself in any access of genital behavior. Sometimes motivational sets that have only obscurely indicated themselves in the waking life of the patient appear with rather startling clarity in excitement. For instance, if the excitement follows the overloading of a sublimatory way of dealing with the problem of lust, then it will often reveal the thing that has been sublimated. Let us take as an example a person who has not given any striking suggestion of any deviation from a heterosexual choice of love-object. Let us say that fairly early in life he has had slight warnings that he had a barrier to any real attachment to a woman, which had shown itself as an undue interest in members of his own sex, but all of this has been gathered into a sublimatory way of life. As long as lust is the thing that is being sublimated, I rather expect that this person will blow up into an excitement; it may, for instance, show itself in the fact that he engages in his first homosexual affair during the excitement. This kind of course of events might be considered almost pathognomonic for people who have overloaded a sublimatory way of dealing with the problem of lust.

MANIC EXCITEMENT AND SCHIZOPHRENIC EXCITEMENT

In the past this excitement on the collapse of the sublimatory organization was considered the start of a manic-depressive history. Of late—that is, for the past 15 or 18 years—it has seemed to me that this is improbable and that, while the excitement is at first quite apt to be rather typically manic, it gets less typically so as time goes on, and winds up as a definite schizophrenic illness.

This brings me to excitement in the quite young, in the periods of middle and late adolescence, which I surmise may be special instances of the same thing. Again, according to the case reports, such excitements often used to initiate a manic-depressive history. But in my long experience they have *never* initiated a manic-depressive history, but have always initiated schizophrenia. Thus I wonder how carefully these cases were observed in the olden days. I might mention what the course has been of several of these youngsters whom I have seen brought in in manic excitement. I have found that it was only when they were beginning to quiet down that I heard them express very foggy concepts which I felt represented more or less unusual implicit operations. Nonetheless, they would shortly be discharged from the hospital as social recoveries or as being improved, and would go home and perhaps back to school or something of the sort. But possibly a year later they would come back to the hospital in an excited state which no one could mistake for that of a manic-depressive; these were now *definitely catatonic excitements*. Although I do not have a vast amount of data, I have some reason for guessing that these younger people, like the ones I mentioned a moment ago, had pretty extensive sublimatory organization; but in this case it did not particularly involve any patterned type of sexual interest, for they had not yet gotten to this stage. The sublimatory organization which had collapsed had involved such things as hatred and fear of a parent. If you look at some of these people from this particular viewpoint for a while, I believe you can actually see that there have been more and more frantically driven attempts to maintain social approval for unacceptable motivation. And the thing finally gets to be physical overactivity; the person starts a lot of new things before he finishes the others and so on, and you can almost see the excitement develop before your eyes. As I have said, this kind of excitement is not manic excitement; it is the forerunner of schizophrenic illness.

SOME PROBLEMS IN THE CLINICAL MANAGEMENT OF MANIC EXCITEMENT

I would like to mention at this point the unthought-out character of manic behavior. In particular, I want to consider the question of judgment. Of course, the impairment of judgment, in a broad meaning of the term, is necessarily a characteristic of all the states that we justifiably call mental disorder. But the impairment of judgment in excitement and depression is something on which psychiatrists often have to draw pretty careful conclusions on the basis of rather uncertain data. The extent to which manics can exercise foresight seems to me to be practically nil, if only because they cannot consider the deeper meanings of anything; they stay on the surface. Whether they experience a necessity for avoiding serious thinking about anything or whether they are merely incapable of serious thought about anything, in either event they cannot exercise foresight. Often a serious problem for the psychiatrist is to determine at what point in the progression toward full-blown excitement a person's judgment is so impaired that he should be restrained from handling business affairs, and so on—that is, when a guardian or a conservator should be appointed for him or he should be pressed into delegating someone else to take over his affairs temporarily. I have a feeling that as soon as a person is markedly elated—elated, that is, in comparison with the mood which people who know him are accustomed to—the psychiatrist should give serious consideration to the validity of the patient's judgment. However, one should note that early in excitement a person may be able to handle a critical situation, even though he seems to have lost the capacity to deal with run-of-the-mill situations. Thus a person may for the most part be too excited to show good judgment, and be easily influenced by optimistic waves into taking reckless chances; yet if a psychiatrist taxes him with the criticalness of his situation and the probability of his being unable to think in terms of consequences, then he may calm down for a while and make fairly good sense. However, this ability to make some approximation to unexcited thinking in the face of critical demand disappears rapidly. At a certain level of excitement, it is impossible to deliberate calmly; and in the case of a great many hypomanics I cannot imagine any pressure under which they would be able to do so.

Thus I think that excitement is to be taken pretty seriously as an index of grave impairment of judgment. Perhaps its gravity should be judged on the basis of the prevailing economic directions. In other words, if we were moving toward an economic boom, I suppose hypomanic judgment might pay off. But if we were moving toward a general business depression, then I would be very seriously concerned about the business affairs of a person who was getting excited, and I would strongly urge his lawyers to have things put in their hands.

The excited person seems to me to be so driven to be unconventional and to traverse conventions, even when he is amiable, that it looks as if he made it impossible for others to avoid exercising restraint over him. He simply pushes until somebody interferes. Thus it seems almost out of the question to get the excited person into a situation where there will not be definite resistance on the part of the environment. The excited person does, I believe, feel *restrained from thinking seriously about anything;* and if there is any kind of restraint which calls out rage in the manic, it is this feeling that something is preventing him from doing any clear thinking. I must confess that the behavior of the manic does not seem to bear out what I am suggesting; but let me remind you that it is sometimes difficult to see what is going on when there is such a cloud of words and ideas concealing everything. I do know that some manics, even when quite elated, are anything but comfortable; that is, they are really definitely apprehensive and even panicky except when they are in a burst of a fresh excursion of movement, which may be vocal only. Thus I am inclined to believe that the excitement of the manic is clearly related to rage, even though in other people there is not always a clear relation between rage reactions and excitement. Although I am not able to prove what I am saying here, I have been able to observe that even manics who appear quite amiable traverse all sorts of conventions and commit plenty of offenses against others; and those who are not amiable are very willing indeed to hurt others, even by physical violence, at the height of their excitement.

Although the manic's hostility is usually manifest in other ways than physical violence, occasionally a manic becomes actually assaultive, such as the manic whom I have mentioned, who attacked a night supervisor in the hospital at the height of his excitement. Whether or not a manic on a hospital ward becomes physically assaultive, he has a deleterious effect on other patients. In fact, the effects of the hypomanic patient on other patients are always, I believe, strikingly harmful. Occasionally one runs into the belief that a hypomanic personality is able to do good work with schizophrenic patients, but I believe that this is entirely legend. Once a manic begins really destructive work with other patients on a ward, it is very difficult to devise any way to stop it, short of actually using violence toward the manic himself. I have found myself at times in no position to do other than use some restraining force.

In general, however, as I have noted before, the hostility of manics does not show itself this directly. They seem not to be moved to what might be called a biological imitation of negativism. There is a confusion of motives, none of which are developed to any meaningful extent, which may be a partial explanation of the usual lack of physical violence in the manic. This confused motivation seems also to be the explanatory principle of the molar activity; and the verbal activity is rather strikingly directed toward thinking and talking as fast as possible, so that the conversation of some manics is literally made up of all the bromides that can be found in the language culture. They sort of rattle these things off automatically, and nothing else is ever said.

One ought to be able to translate something out of depression that would throw some light on the motivation of excitement. But actually the less one studies the question, the easier it seems. The transition from a manic-depressive type of illness to a settled paranoid state, which sometimes occurs, also ought to be quite revealing. I consider that the paranoid state represents the massive transference of blame onto others. But this formulation does not help me in understanding what the manic has been doing before the paranoid transformation.

The Alternation of Manic and Depressed States

To return to the consideration of the clinical entity, manic-depressive psychosis, I should like to mention the traditional definition of this psychosis by Kraepelin as a mental state characterized by recurrent depressions and excitements, or recurrent depressions, or recurrent excitements—that is, both phases may appear in cycles, or merely one phase may recur at more or less regular intervals. At one time I paid some attention to the interval aspect of it. In some cases the spacing of attacks is rather remarkably regular, which actually gives a little support to the notion of biophysicochemical origins. In other cases, the regularity just is not there; such people may have had pretty difficult manic-depressive illnesses but they do not have the next one until something remotely like an excuse comes along; and when they get over that, they may have another one very soon afterwards or may never have another one that is subject to observation. Thus the regularity of attack is anything but an essential part of the picture, although it is sometimes a characteristic.

The Depressed States

The depression in the manic-depressive psychosis is a true one, by which I mean that it follows my own definition of being a preoccupation of consciousness with a very restricted progression of grief-provoking ideas, and in addition is characterized by a more or less striking reduction of activity. Again, often enough to be rather interesting, in this reduction of activity it is the large joint movements of the skeletal apparatus that are restricted. That is the best reason I know of for believing that agitated depressions are depressions—about all such patients do is operate the tongue and the phalanges. The slowing-up is by no means restricted to the skeletal muscles, just as in the manic the speeding-up is not restricted to the skeletal muscles; in both the manic and the depressive, there is also a corresponding change in the activity of the visceral musculature, at least that of the alimentary tract. In depression the reduction of the activity of the alimentary tract sometimes results in the alimentary tract sinking into an atonic repose which is extremely troublesome.

The grief-provoking ideas of the depressive are viewed by him as an entirely adequate mental state, insofar as he is alert enough to have a view. Any attempt on the part of the psychiatrist to explore what one of these ideas could mean, or what is wrong with it, is, if the patient is still that reactive, treated with irritation or anger; the patient does not welcome anyone's trying to brush aside any part of the content. I have found this to be consistently the case in my quite limited experience with manic-depressives. Although I have not been able to document my observations to any extent, an equally important surmise I would make is that other people must *suffer* from the depression. Sometimes the performance of the depressive is quite clearly punitive. And the troublesome performances of a depressed patient occasionally disappear when it becomes evident that there is nobody who would suffer from them. Even though this cannot be observed in each case, I find it very easy to presume that there is something other than loving kindness in the interpersonal relations of the depressed patient, particularly in the light of the quite impressive tendency toward hostility and convention-breaking found in the manic. In any event, I have always found this definite resentment and opposition in the depressive in any situation in which he is confronted with a well-directed attack on any part of the depressed content.

Homicide and Suicide in Manic-Depression

The gravest events that may arise with manic-depressive patients are homicide in the excitement and self-destruction in the depression. Homicide, I surmise, is as nonspecific, you might say, as the thought processes. In other words, on the rare occasions when a patient does kill somebody in a manic excitement, I think the choice of the victim is not to be considered as unquestionably susceptible to study on the basis of personality factors. It approaches misadventure. And the reason why I think there is a lack of precise personality direction in the assaultiveness of the manic is that the manic cannot think to any purpose—even though he can do nothing else but think and is eternally busy thinking. Thus he may kill somebody who remotely resembles someone he would like to kill if he were sane; but I do not know how much the resemblance and how much the happy chance of his picking up a death-dealing instrument has to do with the event.

And just as I have said at various times that schizophrenics kill themselves by misadventure, I think that depressives do too—the misadventure being that they die in the process of making a supposedly unhealing wound in an enemy. As I have said before, very little goes on in the depressives; and whatever does go on is not responsive to any intelligent approach on the part of the psychiatrist to find out who is the target of his destructiveness, for all that is outside the patient's awareness. Yet all my observations indicate quite conclusively that the depressive always hits the target and usually does this, unhappily, by self-destruction. Although this is, of course, familiar to all experienced psychiatrists, it seems worth repeating. The extraordinary thing about this self-destructiveness is that there is no time when it is so likely to occur as during the period of convalescence from the depth of the depression. When a person is thoroughly depressed, he is not apt to be active enough to kill himself except possibly by the exceedingly tedious process of starvation. But some depressives, when they are convalescent, show a determination sufficient to elude all interference; and they kill themselves. A long, long time ago, before I had really found my way around very much in psychiatric thinking, I worked a little with intensely suicidal convalescent depressed people. It left me with what I believe is a supportable hypothesis—namely, *that a particular person who was a destructive influence in the patient's past is the target of the patient's self-destruction. The intention is that that person shall suffer the rest of his life because the patient has destroyed himself.* But I have not heard a patient agree on any of this. Convalescent depressives still show something of the depressive's so-called poverty of thought. In a queer sort of analogy to the excitement, the depressive will run lots of permutations and combinations of the grief-provoking content, but he will not get very far off it. The psychiatrist finds himself unable to get the patient to the point where a stream of associations runs smoothly enough so that the associations take the patient far afield and, perhaps, into the proximity of really explanatory experience. Thus one finds the manic-depressive very, very hard to convert from being a very risky patient into a psychotherapeutic prospect. Incidentally, I have known of a few instances in which psychoanalysts who were fairly obviously of the manic-depressive persuasion, despite their training according to the most highly formulated requirements for psychoanalysts, eventually took the route out by their own hand. Almost as a sort of ironic footnote on my theory of the target, in each instance the psychoanalysts did not kill themselves until they had resumed treatment with some colleague. Some of them have shown a sense of the dramatic in arranging the event in such a way that the colleague suffered —but not, of course, for very long. The idea that merely killing oneself will leave a *permanent* dent in anybody is really quite fantastic.

Paranoid States and Manic-Depression

I want to mention one further idea, which should by no means be mistaken for scientific observation. It is merely an impression which has, perhaps very unfortunately, tended to substantiate itself in my very limited experience: People in whom the excited phase is the conspicuous thing, and in whom the depressed phase is either brief or not very pronounced, have seemed to have an extraordinarily high probability of winding up in fixed paranoid states. In other words, the excitements, after the first few, get more and more bitter, and the feeling of being persecuted comes more easily. And presently, instead of the excitement, the person has a bitter, active, and really dangerous paranoid state, which goes on and on without let or remission.

In this regard I would like to mention that although manic-depressive states are, on the whole, a very discouraging field to me, there is one related illness which I have been able to work with. This is the swiftly developing paranoid-colored excited state in women somewhere around 35 to 45 years old. I have seen quite a number of these in the course of my hospital work. While the paranoid aspect is distinctly impressive, these people also keep themselves very busy—when they come into the hospital, they usually show practically the manic flight of ideas. You cannot get near anything; they run all over the lot. But because that phase passes so quickly, I have felt that there is real therapeutic prospect in these people and that they cease to have the flight of ideas because they find that the environment is protective, regardless of their paranoid convictions. And as they begin to discuss the paranoid elements of the illness, the excitement becomes less and less striking, although they continue to be very high-keyed and overactive and they sleep little, without ever getting tired.

Involutional Illness in Relation to Manic-Depressive Psychosis

It seems worth while to make a marginal comment at this point on the involutional illnesses. I would like to consider them in two main groups—the agitated depressions and what I call the world-disaster psychosis. In women who have a history of manic-depressive illnesses, the occurrence around the time of the menopause of a depression which has a great deal of agitation in it is too interesting and too frequent to be ignored. But at the same time, it seems clear to me that a person need not have shown what I would call unquestionably cyclothymic habits in order to develop an agitated depression around that time. Like all of the involutional illnesses, agitated depression is some sort of blend of something else with schizophrenia; but it is much further from schizophrenia than is the other type of involutional illness, the world-disaster psychosis, which I will discuss presently. Agitated depressives often have rather panicky periods; in fact, some of them can feel panicky many times during the day or, more commonly, during the night. Their content shows many of the suggestions of poverty of thought which one encounters in the deep depression; the agitated depression is unlike the classical depression, however, in that the patients are quite vocal. But although they can very easily be provoked to express the content, they cannot be provoked to get very far from a relatively stereotyped expression of it. I once pestered one of these patients until I was able to lead her to use new words, instead of the stereotyped ones, to express her conviction that something perfectly horrible was about to happen to her beloved brother. Yet I never found any way of getting her to attempt to depict *what* this disaster would be, and I could never get her to try to picture who else might be involved in it except the beloved brother and, of course, herself—since she was already in it. Thus the poverty of ideas—insofar as such a thing exists—is, perhaps, rather striking in the agitated depression, as well as in the deep depression of the manic-depressive psychosis. The agitated depressive is not nearly so reduced in capacity for communication as is the person in a deep depression. Sometimes agitated people's lives practically consist in the expression of apprehension; they look frightened and wring their hands by the hour, looking more frightened and wringing their hands more at some times than at others. And there is still the intangible but perfectly impenetrable curtain that cuts them off from any psychotherapeutic attack that I have been able to find or have heard anyone else describe. Thus, while we encounter the picture of singularly sustained anxiety or extremely easily recurring anxiety which characterizes agitated depressives, we do not know how to make use of the types of interpersonal situation and approach which have proved useful tools in dealing with all other manifestations of anxiety.[1] In the agitated depression, I cannot get anywhere near either the self or whatever threatens the self, because of the impregnably depressive content.

Very, very occasionally one runs onto a person who has

[1] Another kind of anxiety which does not lend itself to this kind of intervention is what I call the *anxiety states*—that is, anxiety which attacks people in a more or less defined setting so that the anxiety itself becomes the disabling symptom. I have not been able to study these states very closely, and so I do not know as much as I would like to about them.

been alleged to be in an agitated depression, but who, you find when you see him, has what I call the *world-disaster psychosis*. I have not seen a transition occur from an agitated depression to a world-disaster psychosis and, frankly, I strongly suspect that such a transition does not occur. However, there are histories of such transitions, and I suppose that one cannot entirely disregard the possibility by assuming that the other fellow is the bum psychiatrist. I do not consider the world-disaster psychosis to be really relevant to the topic of manic-depressives because the content, down to the most refined details, can appear in 17-year-old male schizophrenics, for instance, just as it commonly occurs in very much older people—namely, women of from 45 to 50. The world-disaster psychosis is essentially schizophrenic, and as such is a fairly important part of the theory of schizophrenic processes. Incidentally, there is one part of Kraepelinian psychiatry that occurs to me in this connection, although I am sure that what I have in mind is quite different from Kraepelinian thinking. Kraepelinian psychiatry states that the hebephrenic form of dementia praecox often begins as a depression. And when I think of this statement, it is in connection with the world-disaster form of involutional psychosis which, in the beginning, often appears objectively as a depression. In the beginning of such a psychosis the patient slows down, is sad, is unresponsive to anything cheerful. And then, after the pattern of schizophrenic things, a frankly psychotic process appears, and the thing is under way. The agitated depression, on the other hand, can grow before one's eyes from simple worry to deeply disturbing worry in which there is no possibility of reassurance; and when no reassurance can be given, the psychotic separation has been effected.

I am unable to explain the psychogenesis of the manic-depressive psychosis, for I have been unable to get any real clues to it. I have heard plausible psychogenetic explanations advanced by others at various times, but they have seemed to me to be purely theoretical, unrelated to any concrete situation or to any real patient. I felt in each case that the hypothesis was arrived at by looking at the smallest possible context, sometimes at secondhand, and speculating about it. While the speculations might be interesting, that is not my idea of the way to study personality processes.

Whereas I might feel that the end state of failure of one after another of the dynamisms of difficulty is schizophrenia, I suppose that it is not true in some cases—for example, the manic-depressives. I presume then that certain people may have a good excuse to become schizophrenic, yet they have instead developed this queer manic-depressive pattern. Thus for those people I have to assume that schizophrenic processes are not an end state of everything. It is just something they cannot do, or in some fashion are protected from. I see nothing in the manic-depressive pattern that can be explained as a simple instance by the theory of interpersonal relations, although I have at times speculated on what might be some differences in the home dynamics—in the manner in which they have been treated by their parents, in comparison to the way schizophrenics have been treated by their parents. I have speculated that, while the parents of schizophrenics are frequently extremely arrogant in their relations with their children, the parents of manic-depressives—or rather the fathers—are more conspicuously the self-righteous fathead types. But, as I say, I must simply accept the fact that the manic-depressive remains a mystery to me. Here let me remark that however forbidding I may sound about the manic-depressive (and how satirical I may sound about the hysteric), that does not mean that I value them less as examples of human beings or as less important tributaries to the sum total of our knowledge of the governing limitations of human personality—which are insignificant compared with the magnificent possibilities of human personality. It means merely that I have discovered, from previous tests of myself as an investigative instrument, my own limitations for learning something about my fellows.

Schizophrenia, Paranoid States, and Related Conditions

PERHAPS I should begin by saying why I lump schizophrenia, paranoid states, and related conditions. Conceptually, pure paranoia and pure schizophrenia may be pictured as two absolute—and, therefore, imaginary—poles. Yet the fact is that every person who gets lost in the schizophrenic morasses has paranoid feelings and can be led to express paranoid content at times; and, on the other hand, every paranoid person that I have encountered has in his history a period of schizophrenic content.

The person who approached pure paranoia would be one who, as an adequate way of handling his difficulties, transferred out of his awareness any feeling of blame in any connection. Since one cannot transfer blame into interstellar space, it is transferred onto the persons making up the environment. Anyone competent enough to accomplish this must necessarily also have some explanation of why the environment is so peculiarly vicious, and the net result is very highly systematized delusions of persecution and grandeur. And I may add that the nearer one gets to the pole of pure paranoia, the more obviously the grandeur becomes an explanation for why one should be so persecuted. Despite suggestions to the contrary that occur here and there in the literature, the persecutory distortion comes first and the grandiose explanation second.

But how few people ever approach the absolute pole of pure paranoia may be suggested by the fact that out of, I suppose, fully three thousand veteran cases with which I had some contact in one of the hospitals where I have worked, only one even raised the diagnostic problem of whether he might be a pure paranoid. But it finally was discovered that even this patient's illness had begun with schizophrenic experience—a fact which emerged only in a subsequent hospitalization. At that time he was led to discuss the first of his allegedly recurring mental states, which actually was the beginning of his continued mental disorder, and it included definitely schizophrenic experience. This confirmed what I had long since decided—that it couldn't happen otherwise.

But why is it that one cannot make a blanket transfer of blame onto the environment without undergoing some of this use of the earlier types of referential process? I have a feeling that there is nothing profoundly obscure about it. Although the self is primarily concerned with anxiety—with detecting the threat of anxiety and developing techniques for reducing anxiety and avoiding the recurrence of it—it also is intimately related in a great many ways to refined verbal thinking, to high-grade referential processes using verbal symbols. This is because the learning of language in childhood coincided with the development of the basic structure of the self, and because nonvalidated thinking—these earlier types of referential process—was something that had to be stamped out in the early stages of life as part of the very building of the self. Now the doctrine of pure paranoia would require that the person was wholly secure in his psychosis; there would literally, I think, from the standpoint of theory, be no necessity for the self, except as a device for keeping track of all the attacks upon one and so on. But so massive a maneuver as practically eliminating the necessity for the self would require something other than operations with the validated verbal symbols which are so intimately related to the self; in other words, the self must be subjected to processes which are not classically of it, and these processes are the early, nonvalidated types of thinking which appear in later life as schizophrenic processes. Thus I think it is safe to say that every paranoid person has at some time been schizophrenic for a little while, which means that the universe has been apprehended and dealt with by much more primitive and less refined referential processes than those which later make up the substance of the paranoid state.

The difficulty that we had in getting at the schizophrenic experience in the particular patient whom I have cited is, I think, suggestive of the difficulty encountered with all markedly paranoid-schizophrenic illnesses in getting at anything which can be used remedially. This patient approached pure paranoia in that he was not, from his point of view, in any sense psychotic; there was only a conspiracy that caused him to be in the hospital again and again. He was litigious and he had, by means of lawsuits, made it extremely awkward for a number of people, including at least one very high government official. Counsel for the people against whom he had brought actions were not at all inclined to minimize the skill with which he could build up very impressive claims on the basis of what a psychiatrist could regard only as paranoid formulations, but which a jury might easily regard as an instance of an extraordinarily capable person's seeing how he was being gypped by corporations, government officials, and various other people. Now, to deal with any of this as possibly psychotic, one would have to get at material about which the patient could not immediately reason convincingly against one. And that material was the material that the patient himself could not understand—namely, the schizophrenic beginning of the thing. So, of course, one could get nowhere near any recollection of that; the patient had a perfect life-history that simply omitted it. But finally, by means of the persistence of a very capable psychiatrist, it was possible to document that such a thing had happened.

Thus, according to my way of thinking, there isn't very much use for the psychiatrist to assume that he is engaged in the cure of a markedly paranoid schizophrenic as long as that patient's history continues to reveal no markedly schizophrenic beginning of the illness. If the patient cannot be gotten to review a period when he was thoroughly schizophrenic, then I do not think the psychiatrist can do much with any of the later content. Only people who are quite gifted in referential operations, argument, and rationalization can sustain so complicated a distortion of reality as is the paranoid position. And so, when you encounter a person who can do so, there is no use in struggling with his interwoven blend of facts, misinterpretations, and slightly fraudulent distortions of events. You might just as well start arguing the validity of the value placed by somebody on the Republican or the Democratic political views, for you do not have the essential data, and so you can go on forever.

Some Misconceptions about 'Categories' of Schizophrenia

Schizophrenia is ordinarily presented in psychiatry courses as a mental disorder, or a group of mental disorders, manifested under at least four or five different categories of symptoms. All of these, I believe, were regarded as independent mental disorders until Kraepelin executed his marvelous synthesis, the miraculous nature of which has been somewhat increased by the awkwardness which has attended its use. I refer to the fact that, in the two or three years subsequent to his synthesis of dementia praecox, the experience at the Heidelberg Clinic became more and more troublesome. But by that time, the synthesis had been seized upon as great truth by many psychiatrists, who were much too busy with their own troubles to notice those of the Heidelberg Clinic. And Kraepelin, whom I knew very, very slightly, was not the sort of person who would feel that his scientific stature would be increased by announcing that what he had said in a previous year had been somewhat of a mistake and needed a good deal of refinement. The nearest he could come to it was that, from its original announcement to the last edition of his book, his synthesis underwent quite a growth of complexity.

In the pre-Kraepelinian days we had *catatonia*, which was quite ancient and honorable; that is, it had been a recognized entity for a good many years. It was supposed to be a mental disorder of the early years, the teens and thereabouts, and was rather outstandingly characterized by disturbances of motion, of skeletal activity, and by such phenomena as mutism, the refusal of food, and neglect of the toilet habits, so that these patients were apt to be wet and soiled, and so on. And they showed such phenomena as cerea flexibilitas—which, I believe, teaching psychiatrists used to be very happy to demonstrate to their classes—and "command negativism." Many amazing things were noted about catatonic patients and duly recorded by psychiatrists, I think chiefly for the astonishment of less experienced psychiatrists. That was in the days before Freud had suggested that mental phenomena might be susceptible of understanding, and therefore there was no great need to add speculations to the reports of marvels about catatonics.

Some years after catatonia had been created as an entity, there came *hebephrenia*. According to the classical picture, it started out as a depression, apparently not very deep, which gradually passed over into dilapidation of social habits, seclusiveness, and irregular episodes of incredibly purposeless destructive excitement. Catatonic excitements, which did not occur very often, came in for attention mostly in contrast to the blind, purposeless, destructive episodes which could occur at any time in the hebephrenic.

Then there was added a simple deterioration which got itself called later the *simple form of dementia praecox*, in which nothing much seemed to happen except that the patient got more and more fantastic in his thinking and less and less interested in, and capable of, social refinements of behavior. Another group appeared which, in the later edition of the Kraepelinian system, was divided into the *paranoid form of dementia praecox* and *paraphrenia*. These were considered separate from paranoia and the paranoiac and paranoid conditions, which were regarded as making up a clinical entity quite distinct from dementia praecox. The essence of paraphrenia, according to Kraepelin, was that the person settled down to a chronic, relatively static course of persecutory ideas without marked deterioration.

SIMPLE DEMENTIA PRAECOX

Before I present my own views on schizophrenia, let me say something about simple dementia praecox, which I do not include among the schizophrenic illnesses. There are some people who, rather astonishingly early, perhaps at the age of 14, 15, or 16, get more interested in philosophizing about good and evil, the nature of God and the Universe, and one thing and another, than in how to make the grade in school social affairs. Gradually they become more and more preposterously unrealistic in the statements they make about the nature of God, good, and so on, and less and less interested in their appearance and their activities—in fact, in living. They seldom lose their appetites, however; in fact, they quite often take on a good deal of weight, thereby suggesting the movement which we see in hebephrenia toward an exclusive interest in the orifices of the body. In general, these people simply gradually fall apart, in a sort of caricature of a regression—a very crude caricature because there are no definite steps in it. They eventually reach a deteriorated state which is reminiscent of the late condition in hebephrenia, but without anything very dramatic ever having happened, without any particular tendency to destructive excitements, and certainly without any peculiar involvement of the activity of the striped musculature and so on.

I believe that these people suffer some kind of organic deterioration. I have seen a few of them, and wasted some time with some of them. I have not been able to find anything except the grossest appearances which seem to have anything to do with what I know to be schizophrenia. Especially since the course called simple dementia praecox is shown by some people who are obviously defective in the sense of having very low intelligence—whatever the factors are that go to make up intelligence—I am quite willing to think that here we may have an hereditarily determined deterioration, or at least a deterioration which is determined very early. I think, however, that the actual appearance of the deterioration is likely to coincide with puberty, and I suspect that it may be set off by whatever physiological changes of balance are connected with the maturation of the genitals. Long before being tolerant of any such theory, I was interested in the possibility that it was connected with the interpersonal rather than the physiological changes of puberty. I tried to explore the possible significance of defeat in the social aspects of the sex life; but, in the few patients that I spent considerable time with, I was entirely unable to discover anything in the background of their increasingly vague thoughts about this and that which I would regard as even rather indirectly suggesting preoccupation with sexual problems. On the basis of this sort of experience, simple dementia praecox may be deleted from the schizophrenic illnesses so far as I am concerned.

CLASSICAL CATEGORIES OF PARANOID SCHIZOPHRENIA, PARAPHRENIA, AND SO ON

I think that Kraepelin named paraphrenia because he needed a term for something that did not fit with the usual observation that dementia praecox ought to begin early, which had always attracted him very much. It is true that paranoid-schizophrenic illnesses—that is, schizophrenic illnesses that are apt to wind up as chronic paranoid states which are in turn more or less schizophrenic—are statistically apt to date their onset from much later in chronologic age than is the case with the durable catatonic states or the hebephrenic. But there is a perfectly good reason for this which does not require the postulation of any separations in these things. The distinctions between paranoid schizophrenia, paranoid states, and paranoia will not, I am sure, stand up under any very intensive study of individual patients. I have gone to trouble enough to convince myself of that; and since I do not believe that my conviction suits any inner need of mine, perhaps I am right. The notion that there are these separate forms, amounting very nearly to separate entities, even as Kraepelin recites them, is, I think, an instance of certain culturally conditioned habits of thought having defeated a man of far, far more than average psychiatric ability. Even if Kraepelin has been one of our greatest headaches, he also was a very, very able man. He observed a good deal, and he permitted observations to go on in his environment. Otherwise, the Heidelberg Clinic would not have had so much trouble with his dementia praecox in the succeeding years. I believe that Kraepelin was unfortunately driven by a certain obsessional necessity for completeness that made naming things and juggling with nosological entities one of the most superior forms of human activity, which I think was possibly an attribute of a certain type of German intellectual. Thus even though he made the great central dementia praecox synthesis, he failed to notice that these things that come very near being separate diseases are rather strikingly functions of the personality structure concerned and that such characteristics as age of onset, and so on, point in that direction rather than in the direction of almost separate entities. But that would have been awkward. That would have been recondite and unclear. And so, we got dementia praecox.

The Catatonic: The Essential
Schizophrenic Picture

RELATION OF HEBEPHRENIA AND CATATONIA

Now let me try to present my own view of the relationship of remaining classes of dementia praecox, so-called. As I have already suggested, I consider these to be in no sense separate entities, but to be functions of the personality structure concerned. First, a word about hebephrenia and catatonia. Let us assume that one encounters very grave conflicts between one's needs for satisfactions and one's necessity for feeling secure and free from severe anxiety long before there has been a consolidation of intimacy with a fellow being, a real other person. Then, if there is a schizophrenic disaster —that is, loss of the control of awareness, with the eruption into the field of attention of less refined and specific referential processes which might be called dream thoughts or reverie processes ordinarily ignored—this will be followed by a course which quickly eliminates from the manifestations of the self a great many of the recent additions of the self. In other words, there will be a strikingly regressive course in which social habits, communicative utilization of speech, and so on, will be lost very swiftly; and the gross picture of the hebephrenic will manifest itself. It is correct to say that these people deteriorate very quickly, so far as what we can observe is concerned—that is, the very severe dilapidation of social habits and the disappearance of social values in behavior. As to whether the intelligence factors also deteriorate very quickly, let me say very simply that we have no way of demonstrating the validity of such a view. Intelligence factors are measured almost exclusively by the utilization of verbal communicative techniques and the assertion of socially

validated relations, both of which are seriously affected in the
hebephrenic change. Thus the application of almost any intelligence test becomes beside the point.

Now, on the other hand, if there has been a consolidation
of experience of a preadolescent character—in other words,
if the person has experienced the need for, and novel returns
from, intimacy with another person, a chum—then the eventuality of schizophrenic disaster will not bring about so swift a
regressive divestment of the later acquisitions of personality.
Instead, the schizophrenic disaster will follow a course primarily characterized, I think, by its close relationship to the
nightmares which are experienced by adolescents and by some
chronological adults. In other words, the conflict between the
need for satisfaction and the need for security lowers the
threshold of awareness to the point where these processes
escape the excluding device and take the place of the finely
focused referential processes. And this conflict has a great
deal to do with the very thing we see in troubled dreams and
nightmares, which represent the highly sustained application
to the solution of a problem of rather high orders of reverie
processes and subverbal or autistic verbal operations. As long
as this sort of process continues, the patient can be called
catatonic. At any time, other things being equal, he may
despair, in which case the hebephrenic change supervenes;
or he may find the paranoid solution, in which case a change
into paranoid schizophrenia or the paranoid state occurs. Thus
I would say that the catatonic is the essential schizophrenic
picture.

I have no doubt actually that if we had enough information
on any hebephrenic, we would find that the beginnings of the
illness showed what I call the essential schizophrenic condition—catatonia. I draw this conclusion from my investigation of the very, very few somewhat accessible hebephrenic
patients I have encountered—and most of that accessibility
was in relatives who knew what the patient had said in the

very early days of obvious mental disorder, rather than in anything that I could get from the patient. But it seemed that what had happened in the beginning of the mental disorder corresponded to the catatonic picture. That is, the type of content that we are accustomed to was displaced from attention by referential processes carrying the feeling of extreme urgency and importance that are known to the rest of us only in our sleep, although we certainly make use of many of the same processes in waking periods of absent-mindedness, brown study, and so on. But then we do not know what we are doing, so it gives us no data.

Before going on, let me restate the distinction I have drawn between the hebephrenic and the catatonic. If a person has not had any genuinely meaningful experience of the preadolescent era of development, then if a schizophrenic episode occurs, it will be characterized by a much prompter appearance of the hebephrenic development than is the case in a person who has had such experience. I suppose that the reason why the hebephrenic development appears so promptly in those who have not had this experience is that there is nothing of great value which fixes them to the height of personality evolution they have achieved. It is the lack of a tie with what one may call the real interpersonal world which is so conspicuously lacking in the hebephrenic, whereas that very tie is so conspicuously troublesome in catatonics and in those who eventually make paranoid elaborations. Thus one might say that once one has become preadolescent, one has acquired a sort of tie to other people which has a value which conspicuously exceeds anything up to that stage and which is demonstrated in a great many ways—for our present purpose, by the travail which is suffered by the schizophrenics who do not dilapidate at once or very quickly.

THE SPREAD OF MEANING AND THE DISAPPEARANCE OF PERSONAL BOUNDARIES

Now let me try to say something about the phenomenology of so-called catatonic schizophrenia that will be near enough a generality to be somewhat useful. Of course, the content—and, therefore, the behavior of the catatonic, since it is related to the content—can be of a great many forms and varieties, just as the reported nightmares and other dreams of unhappy people are of a great many forms and varieties. But I believe that this generalization can be made: If, for at least several years before the eruption of the schizophrenic condition, a person has lived with a feeling of some success in making communicative reference to reality—saying what he means, as one might put it—then the notion of meaning, the notion of getting something out of what happens and being able to tell another person about it, continues to be present in the schizophrenic episode. But since the referential processes are of a distinctly less focused, less precise character, meaning spreads widely; and a great many things that have not seemed meaningful since early childhood again become important ingredients of the relevant universe of the schizophrenic. Thus the extravasation of meaning over a great many things from which any meaning had long since been withdrawn as a result of previous experience—if it ever was there—is an outstanding characteristic of schizophrenia. Correspondingly, because there is not the neat but often treacherous distinction between *thee* and *me* which is so exquisitely the result of language operations in the interest of the self, the boundary between the patient and the universe, particularly the personal universe, undergoes the same diffusion. And although this diffusion may seem to be a special property of the schizophrenic state, let me remind you that it is simply implicit in this earlier, less focused type of referential process. If all of us were not able to achieve this very diffusion, this loss of boundaries, in our states of reverie or brown study, we would not get some of our sudden, wonderfully useful hunches. But the point is that the schizophrenic tries to communicate in these terms, while most of us never even know that we sometimes think in them. And when the schizophrenic tries to communicate in this way, it sounds as if he has become involved with the whole universe, or as if he has become involved with vast entities whose performance is, as it were, a cosmic drama which struggles to find the solution for a life problem in the same way that a nightmare does.

THE FEELING OF URGENCY

I have suggested that in simple dementia praecox the person gradually settles down to having fun with his thoughts, and the thoughts get less and less related to anything that can be said to have any purpose. Just the opposite is the case in the catatonic; there is no feeling that the catatonic is sitting idly by and speculating in universal terms. Instead, there is an immense and eternal feeling of urgency. Sometimes it is a terrible urgency—a terror which demands escape, even if it be escape from the whole universe. The urgency may show as the expenditure of a simply enormous amount of energy in frantic activity, which may seem to be merely a sort of stereotyped destructive action or a stereotyped noise production. Sometimes it is simply a feeling of urgency about understanding or finding the explanation for things. It is the sort of feeling that any of us may have when we do something odd—a need to explain it, to have some kind of formula for it. It is as if the person thinks, "I must understand this. I ought to understand this. Why don't I grasp it?"

Very often in the early stages this feeling of urgency results in great efforts to do something about this new universe that one has stumbled into, to take action. Sometimes these actions are so nearly commonplace that they are overlooked by other people and can be brought out later only by very careful questioning of informants. At other times they are extraordinarily dramatic, as in the case of a man who suddenly leaped from his desk shouting that his arm was paralyzed, galloped out, jumped into a car, and drove at 70 miles an hour over a desperately dangerous highway—to be found, when the authorities caught up with him, collided with a tree and in a state of mutism and stupor. Thus the feeling of urgency is at the start apt to be carried out in actions, the purposes of which largely escape us because the actions are dictated by a type of process that does not lead to public performance on the part of most of us. We may do things privately under the same type of process, but we do not advertise it to strangers.

What is the sense of urgency about? What, for instance, was the man who drove over the dangerous highway at 70 miles an hour trying to escape? I would say that it is as if the need for security had, along with other motivational elements, been universalized, generalized, to the point literally of being a fixed feature of living. Some schizophrenics go into literal, true panic at the inception of the thing, and many of them have very terrifying experiences. It is as if the threat of recurrent terror were always on the fringe of awareness—as if there were something terribly important to do, just as any of us would feel a terrible urgency to get away from an extremely menacing real situation. But there is no way to find out from the schizophrenic what it is that is menacing. His urgency has such a sort of totality that good clear thinking cannot be done about it, for it is more real than thought. I think it is quite like the component of urge to escape which appears in fear, except that the urge of the schizophrenic is to do something. And while sometimes it looks very much as if he were escaping, the urgency is seldom present in awareness in that form. Even if he charges off at 70 miles an hour from a very morbifying situation which has literally precipitated his attack, he is almost certain to have in mind something to do when he gets somewhere; the purpose is not just to get away, although getting away from the situation would have been the sensible thing for him to have done several years before.

Thus the vague but driving urgency which the schizophrenic feels is a necessity to do something; to think something; to accomplish something. And the urgency is rather awful, in the sense of always being somewhere around the fringes of awareness. It comes back in the morning when he wakes up, and stays with him until he has fallen asleep. Sometimes, in fact, it makes it extremely unsatisfactory to feel that he will fall asleep, for there isn't any time for sleep. I suppose if one had to try to put such a thing into words, one might say that the schizophrenic suffers an almost unceasing fear of becoming an exceedingly unpleasant form of nothingness by collapse of the self. Incidentally, even if the self is not effective in achieving security, the schizophrenic still has a self, as shown if he falls into the paranoid type of maladjustment. For example, schizophrenics talk occasionally of exploding, or something of that kind. And the urgency also shows in some of the questions a schizophrenic may ask when he is in the later stages of stupor and is fairly free in speech. He will be distracted by your movements and want to know what it means when you rub your eyelids. Everything ought to be understood, you see; it isn't just that he is idly curious; he feels that he ought to understand, and he is sorry that he doesn't understand, and he is almost apologetic for asking you to tell him. Clearly, there is an urgency in the thing. Something ought to be done; and there is no finding out what.

The reason why we cannot find out what the urgency is about goes back to the conception of referential process and to the fact that it is difficult to talk about things that are pretty well out of the experience of the waking life anyway. Perhaps I can give you an idea of what it is like by comparing it to the feeling of duration which we all have. Any of us, if we look into our state of mind, will find that we have a feeling of duration, in addition to verbal processes which have more or less adequate reference to something or other. We know that we were here yesterday, will probably be here tomorrow, and so on; but we could not say what this feeling of duration is about. The state of mind of the catatonic, if he were to observe it, would have not only some verbal processes, at least now and then, and a feeling of duration— but it would also have a feeling of urgency. But as to what the urgency is about, it would be as impossible to say as it would be for any of us to say what our feeling of duration is about.

At the beginning of their illness, catatonics quite often have some very lurid ideas about what ought to be done, but these ideas miscarry so badly and are so obviously mistakes and misapprehensions that after that there isn't very much to talk about. The sense of urgency does not show as something one can deal with as such, any more than I would know how I could make much sense in talking with any of you about this background of feeling of duration, even though it is, I suppose, possibly the only durable and eternal characteristic of what we call consciousness. But the urgency shows in everything the catatonic does that one can talk about, and it should always be assumed to be there, just as in all our talk with our patients we assume that they have the feeling of duration—that memory will document the thing any time we wish.

The feeling of urgency shows even when the catatonic is being amazingly satirical, as some of them can be—really, I think, catatonics are the original source of bitter humor. It is awfully beside the point to feel that the catatonic's state of mind corresponds to what our state of mind would be if we pulled off such cynical comments to a friend or enemy. Instead, the catatonic is doing something that has to be done. It is true that he is being cynical and that he often gets a kick, I think, out of seeing the other person wince. But it is for some purpose. He doesn't know what the purpose is; he doesn't need to know. But if you are dealing with such a patient, you must not assume that he is just having fun at your expense, or something of that kind.

I suppose that if we had two or three of our most gifted schizophrenics here now, and I should turn to them and ask, "What is this urgency for?" one of them might say, "Well, we are really a little interested in getting back to being human beings. It seems quite imperative. I guess that must be what you are talking about." In other words, the urgency is to get together again, to have the world remain, you might say, at peace instead of undergoing the unearthly intrusions and extrusions and divagations and one thing and another that the rest of us experience mostly in our nightmares.

CATATONIC STUPOR

I have already mentioned that the feeling of urgency, coupled with the impractical referential processes, often brings about initial bizarre action of some kind. Now this action is observed by the person himself, for most of the time there is nothing that prevents a schizophrenic from noticing what he is doing, although certain types of observation are interrupted at unhappy moments. But most of his unsureness is in thinking out *why* rather than in merely observing; he has functioning sense organs, and so on, like the rest of us. And the thing that strikes most schizophrenics, as a result of their observations, is that they are crazy. With the clearest and most impelling of motives, they take some action; but this action miscarries appallingly, and it shows them that they are crazy. Take my case again of the man who, after driving 70 miles an hour over dangerous roads for a remarkable distance, hit a tree, and was, by the time the following car caught up, mute and immobile. What had happened was that he had traveled over these roads, missing mountains and taking turns on two wheels, with a feeling that he was under almost divine protection, alone in a universe without trees and other obstructions, perhaps with the feeling that he was traveling over a straight line. But the collision with the tree deleted all of this; it showed that what he had done was crazy, that it just didn't fit any of the patterns which are usually useful in making sense of things. And it is the discovery that these intensely impelled details of behavior do not get one any nearer an urgently desired goal—that, in fact, they very often get one to anything but the goal—that ties up the skeletal activity in the fashion which we call stupor. Incidentally, this stupor is a very active postural business, and anything but the inhibition of all postural tensions.

Here I am offering an explanation that is quite different from Hoch's ruminations about benign stupor,[1] and different also from anything else I know on the subject of stupor. But I believe that stupor is precipitated in almost all cases very much as it was in this case I have described. Something is done under great pressure—under a simply unearthly pressure of necessity—and it is obviously not effective. Something else may then be attempted, but it presently becomes apparent to the patient in his more lucid moments that something is terribly wrong, that he is getting nowhere. And he ties up the whole skeletal apparatus in what starts out, I suppose, to be an intensely alert readiness awaiting for some motivation, some pattern or activity, to appear, but which gradually settles down to be the thing in itself. Such patients do relax in sleep, but the tension accompanies awakening. Sometimes a patient who has been stuporous for months may awaken abruptly one night and do something very active and carefully focused, such as attempting to strangle somebody or making an effort at self-destruction.

The paranoid development can appear under cover of the

[1] August Hoch, *Benign Stupors: A Study of a New Manic-Depressive Reaction Type;* New York: Macmillan, 1921.

stupor. One occasionally sees a transitional situation in which a person who was obviously catatonic comes to look more and more malignantly at the people around him and presently bursts into speech, whereas the typical catatonic says little or is definitely mute.

I can tell you from plenty of experience that stuporous people are extraordinarily alert in their stupor, but they are not having any action; they have had enough action. If, however, they fall asleep, they may be aroused from sleep by another of these impelling drives and again engage in action. They will do something then, only again to be convinced, without much clear thinking about it, that it is just crazy. And so they literally tie themselves into immobility. This might be interpreted, if they thought as we think, as a fear of what they might do. In fact, it is very easy to lead them into explaining the whole thing as a fear of what they might do. But I do not believe it is the case. It is not to keep from making mistakes that they have tied up all of their skeletal muscles; it is distinctly more—as you would suspect from what little we know about dream processes—as if a *power* fixes them. The self and such things have become practically universal. These people are almost a universe of their own, and so of course it is not that "I am holding myself from action"; it is that a power, some great cosmic force, ties up the muscles and prevents action.

Much of the confusion about the catatonic state comes about from what people tell you later. I can say from considerable data that one of the many interests of the schizophrenic in convalescing, with or without the aid of a psychiatrist, is to seem as little 'crazy' as possible. Therefore he is likely to agree with any explanation that anybody hands out that sounds plausible and does not seem very strange. He will document it in the same way that we can document all sorts of fool explanations that protect us from discovering how little we know.

CATATONIC EXCITEMENT

So far I have tried to describe the spread of meaning, the feeling of urgent need for a solution—which may approximate an absolute cosmic necessity, something as driving as if one were God—and the initial bizarre activity, followed by what we call stupor. This stupor, or striking degree of tense inactivity, is sometimes interrupted by eruptions of activity, generally related to sleep, which we refer to as catatonic excitement. This is unlike the initial schizophrenic excursion into activity. The person still feels the urgency, but he has tried something at the start and has given it up and become catatonic —that is, tense and inactive. But this tense inactivity is not enough; the urgency calls for something more than that. So instead of feeling that a power has hypnotized him, or however he might try to describe it later on, now he *becomes the power*. By gestures of power and magical operations involving the whole body, he seeks to affect the cosmic drama in a desirable fashion. This leads to statuesque posing and all sorts of things. This behavior, which has been described as archaic, looks as if it were related to the ritualistic aspects of medieval magical practices, and so on. It consists of intensely meaningful but verbally indescribable gestures, postures, and so on, sometimes carried out with a remarkably slow type of movement suggestive of a high-speed camera movie projected at ordinary rates. I have even at times seen feats of balancing and so on done in a slow sort of ritualistic dance that represented not only the expenditure of an enormous amount of energy in a very quiet way, but also a very remarkable manipulation of balance which many a dancer would be glad to be capable of.

Many of these patients are driven to using speech by this same urgency, and they produce anything from quite reliable statements—in the sense that words are used with consensually valid meaning—to profoundly obscure autistic utterances. Because of the disturbance of reference, they undergo the oddest kinds of experience with speech in the sense that the meanings of words are as widely distorted as could possibly be imagined. Many a catatonic has said things which equaled in every sense the alleged import of the spells cast by our medieval wizards over the Devil, or something of the sort. In general, the schizophrenic has a very terrible time; a good deal of his life is like a horribly important and often dreadful nightmare. Yet part of the time he is much nearer a state of mental health than we would perhaps think. When a patient is in a tense, inactive state or when he is in the activities of the excitement, we may assume that nothing but the schizophrenic processes is getting any attention at all. But at *all other times* we should entertain the possibility that he is not very far from the capacity for verbal communication.

Problems of Eliciting and Interpreting Communication in the Schizophrenic Illness

It is the common experience of psychiatrists with their convalescent or recovered schizophrenics that these patients do not remember the events of the illness. More precisely, however, the point here is that whatever they can recall of these events is not intelligibly communicable to others because it is the type of experience that has never been talked about by any of us. It is like the experience that all of us have had in our early years, before we could use language for referring to our mental states—the type of referential process that is ordinarily excluded from consciousness from midchildhood onwards. Thus the psychiatrist should not be too deeply concerned over the things which the patient apparently cannot recall of his illness; nor should he necessarily struggle to overcome this inability on the assumption that it indicates an unwillingness to look back at what happened. Instead, he must realize that there is no use in trying to say, for instance, what certain things meant; it cannot quite be done. Therapeutically, I think, it is extraordinarily useful to these patients to be reminded that whatever happened to them must be made up of things that everybody could experience, and has experienced; in their case, these things simply took on a rather novel pattern for their time of life.

A great many of the evils that follow the appearance of the schizophrenic dynamism in an interpersonal situation come from the *other* person in it. The ease with which anxiety is aroused—the readiness with which we grow insecure in relations with our fellows—is perhaps never so luridly shown as in the relations of a supposedly healthy person with an unsuspectedly schizophrenic person. The distress of the supposedly healthy person—his discomfort, his desire to depart, to overwhelm the disturbing other person, to correct him, to do *something*, all without any idea of what has happened to make him feel so insecure—is enough to explain much of the aggravation that schizophrenic patients undergo rather swiftly after the first appearance of the schizophrenic phenomena.

Now, aggravating the schizophrenic's condition is, of course, something that the psychiatrist might well avoid doing. One thing that, I believe, only parents and psychiatrists are apt to do in the way of aggravating schizophrenic patients is to permit the appearance of schizophrenic processes in *their own* activities with the patient. Other people who encounter the patient are so disturbed by the caving-in of the tenuous bridge of verbal communication that they may become almost randomly active, and may perhaps frighten the patient to death or enrage him or something or other; but they are so intensely anxious that they are quite unlikely to have schizophrenic processes. Instead, they are going to get out of the situation in some way or other, even if they have to reduce the patient to a pulp before leaving. But the psychiatrist and the parent are so deeply involved with the patient and with their own roles in relation to him that they may try to tail along with him in his schizophrenic processes—the parent, because the patient is part of his family, 'my son' or 'my daughter,' if for no other reason; and the psychiatrist, because he conceives his role to be a sort of mixture of Christ and the Delphic oracle. And so these two people sometimes, I think, outdo the patient in being schizophrenic. In other words, they enter into, and have a feeling of initial success in, departing from communicative use of speech and pursuing all sorts of elusive will-of-the-wisps of reverie that they find sneaking into the edges of their own minds. Thus the parents, quite utterly blamelessly, and the psychiatrist, somewhat less simply, sometimes confirm the reality of the patient's schizophrenic distortions and actually convince themselves that these things are valid by their own extraordinary use of autistic thought processes.

But what *do* you do when a schizophrenic is making an attempt to communicate with you? You may expect, unless the patient is very badly deteriorated in his social interests, that some of the things he says will be simply communicative; that many of the things he says will seem communicative but will be of indeterminate meaning; and that some things he says will seem to be completely meaningless. To take up the first of these categories, I think you may wisely assume that it is impossible to find a person who is utterly schizophrenic, which is preposterous on the face of it. You may assume that in the most schizophrenically disturbed interpersonal relation there will probably be occasional statements that have as simple a meaning as the statements that ordinarily make up meaningful exchange of intelligence. Therefore, you never know when you may hear something that will be simply illuminating and that may well be treated as such. In other words, when something is said which in all probability means just what it says, *that is data*. It doesn't call for either applause or immediate action. But it does justify a mental note being made about it.

The second group—the things said that sound as if they were intelligible, but are not—will not be recognized by a psychiatrist who is inattentive or by a psychiatrist who is certain that one cannot follow schizophrenics anyway. The very existence of this second group of things is the best reason for not galloping into applause when the patient says something you can follow. Some of the things that you can follow, you see, do not mean what you follow. Reasonable patience to observe the context will usually tell you whether communication has occurred or whether the use of autistic verbal operations has occurred. If the patient needs some reassurance—if he begins to wonder what he is doing, and says, "Do you understand?" or something like that—you can always say "Perhaps, in a way; I think so," or something like that. You don't unduly stress the "perhaps"; that would be cruel. But you indicate that you are not too certain, that you will see. After all, that is what happens in all communication; in your interchange with any stranger, you have to wait and see whether you follow; you can't just guess it from the way the sentences are put together. And sometimes telling a schizophrenic just that helps him a great deal.

The last group of things I mentioned are those which seem to be completely meaningless. Now, people don't say meaningless things. But a vast number of communicative efforts are meaningless in terms of the interpersonal situation. When you get no suggestion of transfer of intelligence, it is, I think, extremely unwise for you to join in the psychosis by making use of words in God knows what sense which will be utterly meaningless and uncommunicative to the patient. However, some people have a gift for sensing the reference of essentially uncommunicative operations set in words. A psychiatrist who has such a gift can say quite sincerely, "I think, perhaps, I am following you. Do you by any chance mean so-and-so?"—

recasting it somewhat. And it works. But there are other people who have considerable fun getting lost in the schizophrenic woods with their schizophrenic patients. My own observation is that patients do not seem to cotton to them. I have noticed that the psychiatrist who engages in this sort of thing gets into physical entanglements with patients now and then, from which I conclude that schizophrenics are not entirely hopeless human beings either.

CHARACTERISTIC DISTURBANCES IN COMMUNICATION

The disturbances in verbal communication which one encounters with the schizophrenic include mutism, blocking, the use of neologisms, and the use of other language processes which are effectively meaningless to the hearer. In some cases of *mutism* we can get some information from the patient; in others, we are left entirely in the realm of speculation. The thing always to remember with the schizophrenic is that, while he is alert at all times, under certain circumstances the referential processes that are called out by events are of a type which is so very early, so cosmically undifferentiated, if you please, that there is no expressing the content in words. At such times, the patient's notion of another person to whom he might communicate is certainly no more clear to him than is the notion that many people have about God—the notion of someone who is everywhere and perhaps nowhere and who is able to know one's most secret thought as well as to hear one's most tediously verbal prayer.

The term *blocking* should perhaps be defined here since people may mean any one of many things when they use it. By blocking, I mean an abrupt interference with what the person planned to communicate, so that it is cut off, and there is no way of getting it to go on in the immediate context. The sentence stops, and the person looks blank or looks unchanged, depending on how sick he is. From the psychoanalytic viewpoint, the readiest assumption is that some other thought must have collided with the thought that was being expressed; and in the earlier years of a psychiatrist's work with such patients, he is likely to try to get the interfering thought. But the difficulty is that the colliding thought—if there was a colliding thought—may be essentially incapable of expression in words; there has been a shift in the level of consciousness, and a preverbal or extraverbal type of mental process has intervened. Instead of another thought having collided with the thought that was being expressed, what seems more nearly the case usually is that consciousness has been disturbed, and what was being said is no longer there.

It is nice to suppose that there must be a 'psychic cause' for the timing of blocking and that the psychiatrist should be able to discover it. Presumably there are perfectly adequate explanations for the schizophrenic disturbances of the level of referential process; but unfortunately these explanations, again, are often in terms which are essentially incommunicable, and so they are unlikely to be obtained by inquiry. Occasionally the psychiatrist may notice something about the events at the time the blocking occurred which gives him a clue as to what could be the case. It is improbable, however, that the patient will produce anything very spectacularly revealing which is at a level of awareness that makes for good communication. Thus if a psychiatrist is wise, he does not hit his head against the impassable barrier that he may find in a patient in the form of sudden and almost incredibly great shifts in the type of thought process, or referential process. Such shifts go on in the patient who is badly involved in schizophrenic processes—perhaps in a stupor, or in a condition where stupor is impending.

This may sound discouraging, but I do not consider it so. Various classes of referential processes serve humanity at every stage of development and are of the essence of human living. The fact that a person has, in the presence of another person, a very unstable level of these classes of thought process does not mean that he is completely removed from living and dealing with life. It does mean that his communication is different from ordinary, highly abstract, communicative speech and that a psychiatrist who is attempting to deal with such a person cannot succeed in the type of operation that may be spectacularly and dramatically successful with the hysteric. But then he cannot with an obsessional person either. He may think that he can, because the obsessional can always produce words, and the amateur thinks that these words mean what they would if he used them, which is often not the case. The schizophrenic is just a little bit worse off, or better off, depending on the viewpoint, for he cannot produce even the words in a good many contexts.

Besides these abrupt interferences that we call blocking, there are also disturbances which are seen in what I think are the most illuminating of all the minor subvarieties of schizophrenic conditions—that is, the schizophrenic perplexity states. The essence of these states seems to be, again, that shifts occur in levels of reference. However, these shifts are not nearly so startling in the number of classes of process they may traverse as are the shifts in blocking, but are rather more step-by-step. The person drifts from communicative speech, let us say, into autistic speech, and from autistic speech into preverbal use of articulate noises, and from there into some level of wordless thinking. Sometimes a sentence will undergo change in the process of being said. On such occasions a psychiatrist who is very alert and quite used to the patient can sometimes actually rouse him, as it were, just as one might rouse a person who is falling asleep, so that the patient comes back to a communicable level of thinking and goes on with what he was talking about. This does not happen very often; but on the rare occasions when it does, it conveys a feeling of reality to this conception of shifts in the levels of awareness which could never be conveyed merely by my talking about it.

Another of the disturbances in communication is the use of

neologisms, which are autistic, as all neologisms are except those which are defined, such as the neologisms of scientific terminology. The only reason why the schizophrenic's neologisms sound like such a very special class of things is that we do not pay enough attention to the richly neologistic private speech of children. Children use a great many neologisms, and they serve the same purpose with children as they do with schizophrenics. A neologism of a child carries a lot of meaning —more than one ought to crowd into a word, particularly a word that nobody else understands. But that is simply one of the steps in the learning of language.

The psychiatrist who attempts to work with a schizophrenic must realize that not only can the patient often not communicate, but the psychiatrist himself cannot, by carefully expressed verbal statements, communicate with the wordless levels of awareness in the patient. It works both ways, you see. While the patient may be alert and in touch, this does not mean that he knows what the psychiatrist means or that he may not get very strange distortions of what the psychiatrist says. To draw a parallel with a more commonplace situation, you may feel that you have a rather good idea of what I mean at a certain point, but then be very sadly confused 15 minutes later when you discover from something I say that I did not mean what you thought I meant. And the hurried effort to retrieve the past is practically enough to confuse it hopelessly. That is nothing compared with what schizophrenics have to put up with in all stressful interpersonal situations. So, of course, there is no earthly sense in assuming that they can follow you any more than you can follow a good many of their expressed propositions.

Yet we have some reason to believe that human personality has a fairly adequate account of a great many of the events that impinge on it, even though that is quite a different thing from having an adequate content of consciousness about such events. Therefore, there is every reason for being quite careful to be valid in informative statements made to a schizophrenic patient, because no matter what the statement may mean in consciousness at the time that the patient hears it, it may come back at a more lucid time and take on a good deal of useful meaning. The same thing can be observed in working with any patient, from hysteria up or down; some of the things that you offer, and some of the things that the patient experiences in the therapeutic hour, really become meaningful only after the hour is over, after the patient is out of the interpersonal situation where the events transpired. He may, for instance, see through it between that interview and the next. Sometimes I have offered an interpretation to an obsessional patient who has received it with polite gratitude, but without the faintest signs of anything happening. But several weeks later the patient has happened upon this insight into what has been going on, and it has been very helpful then.

Thus if your interpretation is very adequately expressed, and is as simple and unambiguous as possible, the chances are improved that the patient will eventually get a very adequate insight into the thing, even if nothing happens immediately. With schizophrenics that is especially the case because there is no certainty of when or where a thing may show up again or how it may be useful or harmful. Remember that if one seems to be almost identical with the universe, and to be living within oneself some of the great struggles that are fixed in the mythologies of sundry peoples, or something of the sort, needless to say the doctor who shows up once a day or so is apt to fit into the cosmic pattern, to be one of the gods or devils of the mythological thinking, or to tend to be part of oneself, struggling with perhaps another part of oneself. For this reason, if no other, it is well to be somewhat circumspect in what you give the schizophrenic in the way of example by action and so on.

THE MEANING OF THE RETENTION OF SALIVA

Aside from their disturbances of communication, schizophrenics show further features which seem pretty thoroughly psychotic, despite the fact that the schizophrenic is much more like than unlike the rest of us. One of these features which appears very often in the history of a schizophrenic patient, or which may be observed in the depth of stupor, is the retention of saliva. The saliva is not swallowed and is not expectorated, with the result that the mouth gets pretty full of it and drips. There has been so much speculation about this that I dislike to add my own ideas, which are also relatively speculative. My speculations are based on what patients have told me some months after the stupor had ended. But this does not necessarily mean that I have understood what they told me; it may have been more autistic that I realized. And also, just as dreams are often distorted in the act of ordering them to tell them to the psychoanalyst, so it is quite possible that the significance and necessity and so on which led to a piece of behavior some months back in a stupor are distorted and lose their most highly meaningful aspects in the process of being formulated in words and told to the doctor subsequently.

In the cases where people with a history of retaining saliva have later told me anything about it, their remarks suggest that the saliva is not swallowed because it is dangerous. It is in some fashion menacing to the patient, perhaps menacing to his life. I have not been told, but I assume, that it is not expectorated because expectorating saliva is a type of activity which requires something like a calm mental state or a state of comfortable detachment. Expectoration is not an inborn trait shown by the infant. It simply never occurs to these schizophrenics to spit it out, and if you tell them to spit it out, which would seem to solve the problem, they don't know what you are talking about. They have other things to think of than saliva. The retention of saliva is empirically closely related to the refusal of food—that is, these thoughts about the saliva's being poisonous or dangerous seem to attach also to the food that is offered the patient or perhaps forced down him. There is an especially rich field for speculation in the instances where patients, as quite frequently happens, seem to mix up their ideas of the saliva and the food with the semen. One can speculate at great length about this. But it is lamentable if one takes this speculation to be of some use in dealing with the patient, because there is no way of handling such massive speculations with a stuporous patient. A lot of our psychiatric speculations require a very considerable attention span to be grasped, and the disturbance of referential level in a patient who is in an intense stupor is such that if you cannot get a thing said in six or seven words, I am not sure that it is worth opening your mouth about.

Incidentally, I have quite often found myself talking to such a patient with great care as to my enunciation, speaking quite slowly and perhaps a little more loudly than the actual distance required, because of my intense feeling of the uncertainty of continued touch between the meaning I was attempting to lay before the patient and his grasp on the communicative processes. However, one should never treat stuporous patients as if they were deaf or as if they were infants or children. At the same time, one ought also not to add to the puzzlement which surrounds them on all sides by throwing in a lot of theoretic junk. About the first thing that happens in a schizophrenic episode is that personal meaning spills over onto all sorts of things that in any ordinary type of thinking would have no particular relevance to the patient or his situation. The psychiatrist who invariably has that in mind in dealing with a schizophrenic will be saved a good deal of asinine misbehavior.

Delusions in Schizophrenia as Differentiated from Paranoia

Sometimes a remarkably good personal mythology, you might call it, appears as a result of the spread of meaning to a great many irrelevant events and the occurrence within awareness of the type of referential processes that characterize our thinking in our very early years of life before there is any very clear separation between one's self and all the rest that there is. This personal mythology has very close connection with myths that have been accepted by large groups of humanity over long historic periods, and it frequently appears in terms of great danger, attack, weakness and strength, and all such things. And so, to use the psychiatric jargon, the 'paranoid coloring' appears—the idea that one is being poisoned, or being manipulated, or having this or that done to him by hostile people. Such ideas can always be found in the mental state of incipient schizophrenia and in early stuporous conditions.

Now the notion that people around one are dangerous and ill-disposed toward one and also the notion that there are transcendental superhuman powers that may be malignant or punitive are often thought of as being, in principle, paranoid ideas. But I think that the term *paranoid* must be restricted to those instances where there is this very conspicuous accompaniment of these ideas of malignant power: the person who entertains them becomes blameless, ennobled, and expanded in worth. This is what we encounter in the paranoid states and in markedly paranoid schizophrenia.

But at the moment I am discussing the schizophrenic who incorrectly identifies—as all of us do occasionally—causal relationships, sometimes identifying a cause as being the malignancy of others, or the power of superhuman entities, or magical operations. The schizophrenic is not concerned with problems of blame. These things which sound like paranoid ideas are a part of the disturbance of his grasp of events, caused by the shifting types of referential process and the loss of boundaries of personality, along with, in many cases, extremely clever attempts to understand what has happened.

Now it is true, I suppose, that I have never dealt with a schizophrenic who had not been happy at some time in his life to find that someone else was to blame for something that he had been blamed for; yet I would say that few schizophrenics have come to their psychosis as a result of shame and chagrin for specific traits which they felt were blameworthy. Theirs is a more massive type of unhappiness. They have, perhaps, been excellent scapegoats for others, in that they were so bothered that they were not at all expert at returning the goat to the other person with thanks. They were people especially vulnerable to having blame transferred to them. And they have had the greatest difficulty finding scapegoats themselves; they just have not understood people, or how to deal with people, well enough to make others scapegoats. They are among the most handicapped at juggling blame around.

Take, for example, my patient who is a Yale graduate, but who cannot get started at anything and eventually becomes a night watchman. And then he begins to have curious attacks of somnolence and so on; things at times look different to him; and he falls upon the thought that poison is being put in the lunch that he brings to work at night. Now what does this represent? By a lot of devious thinking one could say that he is washing his hands of his inadequacy and making somebody else responsible, in the shape of an enemy who is poisoning him. But when one talks with him, one does not find anything particularly like that reflected in any way. One finds that he has not hit upon an explanation for his inadequacies. Instead he is still looking for an explanation, and he is profoundly puzzled and very deeply disturbed. He has what somebody long since called the 'insane mood'; the world is beginning to dissolve into a great many unstable things. And apropos possibly of some trifle of gustatory sensation or some hallucination or illusion, as he is drinking his coffee on a particular night, probably in quite an absent-minded condition, he notices perhaps nothing more than the flavor of the coffee. Then the thought of poison enters his mind; if he has been chronically poisoned, that would account for all this.

For the source of this type of explanation of things, we may look to a lot of more or less trivial fiction that all of us have been exposed to, as well as certain myths that appear both in this culture and in many other cultures. And it doesn't have much to do with blame; like a great many incipient schizophrenics, he has been very busy suffering from conflicts and a feeling of profound inadequacy, failure, and so on, but he has not really been blaming himself for it, and this mistaken explanation that he has hit upon has not particularly transferred blame from himself. Thus I do not call this paranoid, and in fact I do not think that it deserves a special name, for, although the explanation hit on by the night watchman is a little startling to a good many of us, it is of a piece with a vast amount of our own incorrect thinking.

In the course of schizophrenic stupor, however, a patient's primitive types of referential process may hit off in the general direction of his being Jesus Christ—the classic case—and the rest of the world, I suppose, then becomes the Jews who are intent on crucifying him. And here we do have a paranoid attitude, unlike the merely mistaken explanations. In other words, here the paranoid dynamism—the transfer of blame —has come into being through shifting the mythological and diffusely focused thinking in the direction of one's being the apotheosis of all that one has wished to be. If this suffices— that is, if the paranoid attitude gives enough feeling of security so that the schizophrenic disturbances of the level of awareness cease—then the person goes into a bitter, highly systematized paranoid state with remarkable speed. But this is quite uncommon. I am inclined to say that if the paranoid development would have sufficed, it would have come rather early.

In other words, I think that those who have in the past had some success at occasionally making somebody else the scapegoat come most readily to the paranoid schizophrenic state—or rather, I should say, to the paranoid state, for they actually do not stay schizophrenic very long. They do a nice job of the transfer of blame and do not have to be very schizophrenic any more.

The fact that paranoid attitudes often do not suffice—that they frequently fail to solve the problems of schizophrenics—is demonstrated by a certain group of patients who show Christ identifications, yet remain catatonic. They grow whiskers, and put up great fights about being shaved, and sometimes they get to look singularly like the artists' conception of the Savior. But they continue to be catatonic; that is, they continue to have postural tension, interference with behavior, and so on —perhaps not as much as they had a while back, when they were just stuporous, but still they are by no means free and easy in their skeletal movements and so on. They do not preach the gospel, and they are not paranoid. They have done everything *but* solve their problem with a paranoid transformation of personality.

A Christ identification may, in the course of human events, progress to a paranoid state, so that the person becomes a more or less well-systematized paranoid schizophrenic. But quite as often, under therapeutic pressure—by which I mean that somebody who really wants the patient to get well pesters him in and out of season, by his presence at least—the Christ identification collapses, and the patient is again lost in the whole welter of universal patterns and is again definitely stuporous. I have had the dubious fortune, but at least theoretically important experience, of having a patient who not only had a Christ identification for a while, but who also was a pretty dangerously systematized paranoid schizophrenic for a while, and whose paranoid system collapsed under alleged therapeutic pressure from me, with the outcome that he was extremely assaultive for years. He is now, I suppose, in a state hospital if he isn't dead of tuberculosis—which is a well-known way out. The fact that the paranoid schizophrenic can sometimes be thrown back into stupor, revert to simple or uncomplicated schizophrenia (by which I do not mean simple dementia praecox), and from that come out quite differently—as a social, if not a real recovery—indicates that the paranoid schizophrenic is by no means always successful in resolving his conflicts by transfer of blame. Such recovery is, I am sorry to say, not too frequent, but is well within the realm of possibility, and has several times been documented in my experience. Moreover, the failure of the transfer of blame to solve the problems of schizophrenics is shown by the shocking character of the persecutions, and so on, that many of them complain of; they are obviously having a very bad time. When the paranoid state becomes a durable maladjustment, it is plenty unpleasant; but it also has its very large returns in the way of security.

I shall not have a great deal to say about the delusions of paranoid schizophrenics. They have been plucked out of the total enigma that any schizophrenic mental state really is to any physician, in the sense that some things have been said which suited the psychiatrist's theoretic slant or personal interest. And so there is a welter of speculation that you can find hither and yon in the literature about the meaning of certain delusion formations. If you are very generous, you may assume that the writer was correct about the particular case he describes; but do not swallow it as an explanation of schizophrenic thinking. There is no explanation of schizophrenic thinking that can be transmitted by speech or in writing because schizophrenic thinking includes a great deal for which those modes of communication are not appropriate. So when you are told that one's homosexual craving leads to this or that, it may be so; you wouldn't know; and neither would the patient.

Pure paranoia, the imaginary state, means that one has become absolutely spotlessly blameless—one is perfect—and the many unpleasant things that one finds oneself engaged in are, of course, the work of the evil world in which one has to live. As a schizophrenic gets more and more to be the almost contented victim of the Masons, or something of the sort, you can assume that the schizophrenic process has probably passed over into the paranoid type of pretty stable maladjustment. It may interest you to try to figure out what signs show when this is to be regarded as irreversible. I know that there are, insofar as people are susceptible to generic classification, some paranoid schizophrenics that it is just perfectly stupid to think of changing. And I know that there are others whose paranoid maladjustment is essentially extremely unstable. I have, in the days when my recklessness was perhaps paving the way for a little sanity later, upset pretty elaborate paranoid systems by nothing more startling than a warm personal attitude toward the patient, combined with sundry attacks on the theories which were most blame-removing, and so on, and inquiries which were disastrous to any peace that the self had achieved. The patients became catatonic again, and we proceeded from there. Some of them, praise God, have been well enough to be out of the hospital for a good many years now, that being over twenty years ago.

Both the so-called paranoid coloring—which is more correctly, I think, identified as mistaken explanations for puzzling events—and the true paranoid attitude originate, I have no doubt, in the schizophrenic disturbance of awareness. But in the case of the paranoid attitude this device of the invention, the discovery, the false causal series, immensely relieves depressed self-esteem; it removes chronic and recurrent anxiety in a particularly neat way in that it makes *them*, not *me*, the source of these regrettable interests, activities, and so on. Now that could not happen—and does not happen, for a long time at least—in people who have been at a great loss as to what ailed them in relation to others—who have been at a loss as to why they could never be quite successfully human, and could not do the sorts of things that other people in their social position seem to have no difficulty in doing. In this case, the element of shame, chagrin, and contempt for oneself is of at least a different character, if not of an entirely different nature, from the feeling that the person has who knows he wants to do things which he regards as beneath contempt. The pre-schizophrenic wants to be human, and cannot find how to do it. The pre-paranoid schizophrenic wants, in addition to that, to be blameless, to be rid of things of which he is profoundly ashamed and which he regards as a part of his handicap in being human.

This may be in keeping with a thing said very emphatically by Kempf [2]—that it is the aggressive, successful people who move rapidly into paranoid development, and the ineffectual, submissive people who do not. I would put Kempf's formulation in these terms: People who are ashamed of certain traits which they are trying to conceal are, I suppose, very apt to make a lot of noise that sounds like aggressive attack on others; and people who are simply profoundly puzzled and who never do seem to make the successful experiment to find out what they want to know are much less offensively evident in their attack on others. The people who develop a schizophrenic episode have been very far from happy for a long time, but many of them do not feel vivid awareness of contemptible traits. They have nothing elaborate in the way of an explanation of their unhappiness; they have had so many hurts, so many rebuffs and frustrations, that they simply do not feel equal to generalizing their experience. They just drop it, one piece after another; you might say that they never have any past, because it is all too painful to look at. They do not blame themselves, and I think that in these people the paranoid development comes much later, if it comes at all. But those people who have a schizophrenic episode and who blame themselves—*really*

[2] E. J. Kempf, *Psychopathology*; St. Louis, Mo.: C. V. Mosby Co., 1920.

blame themselves—for failing because of certain shameful things have a fine chance of paranoid development.

Environmental Factors in the Paranoid Process

The extent to which explanatory doctrines which make other people responsible for one's own shortcomings are utilized varies from family to family. That is, the products of one family will have great ingenuity at discovering how other people are to blame for their sins of omission and commission; and the products of another will be much less clever at discovering scapegoats. If a person always looks to other people as a basis for self-ennobling or self-relieving explanations of things in which these people actually have no genuine causal position, this is, I believe, invariably the work of those adults who gave this person his cultural components. That is, it is not an idea that occurs naturally in the higher animals that I have been fortunate enough to be able to observe. Moreover it seems to me to be beyond any cavil that there is a very important element of the scapegoat in the culture. It is so striking an element that the fear of becoming paranoid seems to me to be fairly close to the surface in people who have enough acquaintance with fairly sound psychiatric ideas in popular form to know something of the meaning of the paranoid states.

EARLY EXPERIENCES THAT ENCOURAGE OR DISCOURAGE THE PARANOID PROCESS

Yet in a culture which seems to encourage the feeling of the transfer of blame from out of one's awareness onto innocent bystanders—in a culture which predisposes its members to such a self-ennobling or self-justifying procedure—the question arises of why only some people go on from schizophrenic beginnings to chronically schizophrenic-paranoid states; and why the paranoid states as mental illnesses are only common, instead of extremely common. I think that this question is answered by the very agency that I have spoken of as determining the paranoid slant of a great many people—namely, the degree to which paranoid explanations, in the sense of explanations involving a transference of blame, have been *de rigueur* and satisfactory in the home environment. But if one parent has on many occasions quite pointedly objected to the other parent's washing his or her hands of blame by moving it over to the neighbors, for instance, then the child who grows up in this home is, I believe, greatly impressed by the attitude of the person who opposes this blanket projection. The reason why this is so impressive to the child is, I think, that it is biological—in the realm of symbol operations—to use simple performances rather than complex ones, if one can—an observation I derive from my experience with dogs, horses, and so on. But in passing from the animal to the social human being, one encounters such a great discrepancy between the processes called out in the interest of feeling secure with one's fellows and the processes directed toward the achievement of more biologically conditioned satisfactions, that there is no one who does not have many complex processes in the sense of more or less conflicted collisions of goals. But in the earlier, formative years, any calm and uncruel questioning of a morbidity is apt to be deeply impressive upon the child—irrespective, I think, of emotional ties. I say this because in some of the material I have gotten from patients—obsessional patients, it is true—it has looked to me as if the parent who certainly did not contribute greatly to the child's feeling of security, who had not seemed warm or close to the child or optimistic about him, had nonetheless, by his sanity, if you please, left perduring impressions and had had beneficial, preventive effects on the absorption of morbidity from the sicker parent. Thus I am very much impressed with our tendency to catch on to anything that is really simple and workable, if we get a chance. So our families produce people with greater or less facility for washing their hands of blame by projection.

A second, and very important, factor which tends to prevent the development of the paranoid slant is that all but the first-born child have very valuable experience in observing the morbidities of the first-born or of the elder children. A sibling no more than a few years removed from one in age is much less terrifically complicated than a parent. Things which would not be open to question in the recurrent behavior of the parent may, when they appear in a sibling, well continue to be open to question, and, in fact, lead to penetrating insight. Thus a paranoid elder brother in a family with a paranoid father would not be a probable source of paranoid tendencies in the third child, let us say, but, on the contrary, might actually act as a cautionary, preventive experience. During the period when this pattern of coming out lily-white because somebody else is to blame could simply become part of this third child, he would instead develop contempt for it in his elder brother, although such contempt could scarcely be felt for the significant father.

The third factor that enters into the thing is the gross character of interpersonal events outside the home. One may have thoroughly disastrous experiences in school or on the playground in trying to pass off blame for one's shortcomings onto somebody else. Since that constitutes a painful experience, it is apt to have some educative value and to appear as a tendency to be cautious, at least, in appraising the people to whom one addresses blame-washing movements. To the extent that this happens, it means that the self-system has developed critical aspects with respect to the free use of transference of blame; while the self-system is the source of the transfer of blame, it also has to protect security by using that device only under certain circumstances. But if, on the other hand, the post-family experience has included some distinguished successes in the use of transference of blame dynamics, to that extent this becomes a more dependable tool of the self-system.

A NOTE ON THE NATURE OF BLAME

I think I have some thoughts about blame that probably are not universally accepted and certainly should be expressed. Blame is nothing inborn; it is not a fundamental characteristic of the human creature. It is definitely a term which applies to a type of experience that one had in childhood, or certainly well before maturity. The character of that experience is perhaps to be approached first by considering, Where does it hit? —that is, Where does the blame-event impinge? Quite clearly, it impinges generally in the region of insecurity. When we are to blame, that means we are unworthy. We have demonstrated an unworthiness that amounts either to an alleged shock to the person who has discovered that we are to blame for something or to distress to some significant person. For example, a more or less cruel parent may get a great kick out of piling blame on the child; or, perhaps more frequently, a teacher may get satisfaction out of making the child suffer for her embarrassments and at the same time conceal her own inadequacy as a teacher by making the child to blame for being stupid or something of the sort. All these blame-expressing statements are of a character which makes one unworthy—that is, which lowers one's self-esteem.

And so, when a person tells me with great solemnity, "I have always felt guilty about doing so-and-so," I prefer to switch into something which, it seems to me, should have an entirely identical meaning. I say, "In other words, you blame yourself for some inferiority or defect, or something of the sort, which led to that action. Is that right?" The person may accept this, or he may protest "No," saying that the reason why he feels guilty about it is that he just didn't have foresight enough to see what the consequences would be to the person who suffered. In which case I say, "Oh yes, you regret that you could not foresee pain for another," which is thoroughly estimable and is scarcely apt to lead to any serious mental disorder. If it is just that one regrets one's lack of foresight, one's inadequacy, either in energy or something else, then at least one is still among one's fellow men. But blame is something else, since it has the individuation which comes from the particular complex of cultural assimilation established by the home and by the pattern of the home and the siblings, and so on, that is less easily associated with the totality of human life. Recognition of defective foresight is the experience of everyone who has the least honesty in appraising life. The peculiar vicissitudes of blame processes, however, are by no means so universal. I think that these same considerations pretty well dispose of the question of guilt and guiltiness, except as a performance by a jury of one's peers, or something of the kind.

PARANOID OUTCOME OF REINFORCING BLAME
PATTERN IN HOSPITAL SETTING

I now want to say something about the handling of the schizophrenic patient in the mental hospital—the environmental pressures placed on him and the extent to which this may have a marked effect in establishing the possibilities of paranoid outcome. I think very emphatically that the handling of the patient has such an influence when it places emphasis on blame and jugglings with blame, somewhat after the pattern that I mentioned of the school teacher. For example, I would expect an increase of paranoid outcomes per capita of schizophrenics in the practice of a psychiatrist who is content to abolish his own feelings of frustration and inadequacy about a given patient with the statement that the patient is not cooperative. The situation from the patient's standpoint is that he hasn't the faintest idea of what the doctor wants and that he can't get the doctor to tell him. And so, finding that he is a total loss, because he isn't doing this mysterious something that the doctor wants, why should he not avail himself of any opportunity to see how the doctor's performances are to blame?

A number of other things are also sometimes done which may encourage paranoid developments in patients. For instance, the notion exists that conflict about homosexuality has some etiologic relationship to the occurrence of paranoia. So some psychiatrists are rather profoundly interested in the importance of this concept of homosexuality, and feel that a paranoid development is very likely in a patient who has homosexual inclinations. I would not be at all surprised if such a psychiatrist's investigation into the schizophrenic illness does not communicate to the patient some notion that he is almost certainly consigned to a life of degraded, perverse interest in members of his own sex, and that this is a risky and dangerous business—in addition to being, of course, awfully contemptible and so on. Of course, the patient does not get this only from the psychiatrist; he has picked up part of it, at least, previously. The tragedy is that schizophrenia does not occur in mature people, but in persons fixed either, I think, at the preadolescent or at the early adolescent level of development. And at those stages of development sex, lust, and the problems of intimacy with others are pressing problems which take on somewhat preternatural importance, and failure at dealing with them seems to constitute a great social liability. So the psychiatrist who feels that paranoid elaborations are a common outcome, and who is perhaps looking for evidences of paranoid attitudes, may actually offer what seems to the patient, in a more lucid moment, a good way out.

Among the most valuable therapeutic activities that I have ever engaged in is the process of dealing with a patient's problems by getting them located somewhere in the time-space pattern of the patient's life. And it is more or less the essential tool for disturbing the paranoid state, if it can be disturbed. For example, I may say to a patient who one day shows that he is particularly disturbed, "Well, this all seems very oppressive today; you were visited by your friend, the padre, this morning I believe." Let us say that the patient can keep track of things long enough to respond, "Yes, I think he got me to realizing how badly treated I was." I then say, "Well, let's not leave it in this uncertainty; do you recall anything he said that connected?" In other words, I am getting nearer and nearer to the context in which some process made its appearance. There is a profoundly sanifying effect in that; and I suppose that this is derived from the brute fact that if a person is oriented, he is usually adequate to deal with the momentary situation. But if, however, he has been brushed out of touch for a while by some emotional business, so that he is not very clear on where he is, or how he got there, then he can go on rapidly piling difficulty on difficulty; and there is no sense in attempting to cure the particular melange of misinterpretations that appears, without first locating the simpler, earlier context.

THE PARANOID PROCESS IN THE MYTHOLOGY OF A CULTURE

I would like to make here a distinction between processes which have the authority of being observed behavior of significant adults, in contrast to processes which have the much less immediate reality that comes to one in the shape of told folklore, read fairy tales, mythology, and so on. I have a theory of myths which is painfully simple. A myth originates with a dream which symbolizes, with peculiar clarity and in a rather vivid statement, a remedy for a vital problem in the culture—that is, something that is gravely problematic to practically everybody in a social area. The solution presented in the dream is likely to be something that is not authorized by the culture, but that is not a major crime—that does not represent a frontal attack on the whole culture complex. It represents a preverbal, or autistic verbal, attack on the problem. When a dream of that kind is told, it appeals very vividly to the hearer, because it attacks a problem which he also is faced with; and so it is then told again, and again catches on. In the process, it becomes refined by the elimination of all the personal trimmings until only the great central action of the dream remains. Then it has become a myth of the people. Now the problems of human life have certain coincidences from one vast area to another—coincidences derived from certain incoherencies and imbecilities in the different cultures—and so there is an overlapping of some of the great fundamental mythological ideas. In the same way, it is not at all strange that in the process of our growing up, any of us may run off, at certain stages, crude imitations of some of these same mythological ideas. Some of us can remember dreams which are, in fact, a great improvement on any existing mythology for the current era. That type of process is primarily related to our sleeping state, for in the course of assimilating culture and learning how to live, we have specifically eliminated, in our conversation with our compeers, free access to that type of thinking. Thus it is of a different order of reality and implication from the type of process picked up from demonstrations in the home. That is, the distinction between *thee* and *me*, which is so of the essence of security operations by the self, is, I believe, not nearly so striking a characteristic of the rest of the personality. It may even be that my very little bid for fame will be that I was so lacking in self that I discovered that human personality exists only in interpersonal relations, except for the noisy self. Anyway, the schizophrenic is less handicapped, if you please, in coming to grips with life by these fantastically impractical mythological thoughts and so on, than he is by such things as the early observation that one can wash one's hands of a feeling of blame by finding that somebody else was responsible. Thus I think that contact with the paranoid attitudes expressed in the culture and represented in the prevailing myths and stories is less important than actual experience in the home. But, as I have pointed out, along with actual

experience in the home with paranoid attitudes, there is sometimes also a corrective actual questioning of the validity of
that type of defense.

Therapeutic and Prognostic Considerations of the Paranoid Process

By the time that the schizophrenic moves into paranoid
elaborations, the travail of the self in attempting to patch up
some kind of security with the persons of the environment—
even if by now these persons are only psychiatrists and hospital attendants—has become almost cosmic. If, along with this
immense insecurity, there has been a family background which
makes paranoid elaborations acceptable—if there has been this
historic success with them—then such elaborations are likely
to appear. Perhaps they are encouraged by a great deal that
can be interpreted in the same way in the mythology of the
Western World, at least; the engrained descendant of such
myths in the preverbal or autistic thinking of the child reap-
pears in the schizophrenic processes. At any rate, the schizophrenic processes take on more and more the coloring of "This
is terrible; it is not my fault; it is the work of so-and-so."

It is by disturbing such paranoid elaborations that one opens
the way to recovery. Before such a patient can recover, I believe that one has to return him to the unhappy, boundless sort
of cosmic existence which makes up severe schizophrenic stress
—which in some cases, where I have succeeded at this maneuver, meant that the patient became stuporous. In other
words, I find no instrumentality for attacking the paranoid
processes *per se*, for this feeling of blameless perfection is a
great improvement on anything else a person can expect in this
world. The way by which I attempt to return such a patient
to schizophrenic stress is by means of a frontal attack on the
convenience of the projection—a frontal attack on the often
transparently unjustified, grandiose explanatory ideas—the
purpose of which is to cause anxiety, to disturb the self from

what little complacency it has achieved in the paranoid illness. And along with this, and much more theoretically promising, is an insistence on finding out when, and under what circumstances, the paranoid convictions rise to the center of the stage, and when their influence over the patient's orientation becomes much less striking. All of this usually collides with some quite terrifying ideas in the patient, which in turn precipitate what I call the prognostic event. This event consists either of (1) the spread of schizophrenic uncertainties—a broadening of meaning, and so on, which makes it impossible for the patient to have anything as neat as even shifting paranoid delusions; or (2) an increase in the amount of time given over to vigorously paranoid ideas, an extension of these ideas, and a firm fixation of them on the physician. So far as I am concerned, this spells prognosis. If the former happens—that is, if the patient does move backward, in the sense of chronologically backward into the more schizophrenic state—then I have hopes, which are very guarded, of course, because I am dealing with a terribly risky, awfully handicapped personality. But if, on the other hand, the reaction to my frontal attack and my attempt to mark the timing of the most paranoid feelings consists of an intensification of those feelings and gets them pretty strongly attached to me, then clearly I am not going to be very successful in my maneuver, and the patient will probably persist in a paranoid schizophrenic condition.

The Nature of the Hebephrenic Change

I have already mentioned that if the schizophrenic despairs, he becomes hebephrenic. Perhaps I should begin this discussion of the hebephrenic by describing what I mean by this despair and showing how it differs from the profound pessimism of the schizophrenic.

Something that is not often mentioned in psychiatry, but is certainly mentioned in military science and is beginning to be mentioned in industry, is a discrimination of states of interpersonal relations—or personality, or states of mind—in terms of high morale, fair morale, some degree of demoralization,[3] and despair. These terms may be said to refer to the extent to which one feels solidarity with others and feels it possible that the group may exercise favorable influence over the course of events. Thus in despair there is a feeling of total, utter isolation and of utter incapacity to do anything that would change an exceedingly undesirable situation favorably.

When we attempt to distinguish between demoralization and despair, we must observe not only the person's utterances, but also his behavior. As a matter of fact, if a person is really in despair, there are no particular utterances, and there is no particular behavior—except that possibly if he is standing and is shoved, he will walk, not very rapidly, for some time in about the direction in which he was shoved. In the demoralized person, pessimism colors his views of things to an appalling degree; but, depending on the degree of demoralization, there is behavior, and the behavior does not faithfully reflect the utter hopelessness which many of the remarks may reflect— often quite the contrary, in fact. And that means that there is a good chance for psychotherapy of a swift and correct kind.

When we are dealing with the schizophrenic, we find a person who is pretty well demoralized, who has little expectation of pleasant and useful developments, and has, in fact, gradually lost all clear hope of such favorable developments. Yet many of his utterances leave the door open to possibilities, however improbable; and there is also some behavior which has to be regarded as motivated by an attempt to alter things favorably, however badly organized an attempt it may be. A certain proportion of these schizophrenics very early leave the field of stress and deep pessimistic expectations and become quite calmly occupied with events pertaining to the preferred

---

[3] Demoralization arises in certain circumstances which are of more than passing interest to us, and which I have discussed in a paper entitled, "Psychiatric Aspects of Morale," [*Amer. J. Sociology* (1941) 3:277-301].

bodily orifice; they then seem no longer to be suffering from the sort of panicky fear that appears in demoralization. This change toward preoccupation with events in the neighborhood of one of the zones of interaction, along with a marked improvement in the stress of the mental state, or the stress of living, occurs, I believe, where the experimentation of early schizophrenia has had the effect of wiping out any thought of success, where the person has literally given up the effort at living and contents himself with existing on a sort of modified autobiological level.

This is what I mean when I say that the hebephrenic has despaired of any effective operation. He has had such disastrous experiences in his initial, rather frantic, schizophrenic attempt at doing something that he has given it all up as a bad job. That is conspicuously shown by the avoidance of interpersonal contacts and the very disturbing effect of interpersonal pressure on the person with the hebephrenic change. On the other hand, the hopelessness of a great many schizophrenics is of a much less finally discouraged character; some of the expressed hopelessness can be discounted, for there is some collaboration, some effectual movement, and so on. This attitude might be compared with my own; it is very difficult to get me to have very pleasant expectations about a patient or about a procedure or something of the kind. That pessimistic attitude has nothing to do with demoralization or despair. It is something that life has provided me with which is quite convenient for me. I do not have the jolts which come from disappointments as easily as some of my more optimistic colleagues do. By having discounted disappointments in advance, I save myself from having to kid myself around them. But this pessimistic slant of mine is very different, indeed, from a feeling that one can do absolutely nothing—that it is all too much.

Thus in the hebephrenic change the element of profound demoralization, of despair of becoming a human being acceptable as such, is rather fundamental. This was confirmed for me by an event which seemed fairly significant to me. We had at the hospital at one time a young man who had certainly been cut off for a long time from much contact with his fellow men by a schizophrenic illness. He spent much of this time in bed, under pressure from his mother, who was away from the house most of the day at work; the father had died some time since, and she was the only person who could contribute much to the support of the family. The young man avoided anything like a close touch with society; in fact, he was hebephrenic to the extent that he was eternally coming up missing if he got out of the house, and would be found wandering around in the remote parts of a large park or some other place where human contact was pretty thin. Finally, by some eventuality which I have forgotten, he came to the hospital; and at this point he looked in a good many ways as if he had been hebephrenic for several years. A very striking characteristic was that he had a silly laugh which repeated itself in and out of season in the most obscure relationship to anything that could be observed to cause it. He was quite seclusive and answered questions, under pressure, with the fewest words possible; usually he simply said, "I don't know."

I spent a good many hours with this boy. He used up a good part of this time taking books out of my bookcase and holding them in front of him, sometimes bottomside up, and otherwise obviously making an exceedingly feeble attempt to deal with me. But still it was an attempt, for if I had not been a nuisance to him, he would not have gone to the trouble of getting a book in between us. We gradually got to the point where our interviews didn't consist chiefly of his evasive action; but still I got very, very little except monosyllables. I was particularly interested in the so-called silly laughter, which had tended to become less ubiquitous in our relationship, although it still occurred frequently. I would carefully keep track of when it did not occur; but probably the next time a similar situation came up, it would occur, and so I wasn't making much progress. One day I had been pressing him about this laughter, offering various hypotheses for it, and when I didn't get anywhere I shrugged my shoulders and prepared to abandon the effort. I suppose I must have seemed particularly down in spirits, for something apparently touched him, and he made the following, for him unprecedentedly long, statement: "Doctor, you mustn't mind me; I haven't much life left." If he had said, "much contact with life left," I think it would have been a perfectly communicative statement.

That sentence did not tell me much about the so-called silly laughter which I was trying to explore, but it did, it seemed to me, express an attitude of resigned separation and true and unalterable hopelessness which I think is the essence of the hebephrenic. Hebephrenics are simply driven to occupying themselves with amusing zones of interaction to keep from being entrapped into very disturbing relations with their fellows. Even if you are badly deteriorated, you cannot cease to have the impulses, and so on, which make up living. But there are some things that you can do with these impulses which are vastly more unsocial than others. You can discharge most of your clear needs for satisfaction without too much difficulty: you can handle hunger by eating everything that you can lay hands on at the hospital table; you can avoid being disturbed by lust—which could be very troublesome in that it might draw you toward another person—by more or less continuously pulling your penis, or doing something of that sort, and perhaps also having a wonderful time with the feces. About the only things that will be conspicuously left, and which you cannot handle, will be the drive of loneliness—that queer emotion built into us, I suppose, to permit us to be social— and the need for security. And it is the need for security which seems to me to be at the very core of the explanation of the so-called deterioration. The hebephrenic deteriorates because the self and the security operations are abandoned, progresssively and rapidly, so that there is left only a rather constant, unchanging feeling that the world regards him with contempt, indifference, scorn, or something of the sort. He gets used to this because it doesn't have any lights or shadows—it is uniform; and all of us can habituate ourselves to a great deal, if there is no prospect of change and no disturbing novelty cropping up from time to time.

I think that some of these ideas on hebephrenics were borne out by Dr. Ernest Hadley's experience with hebephrenics at St. Elizabeths. When I first got acquainted with him, he was a very deeply interested and energetic intern or junior physician. We got quite well acquainted. Those were the days of great theoretic elaborations, when psychoanalysis was in the stage of very rapid evolution. One day Hadley said, "Dr. White has shown a kind of interest in me, and has suggested that if, in addition to my doing my 12-hour-day's work, I want to do a little research, he'd be glad to consider any paper I write." That *was* a mark of Dr. White's appreciation. "What would be a good problem to work on?" I said, "Well, Ernest, the problem that seems to me to be the damnedest one I've ever come across—and one that I certainly would not even attempt because I have no clue—is, What is the nature of the hebephrenic content? What goes on 'inside,' if you please, these chronic, institutional hebephrenics?" Well, he tackled it, and had some truly remarkable experience, which I think reflected a deep benevolence in attitude that would have been greatly to the credit of anybody. He didn't disturb these people as much as most of their environment did. It actually got so that he could sit around during a pseudo conversation among hebephrenics without their all getting up and leaving —which is the way they react to most of us. One of the people with whom he spent a great deal of time was disturbed one morning—not very disturbed, but obviously a little anxious and restless, and just a little frightened—and Hadley was lucky enough to discover that this was connected with passing a very large lump of feces. I do not remember what the interchange was—there was very little said by the patient—other than this information. Hadley had picked up some clue from something said earlier in one of these pseudo conversations in which patients talk to themselves with due regard to the convention of one being silent while another speaks, and so he now cautiously expanded an hypothesis as to some early misunderstanding of anal relationship with some other man. He did it in a friendly enough atmosphere and with enough looseness, or openness, of hypothesis so that the thing could click; and the patient was intrigued in a rather startlingly adult fashion, showing anything but the usual hebephrenic silliness, and improved markedly. I don't think that there was anything like the beginning of recovery, but I know that the distinctly favorable change, which showed itself in a better adjustment to the hospital, lasted for at least the 6 months more that I followed the course of the patient's illness. Here was a person who had been living the comparatively contented life of hebephrenic dilapidation—that is, a hebephrenic can be comparatively contented insofar as he is let alone by anybody who could be significant and disturbing. It was as if he was able to move out of the only occasionally disturbing autonomy of one of his zones of interaction into a relating of this to a time and place in his life which were significant, with rather remarkable results.

Now it seems to me that if it was that easy, it would have happened 'accidentally'—*provided there had been anything much surviving in the way of hope or expectation*—for all of us tend to put ourselves in the way of observing things that are fundamentally of great importance to us, if we get a chance. If there had remained any hopeful expectation, I think the patient would have had a similar fortunate accident long, long before this one, arranged by the, so far as I know, unprecedented event of a psychiatrist spending a lot of time with a hebephrenic patient. Thus I feel that the hebephrenic dilapidation represents the complete demoralization of the schizophrenic, because of the universality of the problem and the utter failure to hit upon any autistic or preverbal processes that offer hope. This explanation is speculative, and I do not know how one would go about documenting it until we know much more than we do now of the content of the hebephrenic. Hadley did find out a good deal about the zonal ideas and so on which lent some emphasis to my conviction about how hebephrenics keep from getting involved with other people. But we still do not know anything about the course of events by which a disturbed schizophrenic begins this downward path.

The course of life gives everyone some experience with everything that I know to be dynamisms of mental disorder. And I believe that one can obtain accounts of experience in remarkably early life which seemed peculiarly to pave the way for schizophrenic development, even though probably only a few of the potentially schizophrenic ever come to the attention of psychiatrists. I can tell you a story which is perhaps as illuminating of my position as any. Years ago I was visiting in the home of one of my colleagues, who had a lovely wife and lovely children. I heard something about one of the children which, I am told, disturbed me deeply; and my colleague, being a psychiatrist, noticed my disturbance and asked me what I was thinking. Apparently I was led into saying that I had been disturbed because the early peculiarity which this child showed was one that so frequently coincided with rather serious mental states in adolescence. All of this has been recalled *to me*, but unhappily is not recalled *by me*. I do know that the event happened, but I haven't a ghost of a notion of what the experience was, or what I said about it. I do remember being disturbed about one of the children in that particular home.

The whole business was called to my attention years later by David Levy, who was treating this boy in late adolescence for a very severe personality disorder. He wanted to know what I had noticed or heard about that evening. And I shall never be able to tell him. But anyway, something had disturbed me, and the history worked out so that it looked as if I had been awfully clever. But I am sure I don't know what it was.

I have said that I think that the obsessional neurosis comes from a pretty definitely patterned family group, which might be described as hypocritical, and I have also said that I feel that the prevailing use of the obsessional mechanism does not guarantee against schizophrenic developments, in some cases at least. And so, if you want to put these two things together, you can say that some people who may have the start toward schizophrenic illness then develop obsessional personality organizations which protect them for a long time from the type of evil that precipitates a schizophrenic illness. I think that is building an awful lot on rather inadequate buttresses, but I wouldn't quarrel with it.

As to any genetic basis for mental illness, I have a very simple attitude there: not proved. If anyone wants to discuss the heredity of eye color with me, I am delighted, except for the fact that it is not a very exciting topic. But I should say that the genetic influences that are strongly conditional of a subsequent psychosis cannot go further than limit the possibility of psychosis, just as they limit the possibility of developments in other directions. There is no shadow of doubt in my mind that mental illnesses arise out of life experience. Many particular patterns of persistent excessive use of dynamism may be established by experience at any time in life. In fact, we can cure patients only because there is nothing fixed and immutably ordained; we cure by improving the adaptation of dynamism to problem, you might say.[4]

[4] *Editors' note:* Sullivan goes on to discuss briefly at this point those mental illnesses which are difficult to intervene with: "I have now and then been able to upset a paranoid-schizophrenic maladjustment and gotten the patient back to the schizophrenic condition, where I feel the field is at least open to the future. And Kempf was able to whip one hebephrenic woman into a durable state of mental health. But there are maladjustments which are even more difficult to intervene with. I am afraid I cannot overcome my conviction that the real psychopathic personality is a very serious miscarriage of development quite early in life, so grave that it makes a very favorable outcome possible only with an almost infinite amount of effort, which in turn, I guess, no one will ever be worth. By and large, I expect to find the psychopathic personality already clearly marked off, and expect it to continue without any great change except for a slow increase in the amount of hostility that it engenders in others and the bitterness, and sometimes alcoholism, which it engenders in the person himself. There is one notable exception: Something that looks very like a chronic—that is, a *real*—psychopathic personality can appear as a resting phase or partial recovery from schizophrenic illnesses under some circumstances, although I am not sure what those circumstances may be."

CHAPTER
15

Therapy with Schizophrenic Patients

WHAT I have said about the essence of the schizophrenic dynamism may be summed up as follows: It consists in a confusion of interpersonal relations by the appearance in awareness of referential processes ordinarily excluded from awareness. The type of referential process which appears is either incapable of being formulated in words, in which case the person does not say anything about it, or it can be formulated only by the use of such autistically unique word-meanings that communication is exceedingly improbable if not impossible. Nevertheless, in the latter case, these verbal processes seem to the person who uses them to be just as proper, suitable, potentially effective, and automatically the thing to do in an effort to communicate as are the highly refined verbal processes which most of us come finally to use with a measure of success by the time we reach adulthood. In other words, the patient feels that these are valid thoughts, suited to communicating to others —they are, of course, valid thoughts to him, but they are not *consensually* valid thoughts—and he tosses them out, to the serious detriment of clarity in the relationship with the other person. His level of awareness is so disturbed that he does not exclude the type of process represented by these thoughts, but looks upon it as if it were a perfectly normal ingredient of consciousness and uses it as such.

Now this theoretical formulation of mine also implies certain things about dealing with the schizophrenic in terms of the tripartite viewpoint. For example, if you acutely exacerbate a motivational system, which always brings intense anxiety, you will very seriously disturb the formulation of the situation as to communication. Let us consider the adolescent who, without finding it at all easy to tolerate the thought itself in his mind, still has unnumbered reminders in the course of a week's life among his fellows that, "I'm probably just a damned homosexual." The "probably" is in its way a measure of what an extremely unhappy mental state this is. He cannot be sure he isn't and he cannot find out that he is. It is just an eternal headache, and a terrible headache. Now if the psychiatrist glibly tosses something at this person which, within his capacity to think, clearly implies that the psychiatrist thinks he is homosexual, then the psychiatrist must realize that the state of awareness and the symbol operations of the patient will undergo the following change: There will appear in consciousness—which means a widening of awareness, in the sense that it becomes more inclusive—mental processes which were natural, let us say, at the age of four, possibly from three-and-a-half to four-and-a-half. In these processes, words are as far from careful referential communicative use as you can imagine. Thus the limits of relevance will now pass from a situation in which the psychiatrist is dealing with a disturbed patient into a situation which may include as relevant everything from the bricks in the chimney to how your legs are crossed and so on and so forth. The situation has been converted from a disturbing clear grasp to the much earlier type of generalization, the nature of which is baffling to an adult mind. And what the schizophrenic has left from the venture is something I defy you to formulate—it can't be talked about because there is no verbal communication of such thought. So that is what you will get if you do anything like that; and so, of course, it is not a very useful thing to do.

Per contra, if you have to deal with schizophrenics, then this formulation of mine implies the importance of carefully putting almost a scaffolding under the patient's self-system in its relation to you—that is, establishing a 'me-you' pattern, if you please, between yourself and the patient which is of an utterly previously unexperienced solidity and dependability. Only then can you get to the point where you can deal with disturbing material without causing this sudden disturbance of the self-function of suppressing more primitive types of mental process, with, as a result, the abolition of communication and God knows what results in the patient, in the sense of what finally comes out as a result of your efforts.

As I have already emphasized, the schizophrenic distortion is one that comes from the very time when the more primitive type of mental process was the natural and only prevailing type of mental process or symbol operation. As a very simple inference from this statement, you could say, if you had to try to describe the essential difference between a person who will have schizophrenia and a person who won't, that the structure of the self-system is concerned. That is the only thing that is in any sense different in the schizophrenic from anyone else; the schizophrenic's self-system cannot control awareness in certain situations where insecurity is suddenly aggravated because of the stirring of what are formulated as extremely dangerous impulses. Then, of course (meaning that it is an extremely simple inference), the self of the schizophrenic is much less adequate as a dynamism for operating with other people than is the self as it is ordinarily encountered.

Now you begin to see my viewpoint about the shocking nonsense, the profound absurdity, of one of our colleagues who devotes or did at one time devote himself to finding out the weakness of the ego in the schizophrenic. That has been blandly swallowed by lots of people who, having refined referential possibilities, seem never to use them. If, by weakness, you mean that a thing of the most incredible efficiency, considering reasonable probabilities, has been evolved out of almost nothing—if making an incredible amount out of very little is weakness—then the ego or the self-system of the schizophrenic is weak. But my dealings with schizophrenics for twenty-five years have impressed me with the fact that in what these people do, they show more simply, consistently, and astoundingly the almost infinite adaptive capacities of man than do all of us fairly successful people. They have, unlike us, never achieved the degree of self-esteem and certainty of ability to get along with other people that makes some major field of interpersonal action safe. Yet they often, till the smash comes, give the impression of extraordinary ability to protect themselves from troublesome people and to go their way in the face of condemnation, criticism, and so on. In fact, think of the weak ego that makes a schizophrenic kid just before the smash get jobs in house-to-house soliciting to make a man of himself. It is a funny meaning for "weak," isn't it? Schizophrenics are the people who suffer most intensely from the horrible problem of "What will the next person be like?" with never a suspicion that he might be pleasant. Yet this boy I have just mentioned exposes himself to every sort of Tom, Dick, and Harry under the worst possible circumstances in order to become a man. So let us not talk about the weakness of the self-dynamism of the schizophrenic. Let us talk about the extreme poverty of favorable opportunity that the schizophrenic has had for building a successful self-system because, early in life, the idea was in some way conveyed inescapably to him that he was relatively infrahuman, a burden of sorts. And in the growth through the juvenile era to preadolescence —which is the nearest approach to happiness and peace of mind with another person that many people ever have—he has headed off favorable experience, partly because he has had no experience with which to analyze favorable experience and partly because he has already developed such idiosyncracies of distance, and so on.

A person who suffers insecurity is driven by a whip—anxiety—that hurts more than any of the individual whips of the biological needs. You will not find anybody pursuing anxiety for pleasure, although people have literally taken much pleasure in being ascetic, celibate, and so on. There is no whip that is so keen and cutting as insecurity—anxiety—in regard to one's dealings with others. Driven by fear, the schizophrenic has looked up practically all the blind alleys there are. In other words, he has gotten all the advice, and in the earlier years has attempted to follow some of it, and has gnashed his teeth at all the possible criticisms of himself and has carried out that type of criticism of others which even at its best is only mildly amusing, and threatens any warm esteem on anybody else's part. He is ready for almost anything except peace of mind and a feeling of security in dealing with his fellows. So, again drawing off conclusions of childlike simplicity: How can a psychiatrist provide a situation of this novel dependability, this relative security, between the self-system of the schizophrenic personality and the psychiatrist?

I can perhaps begin best by answering this question negatively. Being the great physician who holds out the balm of cure is quite obviously not the best approach. If every time that a schizophrenic looks at any of these great people who know the answer to everything, he next finds himself lying prone in a mud puddle as the great pass on, then a psychiatrist can stage no act as to how wonderful he is that is apt to have quite the desired result. And no distillation of wisdom, in the sense of a penetrating realization of the type of difficulties the patient has and the picturing of a way of life by which the patient may avoid some of these difficulties, is apt to have the desired result. Even if it is wisdom, the patient has no background by which to realize that it is wisdom and no longer takes any particular comfort at the laborious prospect entailed in carrying out this wisdom. Furthermore, if the psychiatrist makes a great statement of where the difficulties lie and where peace might be found, he will necessarily formulate things that the self-system of the schizophrenic cannot tolerate, and therefore the schizophrenic phenomena of the earlier type of thinking take over—and neither you nor, I guess, God will quite know where the patient is and what he has gotten out of the psychiatrist's wisdom.

So, clearly, these things are not it. There is another thing that I strongly disadvise as an experiment, although it is an intensely interesting experiment and under certain circumstances might conceivably have a high probability of success. This is, to tamper with your own awareness and the limit to which your self-system will permit primitive processes to wander into awareness, and to try to talk to the schizophrenic on the schizophrenic level. There are moments of inspiration when such things happen, and I wouldn't be surprised if there are some people who could do it. If one could imagine an ideally healthy person who had not come through a culture which includes the necessity of doing vast numbers of things which one cannot understand, he might well bring to adult life access to these more primitive levels in which he could talk to the schizophrenic. But from the definition of how we become what we are, that is at best an exceedingly rarely successful experiment.

Thus we must clearly neither try direct communication of security nor be so superior that it is impossible for an extremely insecure person to imagine being on the same level, but must imagine himself always farther down the stairs. And we must also appreciate this frightful delicacy of the balance between types of thought on which communication is suspended in its practical meaning—even though there is always a vast amount of communication that is not at a practical level. With the schizophrenic you do not know what is communicative, and you cannot always be sure; and if you have a horribly risky thing to do, then you don't depend on these intuitive, empathic contacts. I say this even though I once had an extremely valuable assistant who, I would say, depended almost entirely on such contacts, and with great success; but by the time we have gone through medical school, I am afraid that none of us have saved that much of our personality.

What then does one do? One has to structure the relationship with the schizophrenic by, first, avoiding any avoidable, foreseeable disturbance of the patient's security. Now that does not mean that one has to become far more insane than any patient is, by attempting to create a new universe—even though I have heard of one notable case where a great success was achieved in building a second universe around a very wealthy woman, which in fact wasn't very different from our universe. That is, culture so enmeshes us and is in us and so on, that we can't do anything very fantastic in changing the pattern of the world, past, present, and future. So there are occasionally times when the security of the patient will necessarily receive bad jolts. But an exquisite care in avoiding unnecessary bad jolts—and when you begin to concentrate on it you find that most of the bad jolts people have in interpersonal relationships are avoidable—will at least give you a good chance to maintain communications. This good chance at communicating with the schizophrenic implies, by my definition, that the precise meanings of words in your mind and in the patient's mind are probably by no means identical. In other words, the residual autistic meaning of the schizophrenic's verbal symbols is much greater than yours. It follows that your statements must always be as near the commonplace—as near what everybody has heard and followed somewhat—as you can make them. And then comes the final thing which makes one a psychiatrist instead of a scientific person using a fairly adequate theory. When a patient's insecurity is provoked by all sorts of things which the psychiatrist has no control over, when there are disturbances of awareness and so on, the psychiatrist can still have a feeling of familiarity without the conceit of feeling that he is intimately following what is happening. In the place where the patient has the most profoundly great skepticism of himself and any other person—his 'in pain' area, as we might call it—the psychiatrist is not upset, doesn't start climbing the furniture or calling the police or preparing for battle, but regards it as part of the universe. The schizophrenic must have lost the feeling of naturalness in this kind of thought, as we all do as we pass from mid-childhood to our adult competence. Now he finds somebody who demonstrates that—no, this is not understood but neither is it terribly strange; and the patient begins to realize this during his more lucid moments and by a great deal of fairly lucid reflection. That immediately reduces the gravity of being schizophrenic to the patient, you see. The patient notes that somebody else seems to consider his communications not desirable, something to get rid of, if possible, but by no means fantastic. In addition, there is the positive contribution to the patient's realization that he has at last got to somebody who will be a real help instead of a delusional help followed by a sharp rebuff and disappointment. That, I believe, is achieved very largely by great care in assuming the probabilities from the patient's standpoint as to your operations. Now that in many ways implies everything that I have said, but it also implies something I haven't said quite clearly enough.

Since the schizophrenic has a whole pattern of inadequate security dynamisms, the inadequacy of which has been a terribly impressive aspect of all his previous life, it is a pretty good bet that the instances in which he has succeeded have left very little easily accessible evidence; in such circumstances an occasional success can either throw him into an excitement or is immediately followed by a firm conviction that, "Well, it's probably a mistake on my part—at least it won't last and the next thing that happens will be bad." In many of our very insecure operations in life, if the other fellow obviously expects us not to do what he wants, the chances are we get so puzzled about it that we don't do it. Thus the schizophrenic person practically guarantees a great deal of woe for himself. So the psychiatrist cannot expect to have very ready access to the type of neat, reassuring illustrations which can be used with some patients. With the schizophrenic, I cannot even use the reassurance which I use unhesitatingly on the obsessional at the appropriate time: "Oh, well, I suppose you drink your coffee at breakfast with clarity and impunity, and the only reason I mention that is that I presume you don't think a great deal about drinking your coffee. And for God's sake, don't begin, otherwise you'll drown yourself." But you cannot spring things like that on the schizophrenic; he probably has sputtered in his coffee, or dropped a cup on somebody's lap, or something of the kind, which will then suggest even more painful eating memories.

I would say that a good many of the therapeutic operations calculated to increase the schizophrenic's feeling of security must be done indirectly. But I do not mean that you can possibly justify being obscure with a schizophrenic. There is a difference between being indirect and being obscure. Communication is difficult enough, without your getting so clever that nobody could be quite sure what you mean. I will try to give an illustration of the distinction I am trying to make. The patient I shall discuss had, among the many disturbing aspects of a schizophrenic psychosis, decided that he had never been married to the person who claimed to be his wife. But it is safe to say that the marriage was most certainly clear to this patient. Schizophrenics most of the time have access in awareness to such things as the marriage ceremony they have participated in; it's there; it's an experience, and they can't get rid of it. But the position of this patient was, "I was never married to this woman. She is not my wife." At that point a psychiatrist might say directly, "I can understand that you might be in the mood to deny the marriage." That is a perfectly intelligent remark; but it is so direct that I would expect the psychiatrist to be defeated unless he has already gotten a long way with the patient. It is a clear expression of judgment, and most of the judgment that this patient has ever gotten, you see, hasn't been any good to him, so it doesn't mean very much. But notice what could happen if the psychiatrist instead says, "I can understand your having doubts, or even a tendency to deny the marriage." Notice that the word "doubts" has been pushed into this context; that makes all the difference. The psychiatrist has introduced "doubts or" before the denial of the marriage. That is an instance of what I mean by indirection in dealing with the schizophrenic. I can't expect much of anything to happen from the more direct approach, because these people have learned that all sorts of things that looked promising are just hocus-pocus when they turn their backs. But instead I talk in terms of doubts which were not part of the context—no doubts of the matter were expressed; the patient said flatly, "I'm not married to this woman." After my remark about doubt, I would then go on to other things, for the major movement I make is of no importance except insofar as it carries this addition of the context of doubt, which will get no attention *then*, under the general principle that what you don't follow, you don't react to in schizophrenia— it usually gets you in dutch. But I would hope—which is all I ever do—that presently when things are quite calm and there is no personal pressure from my presence, there will be a tendency for the patient to think, "Why, I *did* marry that woman. Now why do I say she isn't my wife? Oh yeah, that doctor! He said *doubting* or denying! Christ, yes! I suppose that's the fact. I got so used to saying, 'How in hell *could* I have married this woman' that finally I decided I hadn't."

What I am trying to get at is that before the flat denial, there must have been the experience, the state, that many of us have about our disastrous performances: "How *could* I have been fool enough to do that?" It is sort of an inquiring doubt business. Then the patient, without my "having done it"—that's the illusion that I wish to produce—says, "Ah yes, the doctor sees all that. He knows that in a dilemma like this I have long periods of unhappy doubting and so on, and it finally resolved itself into this idea that she isn't my wife." Thus he can draw off the conclusions; you have gotten the notion started in the patient by a minimum positive operation on your part. But an infinity of attempts to do the same thing more directly will often just fail, quite often because any such attempt will recall to the patient very unhappy relationships with some person who might have helped him, but who, unhappily, too greatly disturbed his security so that the schizophrenic processes flowed in.

Consultation on the Case of a Schizoid

Sullivan has already commented on the therapeutic problems of eliciting and interpreting communication in the schizophrenic illness. The therapist's problem in treating schizophrenia is to find a way to relate to what is communicative in the patient's productions. Such communications are, of course, fragmentary, and therefore Sullivan's comments on the problems presented by his colleagues are fragmentary. For this reason, we have included here, as a case illustration of his therapeutic approach, his comments on the case of a schizoid who—while relatively inarticulate—was able to communicate something of her problems to her therapist. Also included in the section immediately following is a fragment from the case of a schizophrenic in which Sullivan ignores the presenting problems—the patient's delusions and the problem of tube feeding—and comments on the occasional communicative remark of the patient's.

The first case is then that of a schizoid—a young married woman who is extremely tense, apprehensive, and inarticulate. Her main difficulty, as she describes it, is that she is an inefficient housekeeper who "lazes" most of the day away. She looks upon herself as a failure. Treatment in the case has bogged down, after several months, and the question raised in the presentation of the problem is, What techniques can be used to get things moving again?

The patient is a product of an extremely traumatic childhood, during which she was deserted by her mother and later abandoned to the care of the maternal grandparents by her father, who was himself unreliable. In the grandparents' home she was treated more or less as a servant; but as she was very gifted intellectually, she managed to finish college and earn a Ph.D. in economics. She married a fellow-student in the same field and became a house-wife. Her husband is extremely critical of her as a housekeeper, and has frequently told her about romantic entanglements with other women, always presenting these women to her as romantic ideals. During the ten years of marriage, in which two children have been born, the relationship has steadily worsened, with the husband threatening divorce and immersing himself in his work, and the wife leading an increasingly inactive and isolated life.

Sullivan: I have a number of considerations in mind, the first of which is to get the patient to notice that, even before her husband's recent promotion, they were perfectly able to afford at least a part-time maid. And as the patient finds herself show-ing, I suppose, unrecognized resentment of the burdens of her life every morning, I would start therapy by asking, "Well, why haven't you a maid?" And I want to *know*, in a fashion that makes it perfectly clear to me why they don't have a maid. If there isn't any adequate explanation, I would then ask, "How about getting one?"

I would go on by saying that her training seems to be rather exceptional for a person who has accepted a purely domestic role all these years and that, under the circumstances, her feel-ing of helplessness to get going in the morning rather en-courages me than otherwise. Has she never heard of a woman who preferred something else to domestic preoccupations? I would ask, "Has this never occurred to you, or has it occurred to you as something morbid and strange?" (I would suppose it had actually never occurred to her at all.) Then I would want to know how it happened that she went through college and took a graduate degree in economics; since women econo-mists are not the most common thing in the world, I would point out that it looks to me as if she must have followed some natural bent. Now of course it may come out that she did it because great-aunt Catherine recommended it, something of that kind, but that immediately excites me about great-aunt Catherine, who seems to have had ideas, you know.

What I am attempting to do here is to get her mind open a little bit to the fact that not only is she in a disagreeable situation, but she finds it disagreeable. And by sort of hounding her to prove that she is an exceptional woman with an exceptional education—and an exceptional inclination to go on suffering an impossibly silent domestic involvement—I am simply hoping to crack the shell that surrounds all her feelings. Until she raises her sights to something, I think that an attempt to get her clear on how much she resents her husband and all that would be merely an intellectual exercise. She would catch on very quickly, and nothing would happen, except possibly that she would feel that things were getting a little worse. But if I start the other way—if I get her to wondering what the hell she has been doing all this time and why she has never felt entitled to object to any of it—then I can anticipate that she will be equal to feeling some very real anger at times.

I would sort of hound her with commonplace things, not because I care too much about the facts themselves at the moment, but because I want her mind to begin to reach a little outside the magic circle of insulation in which she has been living all this time. Otherwise we are just going to get some fine thinking. There must be an outward movement of her interest, a beginning suspicion, "Well, this really wasn't all necessary and inevitable," before I can expect her to do much real observing of the play of interpersonal movement that probably has characterized her, as it does all of us, all her life. The very lack of outward signs of suffering indicates how early she accepted as fit and inevitable that she should be the slavey in her maternal grandparents' home and that she should in some fashion be kept from associations with other people, presumably because she wasn't good enough or trustworthy enough or just didn't have sense enough. I would lead her to talk a little bit about how she explained this tacit ban on her developing ordinary relationships, and I would expect that she would then hint of her acceptance of her unworthiness for a free life. At this point I would ask, "Well, now, how do you explain college and the rather original choice of subject that you carried through so well?" Then, after I had listened to a good deal of that, I would come down like a ton of bricks on economics. "Well, how about economics? Why has that interest vanished from your life without a trace? You take a Ph.D. in economics, marry an economist, and as far as I can discover, from then on research in economics has been left exclusively to him. Did that suit him? Was that what he insisted on? Did you just accommodate his feeling that it was awkward to have a wife who knew something about his business, or what?"

Thus, by that remote route, I hope that I would begin to get to her resentments toward her husband. They will be so far back in experience, you see, that immediate explosive danger will be diminished by the time she gets anywhere near the present. It seems to me that *the* big problem for the therapist in dealing with a person like this is to close in on areas that inevitably must open her mind to a reassessment of what has been taken more or less for granted as a continuing act of God.

The thing I would be determined that this woman should tell me sometime or other is that she has discussed with her husband just what he had in mind in advising her in long, ecstatic letters of his great love for another woman some years back, and I would try to get her to look at that simply as a piece of research or investigation. "Now here is a very interesting research problem," I would say. "One's husband goes off and becomes terribly enamored of some goddess and writes his wife all about it. Now what was he doing? What did he think he was doing?" She doesn't know, of course; she hasn't had any experience in being anybody's husband. Then I ask her, "But why not find out?" Here again, I hope that I would be pushing on something far enough away and essentially intriguing enough so that she will rather calmly ask him a few questions. I think they will be very profoundly embarrassing questions. My notion of why a husband does things like that is not to the husband's credit at all. And maybe she will have the privilege of seeing him quite disconcerted in explaining this, and maybe that will introduce the idea to her, "Well, this bird who has always said he was horribly insecure and so on, *is* horribly insecure. Why is he picking on me then? Why should I be his whipping-boy?" And I am pretty sure that he will respond very hastily to good management on her part. I may be wholly wrong, but he sounds to me like a person who has been getting away with murder because he was fortunate enough to find one of these incredible women to whom it has never occurred that there is any fun in life or any give-and-take; and I think one starts her education in what I call the *middle distance*, before college and through early marriage, winding up with the great love that came into the husband's life and had to be embalmed in letters to his wife. I do not take an interest in current events with her husband, first, because I wouldn't know what on earth they meant, for she is a poor observer and has carefully looked the other way a great part of her life, and, second, because I wouldn't know what foolishness she might think I wanted her to engage in. You see, I particularly don't want her to get the impression that I think she ought to roughhouse him and throw some of the bric-a-brac at him, because the poor man might take flight. He might become completely undone. And I am pretty certain that he is insecure enough so that she will find, to her great astonishment and permanent gratitude, that she can manage with him *if* she proceeds slowly enough along the line I have suggested.

I am not after anything here that is going to be very difficult to recall. It would be well within the realm of reasonable recall for all of us. What I am trying to do with the middle distance is literally to lift her eyes above this tiny little irregular area in which she lives. Part of that will be done by getting her to review this utterly slavey existence that was so convenient for the relations with whom she lived in her girlhood. Why did she never suspect that anything else was possible? Where has she been all her life? What was the doom, the inherent handicap that made her so practically resigned at all stages of her life to what I think is best summed up as an almost complete lack of any fun? There wouldn't be anything at all odd about this woman if she had been born a century earlier in middle New England. She might in that setting have had a placid life. But a hundred little times she seems never to have noticed that life for her in the world of today was a poor imitation of what other people in similar circumstances had been having all this time.

Now I approach the situation in this way because I don't see anything malignant anywhere in it. The husband sounds more like an insecure tyrant than anything else. Maybe he is also schizoid. He also has apparently no better grasp on the principle of fun in life than to have an almost classically autistic love affair every now and then; I wouldn't be a bit surprised if some of the women he has been so enamored of have known nothing about it. Also, I do not feel completely discouraged about his perhaps ultimately finding that psychotherapy for himself, though undesirable, is inescapable. I think that he, too, can lift his sights a little bit without any serious upheaval of personality and without this marital group breaking up. I would hope that together they might even emerge from this sort of numb dullness that almost asphyxiates them at times, and get a little bit of pleasure out of life.

Fragment from the Case of a Schizophrenic

This fragment has been selected as summing up Sullivan's overall approach to both schizophrenia and mental disorder in general, since it seems to synthesize much of his attitude toward patients in terms of both theoretic and human considerations.

Sullivan is asked to comment on the rather discouraging progress of a young schizophrenic boy who is delusional and has to be tube-fed part of the time. The content of the boy's verbalizations is extremely sparse, on the average of one coherent sentence for each therapeutic hour. The staff knows that he has had a love affair which terminated by the girl marrying someone else. Whenever he mentions this girl, it is always in terms of the fact that she is now out of his mind, that the affair with her is of no importance, and so on.

Sullivan: There is a marvelous chance to get at a very severe disappointment of this patient if one uses as a cue these little remarks that the girl is "of the past" or she is "out of my mind," or that she was something "of no importance." If the psychiatrist swiftly comes back with something like "Nonsense, you were happy with her," he may have opened the patient's mind. It is the very speed and directness of a completely unsuspected comment like that which sometimes fixes vividly the involuntary attention of the patient. And if the psychiatrist can then move a few steps further, after he has caught the attention of the patient, he may actually reopen an issue that has in truth been treated rather as this patient's remarks suggest—namely, the experience has been abandoned because it is a source of too great regret and grief. In a situation of this kind, once I have startled the patient into any alertness by some variant of "Nonsense, you liked her," I continue the attack by some such remark as, "And there's no reason on earth why the pleasure you had in her company should be thrown away just because the relationship didn't last forever." And if the patient is still in touch with me, I can then become a bit philosophical and say that in my experience any pleasure one has with anybody, even if it is only for a day, is something that it is good to *treasure*. There will be plenty of pain anyway. And if there was some pleasure before the pain—isn't that something to have had?

What I am really doing here is something of much theoretic complexity. Insofar as he was happy with this girl, he has proved that he can be human and enjoy life. Now that is far too important for me to leave it alone, no matter how ghastly the finish of this relationship was. It indicates that the patient has some asset which can then be extrapolated into the future —that he might again be happy with someone, even if again the relationship might end badly. That is immeasurably better than being haunted by obscure, practically transcendental horrors which probably are the most vivid experience that the patient has now.

Index

Acculturation:
  and early referential processes, 4,
    10, 22–24
  sublimation in, 14, 17, 31
Algolagnia, 84–86, 151
  relation to paranoia, 86, 89
Amnesia, in hysteria, 217–219
Anger, 95–98
  in algolagnia, 85–86
  rage, relation to, 98–99
  See also Rage
Anxiety, 3, 4, 11, 92, 167–169
  in agitated depression, 301
  differentiated from fear, 92–95
  early referential processes, rela-
    tion to, 3, 4–5, 7
  in paranoia, 340–342
  in selective inattention, 55–58, 59
  relation to:
    anger, 95–98, 99
    envy, 128–129
    guilt, 113–115
    rage and hatred, 98ff
  source of, in obsessional neurotic,
    229–234, 238–242
  See also Self-system
Autistic, the, 21n, 22ff, 29–30
  in early referential processes, 20–
    24
  in obsessionalism, 29–30, 232, 248–
    249
  in paranoia, 145–150
  in schizophrenia, 185–186, 330–
    331, 361
Automatic writing, 70
Automatisms, 70–75, 166, 203, 255
Awareness:
  contents of, in schizophrenia, 3–4,
    12–14, 182–185, 361
  control of, by selective inattention,
    38–58
  in dissociation, 65–76
  restriction or suspension of, in
    emergencies, 41–42

in sublimation, 14–18
  See also Self-system

Benign stupor, 321
Blame:
  nature of, 345–346
  in schizophrenia, 335–342
  transfer of, 87, 89, 146–148, 304–
    305, 339–347
Blocking, 328–330
Brown study *see* Revery

Cannon, W. B., 92
Catatonia, as the essential manifesta-
  tion of schizophrenia, 308, 312–
    334
Censor concept, 167
Childhood, mental disorder in, 358–
  359
Christ identification, 338
Chum, preadolescent, 106, 152, 313
  See also Preadolescence
Classification of major psychoses,
    193–194, 284, 304–312
  See also Clinical entities
Clinical entities:
  as an approach to therapy, 193–203
  pragmatic use of, schematized in
    terms of hysteria, 220–228
Clinical examples:
  agitated depression, 301
  hebephrenia, 354–358
  hysteric with amnesia, 217–219
  manic-depressive psychosis, 284–
    285, 286–287, 289–290
  obsessionalism, 242–247, 255, 256–
    259, 261–264, 272–283
  paranoid, preadolescent, 151–153
  selective inattention, 44–48
  schizophrenia, 197, 255–259, 261–
    264, 324–334, 350–351, 361–378
Cognitive distortions, 174
Cognitive processes, 149
Collaboration, defined, 98

379